719 - Juni 1989

VIII, 193 Seiten, zahrl.
  Abb. u. Tab.

Gebunden DM 58,--

Gesamtherstellung: Meister-
  Druck, Kassel

F. Bender · W. Meesmann (Eds.)

Treatment with Gallopamil

Results of recent research on calcium antagonism

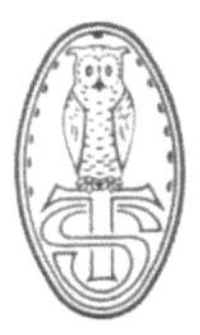

Steinkopff Verlag Darmstadt

III

Prof. Dr. F. Bender
Medizinische Universitätsklinik
und Poliklinik
Albert-Schweitzer-Straße 33
4400 Münster

Prof. Dr. W. Meesmann
Institut für Pathophysiologie
Universitätsklinikum Essen
Hufelandstraße 55
4300 Essen

CIP-Kurztitelaufnahme der Deutschen Bibliothek

Treatment with Gallopamil : results of recent research on
calcium antagonism / F. Bender ; W. Meesmann (eds.). -
Darmstadt : Steinkopff, 1989
   Dt. Ausg. u.d.T.: Therapie mit Gallopamil

ISBN-13: 978-3-642-85378-4   e-ISBN-13: 978-3-642-85376-0
DOI: 10.1007/978-3-642-85376-0

NE: Bender, Franz [Hrsg.]

Type-setting, printing and bookbinding: Meister-Druck, Kassel

IV

Preface

Calcium antagonists are currently the most extensively investigated drugs for the treatment of heart disease. They are used worldwide with great success and a comparatively low incidence of adverse reactions. The most prevalent and threatening diseases in modern industrialized societies – the various forms and complications of coronary arteriosclerosis and arterial hypertension – are amenable to treatment with calcium antagonists.

The pharmacological spectrum of calcium antagonists is highly specific and was supplemented a few years ago by gallopamil, a verapamil analogue. The experimental work reported at this symposium was concerned with effects of gallopamil on the electrophysiology of the heart, particularly in acute myocardial ischemia. New therapeutic features of myocardial hypertrophy and hypertrophic cardiomyopathy are discussed. In medical practice, gallopamil has proved particularly useful for the treatment of angina pectoris. Studies comparing gallopamil with other calcium antagonists are described to profile the properties of the drugs in terms of their specific therapeutic value. There is still a need for more differential therapeutic trials. This first international symposium on gallopamil was attended by experts from institutions devoted to theoretical and clinical research and general practice.

Werner Meesmann
Essen

Franz Bender
Münster

Contents

VIII

Pharmacological aspects of calcium antagonism

H. A. Tritthart

Institute of Medical Physics and Biophysics, University of Graz

My first publication on gallopamil, then still known as substance D 600, appeared about 20 years ago (1). As you know, the first experiments with this new, selective and Ca-competitive group of antagonists were carried out in Professor Fleckenstein's laboratory in Freiburg. From the start, gallopamil was the most potent Ca antagonist and all other compounds were compared with D 600. Since then the number of experimental and clinical studies on Ca antagonists has grown enormously and they are now virtually impossible to review.

In the United States the era of the Ca antagonists only started a few years ago, whereas in Europe we have pioneers like Professor Bender to thank for amassing a wealth of clinical experience. The clinical indications for today's Ca antagonists were also discovered in Europe.

We call this very diverse group of compounds (Fig. 1) Ca antagonists, sometimes known as "Ca-entry blockers", because they inhibit Ca-dependent processes associated with excitation and contraction in the myocardium and smooth muscle.

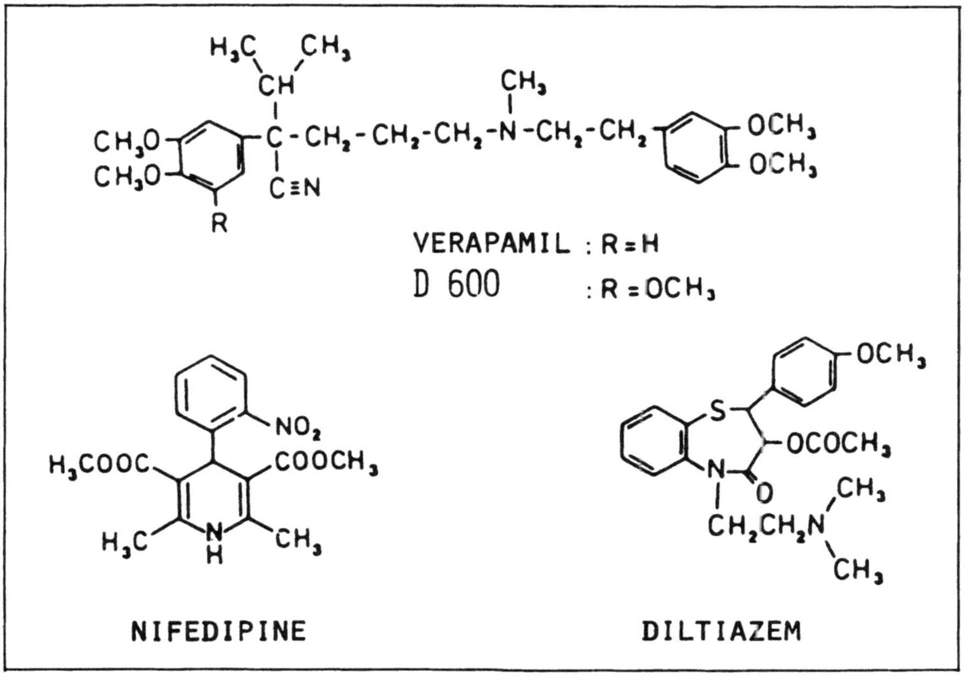

Fig. 1. The structural formulae of the Ca antagonists gallopamil, diltiazem, nifedipine and verapamil.

It was originally reported that the effect of Ca antagonists was similar to that of beta-adrenoceptor blockers, but in 1967 Fleckenstein et al. (2) demonstrated that Ca antagonists do not block the beta-adrenoceptors and this was confirmed in 1968 by Nayler et al. (8). In 1970 we published the first results obtained using smooth muscle (4, 9). This research showed that Ca antagonists inhibit excitation and electromechanical coupling in smooth muscle. The relaxant effect on smooth muscle is also evident with uterine and bronchial fibres.

Table 1. Comparison of the effects of beta-adrenoceptor blockers and Ca antagonists on smooth muscle

Beta-adrenoceptor blockers			Calcium antagonists
Contraction	———	Bronchi	——— Bronchospasmolytic effect
Contraction	———	Arterioles	——— Relaxation
Contraction	———	Uterus	——— Relaxation
Increase resistance in the normal myocardium	———	Coronaries	——— Relax extramural vessels

Table 1 compares the effects of beta-adrenoceptor blockers and Ca antagonists. In these respects Ca antagonists have the same effect as beta-adrenoceptor stimulation and are therefore the exact opposite of the beta-adrenoceptor blockers. A large number of different experiments soon showed that Ca antagonists relax all types of smooth muscle, their most pronounced effects being on the major extramural coronary vessels and peripheral resistance vessels.

As you know, drugs only exert an effect if they are taken up by, or bind with, a specific structure. This receptor theory, which has prompted a large number of biophysical, physiological and pharmacological studies, poses two questions which are now the subject of the most exhaustive research, namely: 1. Where do Ca antagonists bind? and 2. What are their structure-activity relationships?

Gallopamil and verapamil are very similar, but they are very different in structure from the Ca antagonists such as nifedipine and diltiazem which are also widely used clinically (see Fig. 1). It is therefore extremely unlikely that the Ca channel contains a single binding site which acts as the receptor.

Indeed, it is now postulated that the Ca channel contains at least four receptor fields and there is certainly further scope for a corresponding number of naturally occurring substances, some of which may not even have been discovered yet. Hypothetically, binding sites for Ca antagonists may also be divided into different channel types, such as voltage-dependent channels or receptor-operated channels, and there may be also subtypes of Ca channels and inactive precursors. It would be of major medical significance if we could understand the important pathophysiological factors which affect the channel system of the membrane, or in other words receptor density or receptor turnover in the membrane.

Interestingly enough, in phylogenetic terms Ca channels were the earliest system in excitable cells, predating the sodium channels and, in the nervous system of molluscs for example, the calcium channels are the system responsible for excitation. Ca channels are therefore to be found in an extraordinary number of systems and they are involved in a great variety of functions; there are even Ca channels in plant cells.

2

Table 2. Effects of Ca antagonists in vitro

- Release of neurotransmitters from presynaptic nerve endings
- Catecholamine secretion in chromaffin cells
- Release of vasopressin and oxytocin in the neurohypophysis
- Stimulation of secretion in the adenohypophysis
- Glucose-induced insulin secretion in the beta-cells of the pancreas
- Collagen-induced platelet aggregation
- Aldosterone secretion in the adrenal cortex

As Table 2 shows, a large number of cell functions are dependent on transmembrane Ca influx and can be blocked in vitro by Ca antagonists. We do not know what new, selective effects may in the future be offered by other compounds, but as regards the Ca antagonists in clinical use today, only two of the many effects listed in Table 2 are important clinically. According to results published by Hiramatsu et al. (5), nifedipine can inhibit aldosterone secretion. The second relevant factor is a slight, but significant, reduction of platelet aggregation and prolongation of bleeding time, probably as a result of inhibition of Ca influx into the platelets. Although there are numerous binding sites for Ca antagonists in neurons and in skeletal-muscle cells, these cells are not affected by therapeutic concentrations of Ca antagonists; their inhibitory effect is confined mainly to Ca channels in the heart and smooth muscle. There is also plenty of evidence to suggest that, except at excessively high concentrations, Ca antagonists do not inhibit the movements of calcium in intracellular organelles such as the sarcoplasmic reticulum and mitochondria. These results, and the fact that Ca antagonists have no effect on membraneless myocytes, indicate that the site of action of these drugs is the cell membrane; Ca antagonists bind to the protein macromolecule which forms a tunnel through the double lipid layer of the membrane and acts as the Ca channel (Fig. 2). Ca-channel function can be seen as analogous to enzymes. The task of the Ca channels is to reduce the energy required for the transmembrane migration of Ca ions, thereby increasing the diffusion rate by a factor of about 10^{30}. In fact the Ca channels also exhibit substrate specificity, that is to say they exhibit ion selectivity and competitive inhibition by substrate analogues such as ions (manganese, lanthanum, nickel, cobalt etc.) or inhibition by blockers, namely Ca antagonists. Finally, again like enzymes, the Ca channels are capable of rapid changes of conformation in that they can jump backwards and forwards between open, or permeable to ions, and closed (Fig. 3). The factors which affect the opening of Ca channels are 1. The membrane potential (voltage-dependent channels), and 2. The binding of transmitters to receptors (receptor-operated channels). Finally, opening of the Ca channels can also be affected by 3. Specific phosphorylation of the channel by, for example, cyclic AMP. It must be assumed that, when open, the permeability of an individual channel is constant and that the factors listed above modify the influx of Ca by altering the probability of a particular channel being open.
Cyclic-AMP-induced activation of protein kinase and of channel phosphorylation increases Ca influx, presumably by increasing the probability that the Ca channel is open. Ca antagonists have the opposite effect, that is they reduce the probability that the channel is open (see Fig. 3). The summated activity of many channels determines the overall flux for a cell and the lower the probability that many Ca channels in the cell membrane are open the lower is the transmembrane influx of Ca in the heart or smooth muscle.
The ion fluxes across the membrane of isolated myocardial cells can now be measured accurately (Fig. 4), but unfortunately similarly accurate measurements are still difficult to

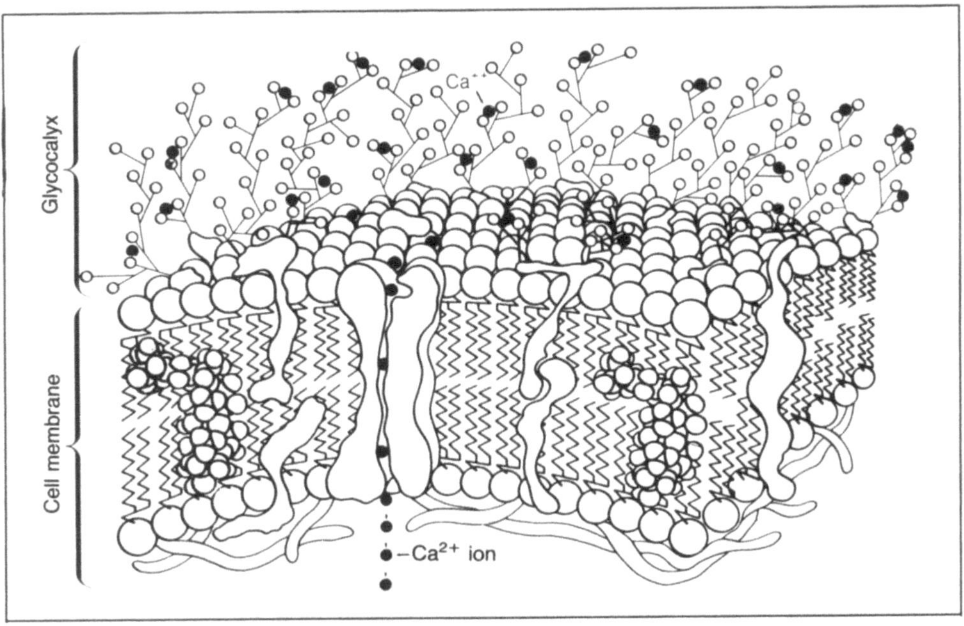

Fig. 2. Diagram showing how the Ca channel is arranged in the cell membrane as a transmembrane tunnel protein.

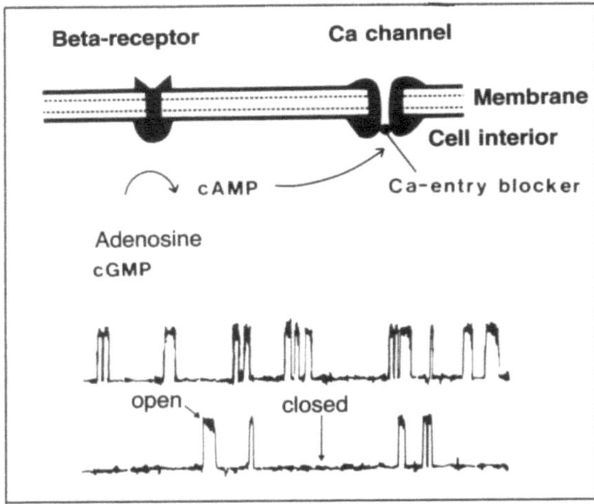

Fig. 3. Diagram showing the Ca channel (top), and how Ca antagonists block and cAMP stimulates the stochastic opening of the Ca channel.

obtain from non-striated myocytes. Sodium influx and Ca influx can be measured by voltage-clamp experiments, as shown on the right of Fig. 4. Ca influx was completely blocked after adding gallopamil. Fig. 4, bottom right, shows the analysis of experiments

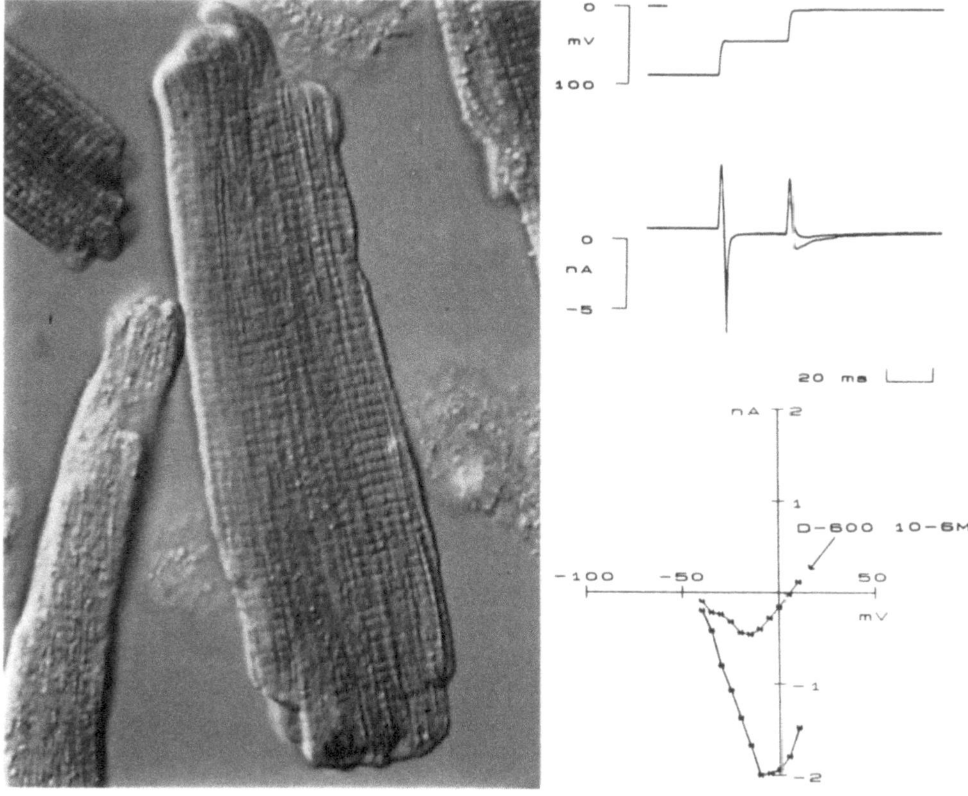

Fig. 4. Isolated myocardial cells in culture (left) (Nomarsky interference contrast, magnification about × 600) can be used to obtain an accurate measurement of transmembrane ion flows. The trace in the top right shows a voltage-clamp experiment to measure the influx of Na and Ca. Gallopamil inhibited the Ca influx. The graph (bottom right) shows the analysis of experiments of this type (n=6, 1 Hz, 36 °C, 10^{-6} M gallopamil allowed to act for 10 min). If the drug is allowed to act for longer Ca influx cannot be stimulated at all.

such as these carried out on single cells. At a concentration of 10^{-6} M, within 10 minutes gallopamil had almost completely inhibited Ca influx. Ca influx was completely blocked after gallopamil had been allowed to act for a longer period. Na influx (not shown) did not alter. Using human papillary muscles, Nawrat and Zong (7) found that, even at a higher concentration, gallopamil does not inhibit sodium influx and thus it does not have a membrane-stabilizing or quinidine-like inhibitory effect.

When Ca antagonists of the gallopamil type are given by the intracoronary route their action in inhibiting Ca influx has the following effects on the heart: 1. it reduces the heart rate, 2. it slows AV conduction, 3. it reduces the contractile force and oxygen uptake of the working myocardium, and 4. it causes vasodilation, particularly of the major extramural coronary vessels. However, when gallopamil is administered systemically, these direct effects on the heart are accompanied by peripheral vascular effects and so, depending on the circulatory picture, the direct cardiac effects are masked by reflex compensating responses. This reflex

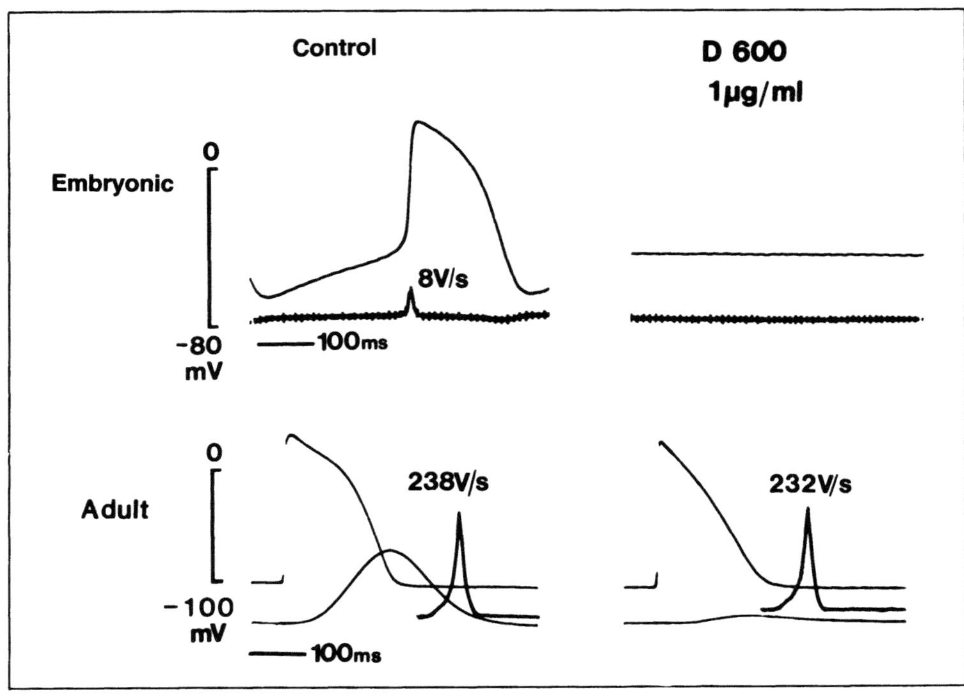

Fig. 5. In an early phase of development the embryonic ventricular myocardium exhibits Ca-dependent pacemaker action potentials which are completely blocked by gallopamil (D 600). As the resting potential increases and stabilizes and the ventricular myocardium becomes increasingly differentiated, fast Na channels take over the task of impulse propagation. In the adult ventricular myocardium gallopamil has no effect on the depolarization phase of the action potential (cf. dV/dt in V/s) or on impulse propagation, but it flattens the Ca-dependent plateau phase and reduces the contractile force.

control of the direct cardiac effects of the Ca antagonists may itself be modified by the Ca antagonists (6). The effects of gallopamil in patients may be summarized as follows: it reduces the heart rate during and after exercise, it reduces preload and afterload, and it reduces O_2 uptake and contractility to a minimum consistent with normal pumping function. Thus, the overall effect is to ensure that the heart operates more economically. With nifedipine the reflex compensating responses are often excessive and the heart rate rises. The marked coronary vasodilation elicited by Ca antagonists together with the improvement in the external conditions in which the heart has to operate more than compensate for the reduction in left ventricular contractility, with the result that less oxygen is consumed; cardiac output remains the same or actually increases, even in patients with compromised pumping function (10).

Gallopamil affects the heart rate and AV conduction by acting on regions of the heart in which impulses are generated or propagated. Typically, these areas have a low membrane potential and are capable of spontaneous impulse generation. Both are comparatively poorly differentiated areas in which we find primitive forms of impulse generation and conduction, in other words Ca-dependent action potentials. Ca-dependent potentials also occur, for example, in embryonic cells of the working myocardium as shown in Fig. 5. In

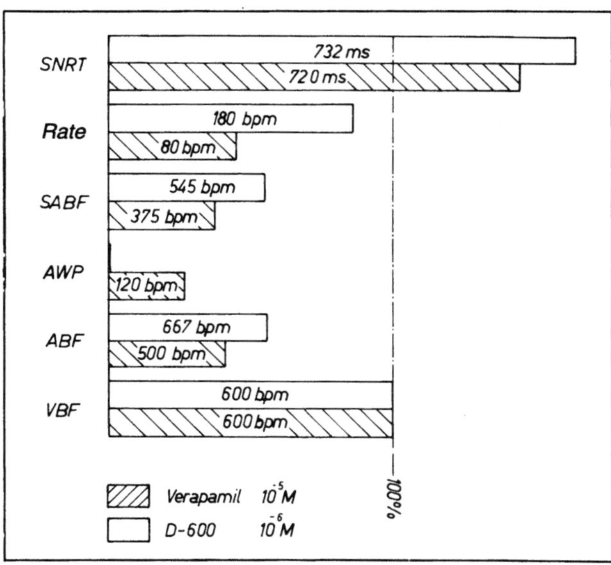

Fig. 6. Standardized changes in sino-atrial node recovery time (SNRT), heart rate, sino-atrial border frequency (SABF), atrial (ABF) and ventricular (VBF) maximal pacing frequency and anterograde Wenckebach periodicity (AWP) after adding high concentrations of gallopamil (open bars) or after verapamil (hatched bars). Experiments carried out on the Langendorff perfused guinea-pig heart preparation, comparison with control values (100%) made 10 min after continuous perfusion of the stated concentrations of the Ca antagonists (34 °C, Tyrode solution, n=3).

these cells gallopamil completely inhibits Ca-dependent excitation, whereas in the adult myocardium, in which the membrane potential is more negative, the sodium flux is responsible for perpetuating the impulse. If the membrane potential is reduced far enough by, for example, an increase in the potassium concentration or by an electrical current, even the normal working myocardium can be depolarized to such an extent that its ability to generate impulses spontaneously, which depends on Ca influx, re-appears. Ca antagonists have a selective effect on Ca action potentials both in areas in which the membrane potential is naturally low, namely in the sino-atrial node and AV node, and in areas in which it has been reduced artificially. Along the route taken by a normal impulse, from generation in the sino-atrial node via the AV node into the ventricle, we find Ca action potentials in the P cells of the sino-atrial node, which are responsible for impulse generation, and in the N cells of the AV node, which are responsible for slowing conduction. It is important from the clinical point of view to know the preferred nodal sites of action of the Ca antagonists, the nature of their action and the extent to which such effects can be offset by compensating reflex responses. The direct action of Ca antagonists on the sino-atrial and AV nodes can be studied in isolation, that is to say without reflex compensating effects, by using the Langendorff perfused heart preparation. In this preparation, in which all Ca antagonists exhibit a dose-related bradycardic effect, the effects of Ca antagonists can be demonstrated by stimulation.

Figure 6 shows the analysis of stimulation studies and compares the effect of gallopamil with that of 10 times the concentration of verapamil. Both compounds definitely prolonged sino-atrial node recovery time, reduced the heart rate and reduced the sino-atrial border frequency. Both compounds also caused a clear-cut reduction of atrial border frequency, whereas ventricular border frequency was unchanged. The much more powerful effect of gallopamil is illustrated particularly well by the anterograde Wenckebach point, or in other words by the reduction in the border frequency for conduction through the AV node. However, the inhibitory effect of gallopamil and of verapamil on the N cells of the AV node is identical in type: Ca influx declines, the rate of depolarization falls and the conduction rate diminishes. Typically, this inhibitory effect is markedly rate-related, in other words after inhibition and a sufficiently long pause there is an almost normal impulse and the next impulse is conducted much more slowly, or depolarization is much slower and so on, that is to say there is a typical Wenckebach-like conduction block. In the final analysis, the effect of gallopamil is rate-related because the phenomenon is markedly potential-dependent; typically, this is demonstrated by the fact that, when the pacemaker cells have been inhibited, the gallopamil-induced arrest can be temporarily abolished by membrane hyperpolarization. This is illustrated by the experiment on cultured pacemaker cells shown in Fig. 7.

Although all Ca antagonists inhibit Ca action potentials in the AV node to some extent, only the group represented by gallopamil, verapamil and diltiazem has a markedly rate-dependent and potential-dependent action in prolonging the refractory period of Ca-dependent excitation processes. This difference in inhibitory effect has an important bearing on the clinical use of Ca antagonists. Gallopamil, verapamil and diltiazem slow AV conduction by prolonging the refractory period of the AV node, whereas nifedipine does not.

In recent years we have learned some vital facts about the key role of Ca ions in the chain of events involved in ischaemia and in the reperfusion of ischaemic areas. These events are

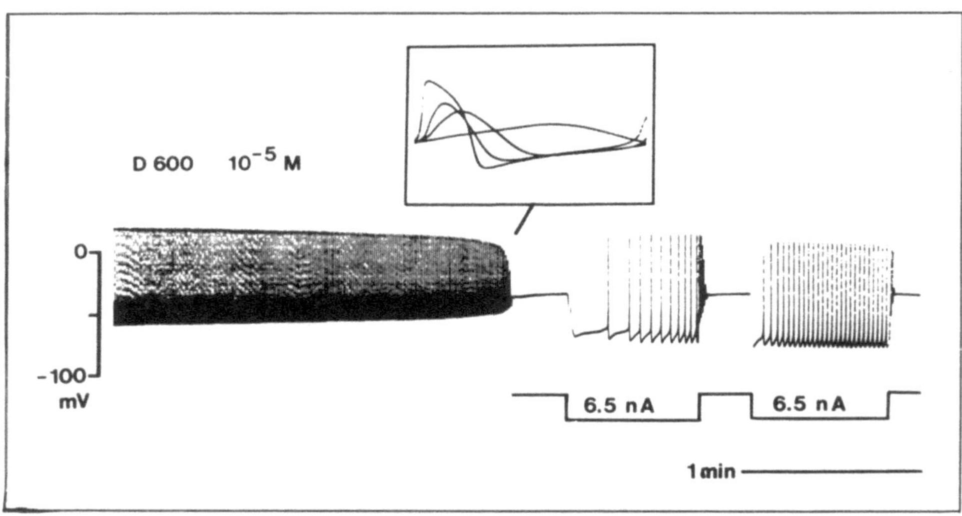

Fig. 7. The inhibitory effect of gallopamil on isolated, cultured pacemaker cells (from 11). The inset shows superimposed action potentials recorded as the inhibitory effect of gallopamil developed. The tracing (centre left) shows the transition from spontaneous impulse generation to gallopamil-induced arrest of Ca-dependent impulse generation. This effect was reversed by membrane hyperpolarization (applying a current of 2 nA and 6.5 nA, right).

associated with gross overload of the myocardial cells with Ca ions, which destroys their function and structure. The high concentration of calcium in the cytosol coincides with high levels of inorganic phosphate produced by ATP cleavage. Both factors seriously imperil the structure and function of the mitochondria, for mitochondria assiduously store Ca ions, but this calcium jeopardizes their ability to synthesize ATP. The high levels of inorganic phosphate cause the mitochondria to swell, and inhibit oxidative phosphorylation. However, the rise in intracellular Ca also activates phospholipases, which threaten the cell membrane, the mitochondrial membrane and other membranes. Phospholipid hydrolysis initially renders the membranes more permeable and finally destroys them with the production of free fatty acids, which may be a perilous arrhythmogenic factor. Ca-dependent activation of phospholipases is a fatal vicious circle: calcium levels in the cells and mitochondria continue to rise, posing the threats described above, the cell membrane becomes completely depolarized and even macromolecules escape from the cells. The simplified series of reactions in Fig. 8 shows how the rise of Ca ions in the cytosol leads, via a number of intermediate stages, some of which are not shown, ultimately to cell damage and cell death. Like the myocardial cells, smooth-muscle cells also depend on Ca ions for excitation and electromechanical coupling. Activator Ca for contractile processes passes through the membrane via voltage-dependent and receptor-operated channels. There are numerous intracellular sources of activator Ca including the sarcoplasmic reticulum, a membrane-associated Ca fraction and possibly the mitochondria or perinuclear cisternae. The range of receptors or voltage-dependent Ca channels present can vary enormously and is contingent on the function of the cell and its parent organ.

In pharmacological tests, the stimulus which causes smooth muscle to contract is either membrane depolarization (typically this is achieved by raising the potassium concentration) or the addition of a transmitter such as noradrenaline (Fig. 9). The typical mechanical response to membrane depolarization is tonic and depends very much on the extracellular Ca concentration, since under these conditions activator Ca flows in through the channels in the membrane. The mechanical response to transmitters is often phasic and less dependent on the extracellular Ca concentration, which indicates that activator Ca is mobilized predominantly from intracellular sources and that changes in membrane potential are a less important factor. For example, if the bath solution is depleted of Ca ions during membrane depolarization, the smooth muscle relaxes completely. Basically, the Ca antagonists have analogous effects: they inhibit the opening of membrane channels during depolarization, thus preventing the influx of Ca, and they may cause prompt relaxation even though the membrane is depolarized. On the other hand, Ca antagonists only block transmitter-induced contractions of smooth muscle to the extent that such a contraction of the particular muscle is itself Ca-dependent. This varies enormously even within a vascular bed and depends on the number and type of receptors on the cells.

The initial experiments with gallopamil (4, 9) in which the electrical and the mechanical activity of smooth muscle were recorded simultaneously, showed that gallopamil is also a powerful blocker of the electrical activity known as "spike activity", that is to say the number and frequency of the action potentials. Thus, in addition to causing smooth muscle to relax, it also largely suppresses the muscle's spontaneous electrical activity. These findings are interesting as regards the clinical use of Ca antagonists because the coronary artery and, for example, the basilar artery exhibit large-amplitude spasms in response to a variety of stimulants including ergotamine, serotonin and acetylcholine (3). This vasospastic activity is markedly Ca-dependent and is probably evoked by pronounced spontaneous

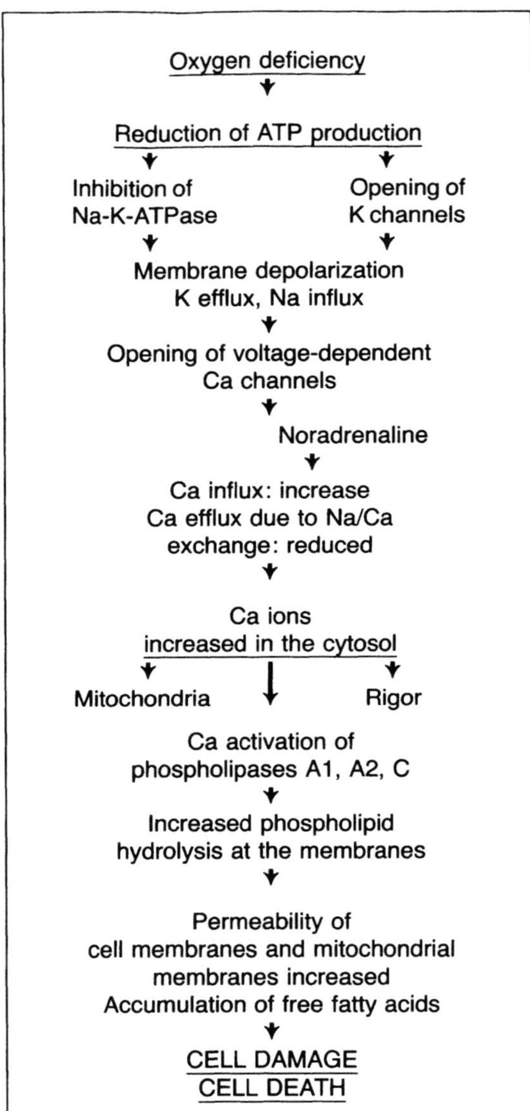

Fig. 8. Synopsis of some of the sequential reactions and Ca-dependent processes which take place in the hypoxic myocardium.

electrical activity. The spontaneous electrical activity detected in many smooth muscles is controlled by the opening of voltage-dependent Ca channels in the membrane. A feature of Ca antagonists is that, at threshold concentrations for abolishing potassium-induced contracture, they can completely block the vasospastic activity. These results, obtained experimentally, correlate well with clinical data, obtained from various disciplines, which indicate that Ca antagonists are the drugs of choice for preventing coronary spasm in patients with unstable or Prinzmetal's angina. Ca antagonists are being used with increasing

10

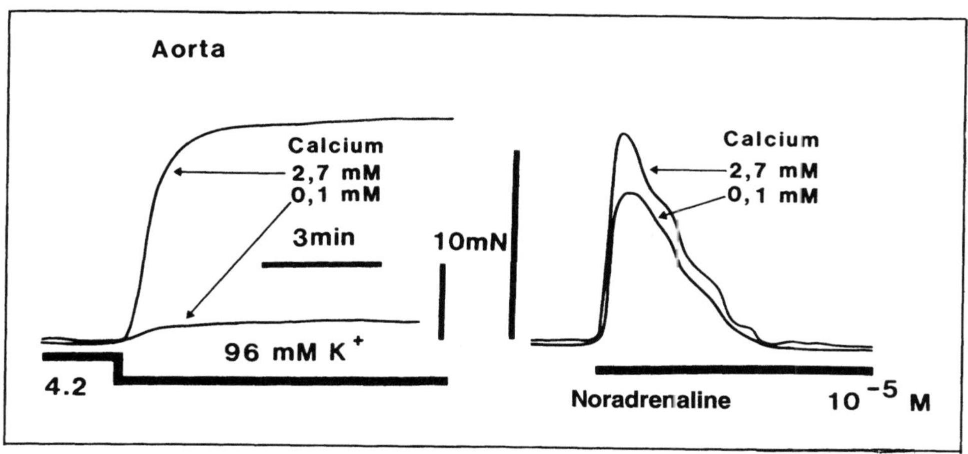

Fig. 9. Diagram showing smooth muscle contraction stimulated by membrane depolarization (adding potassium) or by a transmitter, and the effect of altering the extracellular Ca concentration on these two types of contraction.

success for treating hypertension particularly in elderly patients and their relaxant effect on the smooth muscle of the airways is of benefit to asthma patients.

References

1. Fleckenstein A, Tritthart HA, Fleckenstein B, Herbst A, Grün G (1969) Selektive Hemmung der Myokard-Kontraktilität durch kompetitive Ca^{++}-Antagonisten. Naunyn-Schmiedebergs Arch Pharmak 264:227
2. Fleckenstein A, Kammermeier H, Döring HJ, Freund HJ (1967) Zum Wirkungsmechanismus neuartiger Koronardilatatoren mit gleichzeitig sauerstoffeinsparenden Myokardeffekten, Prenylamin und Iproveratril. Z Kreislaufforschung 56:716–744, 839–853
3. Ginsburg R, Bristow MR, Harrison DC, Stinson E (1980) Studies with isolated human coronary arteries. Chest 78:180
4. Grün G, Byon KY, Tritthart HA, Fleckenstein A (1970) Inhibition of automaticity and contractility of isolated human uterine muscle by Ca-antagonistic compounds. Pflügers Arch Eur J Physiol 319: R 118
5. Hiramatsu K, Yamagishi F, Kubota T, Yamada T (1982) Acute effects of the calcium antagonist, Nifedipine, on blood pressure, pulse rate, and the renin-angiotensin-aldosterone system in patients with essential hypertension. Am Heart J 104:1346–1350
6. Millard RW, Gabel M, Fowler NO, Schwartz A (1982) Baroreceptor reflex sensitivity reduced by Diltiazem und Verapamil. Fed Proc 41:57959
7. Nawrath H, Zong Xian-Gang (1983) Elektrophysiologische Untersuchungen mit Gallopamil am Ventrikelmyokard des Menschen. In: Kaltenbach M, Hopf R (eds) Gallopamil, Springer Berlin Heidelberg New York Tokyo, pp. 69–74
8. Nayler WG, McInnes I, Swann JB, Price JM, Carson V, Race D, Lowe TE (1968) Some effects of iproveratril (Isoptin) on the cardiovascular system. J Pharmacol Exp Ther 161:247–261
9. Tritthart HA, Grün G, Byon KY, Fleckenstein A (1970) Influence of Ca-antagonistic inhibitors of excitation-contraction coupling on isolated uterine muscle. Studies with the sucrose gap method. Pflügers Arch Eur J Physiol 319:R 117

10. Winniford M, Markham R, Firth B, Nicod P, Hillis D (1982) Hemodynamic and electrophysiologic effects of Verapamil and Nifedipine in patients on Propranolol Amer J Cardiol 50:704
11. Koidl B, Tritthart HA (1982) D 600 blocks spontaneous discharge, excitability and contraction of cultured embryonic chick heart cells. J Mol Cell Cardiol 14:251–257

Author's address:

Prof. Dr. med. H. A. Tritthart
Karl-Franzens-Universität Graz
Institut für medizinische Physik und Biophysik
Harrachgasse 21
A–8010 Graz
Austria

Discussion

BENDER

Dr. Tritthart, you did not once use the word calmodulin. Entire conferences and congresses have been devoted to calmodulin and for a long time now it has had a high profile in the literature. Is there such a thing as calmodulin, do we need it, or is it simply a word for the functions you have described?

TRITTHART

That is a difficult question. Of course there is such a thing as calmodulin and there is no doubt that we need it. Within the cell calmodulin is the mediator of calcium-dependent stimulation processes and it is important particularly in smooth muscle. Its role in the myocardium is at the very least questionable and it may be irrelevant. That is the current position. Inhibitory effects of calmodulin can be measured very accurately in vitro, but the prominence of these inhibitory effects in cell function is unclear. Not only is calmodulin partly responsible for activating myofibrillar ATPase, but it also stimulates the calcium pump and thus it is also responsible for calcium efflux. On the other hand, it stimulates the re-binding of calcium. I deliberately did not discuss calmodulin because intracellular effects of calcium antagonists are now also a topic of much debate and some very interesting results have emerged, but basically we still know very, very little which might be of help to the clinician.

Comparative effects of calcium antagonists and of inotropic agents on the development of hereditary cardiomyopathy in the hamster

G. Jasmin, L. Proschek

Department of Pathology, University of Montreal

Introduction

The pathology of hereditary cardiomyopathy in the hamster has been well documented in recent years (1–10). This primary congestive type of cardiomyopathy develops in characteristic, well-defined and predictable stages, namely: 1. a necrotic phase with multifocal cardiac lesions, which develop in animals between 30 and 120 days of age; 2. a healing phase with scar formation and progressive dilatation of the atrial and ventricular wall, occurring between 120 and 200 days and, finally, 3. a terminal phase with moderate to severe heart failure between 200 and 300 days (2). The changes in the heart are not visible under a light microscope until the animal has reached 30 days. These lesions reflect a more generalized myopathic process and they probably derive from the same genetic molecular defect.
The prevailing hypothesis that this condition is due to defective calcium metabolism (11–14) led the authors to investigate the effect of cardio-active drugs on the development and progression of this hereditary form of cardiomyopathy. Therapeutic studies were carried out in an attempt to interfere with certain critical phases of inner cell metabolism possibly involved in the necrotizing process of the myocardium. The main substance of this report is a quantitative and qualitative assessment of degenerative changes in the heart.

Material and methods

Animals

All the experiments were conducted with male and female Syrian hamsters with cardiomyopathy. The animals were of the UM-X7.1 strain aged between 27 and 30 days. They were housed under controlled conditions (26 °C, with a 12:12 h light-dark cycle) with free access to Purina laboratory food and tap water. Animals of the same litter (± 10) were distributed evenly amongst the various groups, taking into account sex and body weight. After a few preliminary tests, in most cases the experiments were repeated several times. The drug substances were dissolved in physiological saline solution or in a suitable vehicle and administered systemically, twice daily. Data on the dosage, formulation and total number of animals used are given in the Tables. Except for the gallopamil (D 600) study which lasted 200 and 300 days, all the studies were carried out over 28 days so that the animals would reach the critical age of 55 days at which time the necrotic changes become fully expressed in untreated animals.

Autopsy

At autopsy a gross pathological inspection of the hearts was carried out to determine the total number of necrotic foci. After dissecting out the heart and removing the atria, the remaining ventricular tissue was rinsed, blotted and weighed. The septum and adjacent segments of ventricle were fixed and prepared for routine histological examination. The residual fragments of the ventricles were homogenized and their calcium content was determined in acid extracts by an atomic absorption technique (14). After isolating the mitochondria, oxidative phosphorylation was measured by polarography (14). The protein concentration was determined by Lowry's method (15).

Assessment of the cardiac necrosis by microscopy

As mentioned above, cardiac lesions are predictable after the animal is 55 days old. Irrespective of whether it was myolytic or coagulative (2), the necrotizing process was scored from 0 to 3 according to the severity and extent of the ventricular lesions. The sections were examined under a microscope using a double-blind procedure. The degree of damage was rated 1, 2 or 3 (with half marks if necessary) to designate slight, moderate and severe necrosis respectively. The highest score corresponded to 50% damage to the ventricle. The average score for the microscopic findings in 60-day old hamsters with cardiomyopathy was 2.2 for a minimum of 10 animals. A score above 2.2 indicated "aggravation", whereas a score of less than 1.4 in 80% of the animals represented significant "cardioprotection". The statistical significance of the results was determined using Student's t-test. Differences of $p < 0.05$ versus the untreated group were regarded as significant.

Results

Comparison of the effects of calcium antagonists

Our first results go back as far as 1972, when my colleague Bajusz and I first observed that verapamil prevented the early necrotic changes in the myocardium of UM-X7.1 hamsters with cardiomyopathy (11, 16, 18). Later on, we found that gallopamil, at a lower dosage, was just as effective and better tolerated (19, 20).
Table 1 shows that various calcium antagonists had little effect on the body-weight gain or on the increase in ventricular weight, except for verapamil, which caused a significant increase in myocardial weight. However, it was clear that the calcium antagonists were not all equally effective in preventing the necrotizing process (Fig. 1). Apart from verapamil and gallopamil, only diltiazem and prenylamine significantly reduced the severity of the cardiac lesions, whereas nifedipine and bepridil were virtually ineffective. There was a close correlation between the calcium content of the heart and the severity of the necrotic changes. It should also be mentioned that none of the calcium antagonists we tested ameliorated the skeletal muscle lesions.
Preliminary studies with anipamil showed that it is well tolerated when injected subcutaneously. It caused a slight increase in ventricular weight, but there were no necrotic changes (Table 2). Like verapamil and gallopamil, anipamil did not prevent the skeletal muscle lesions or the rise in the serum creatine kinase (CK) level.

Effect of gallopamil on ventricular heavy-chain (HC) myosins

It has recently been demonstrated that the distribution of heavy-chain myosin isoenzymes alters as the hamster cardiomyopathy progresses (5, 6, 21). We attempted to prevent the

Table 1. Bodyweight gain, heart weight and ratio of heart weight to body weight of hamsters with cardiomyopathy, after treatment with calcium antagonists

Treatment (number of animals)	Dose (mg/kg/d)	Bodyweight gain (g) (initial weight 48 ± 2 g)	Heart weight* (mg)	Heart weight* (mg) Body weight (g)
Untreated (38)	Saline solution or vehicle	30 ± 1	243 ± 5	3.17 ± 0.06
Gallopamil (28)	2 subcutaneously saline solution	29 ± 2	259 ± 6	3.29 ± 0.07
Verapamil (35)	20 subcutaneously saline solution	28 ± 1	276 ± 7 $p < 0.001$	3.68 ± 0.06 $p < 0.01$
Diltiazem (14)	150 orally saline solution	27 ± 2	245 ± 5	3.21 ± 0.08
Nifedipine (21)	20 orally 30% DMSO	28 ± 1	247 ± 7	3.10 ± 0.12
Bepridil (17)	150 orally 2.5% ethanol	27 ± 1	235 ± 9	3.11 ± 0.07
Prenylamine ** (14)	100 orally aqueous solution	15 ± 2 $p < 0.005$	211 ± 5	3.26 ± 0.08

Means ± SEM

* Ventricle alone;

** Treatment with prenylamine, 3 weeks. Bodyweight gain, heart weight and ratio of heart weight to body weight in the corresponding control group: 24 ± 1, 210 ± 5 and 3.23 ± 0.06 respectively; $P > 0.05$ versus the untreated control group is regarded as not statistically significant. In other cases the level of significance is stated.

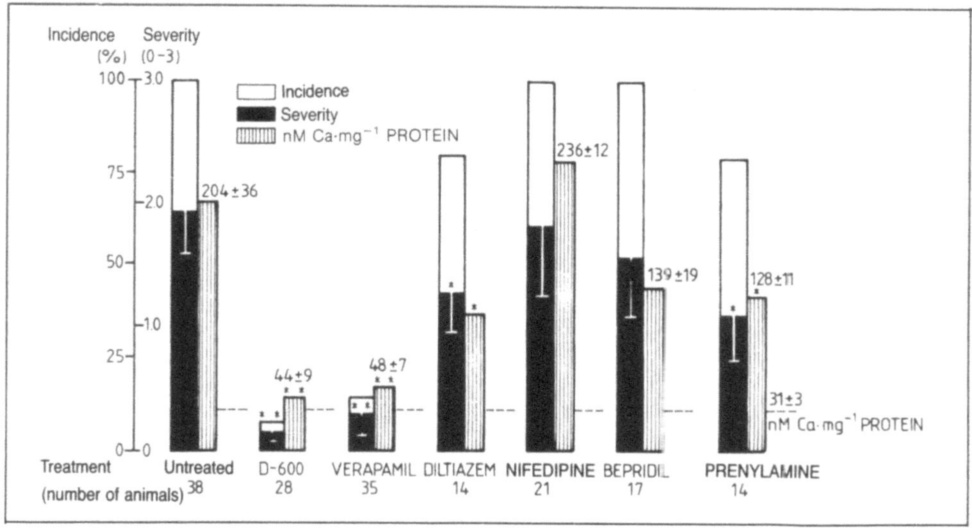

Figure 1. Comparison of the effect of calcium antagonists on the development of necrotic changes and on the calcium content of the heart of UM-X7.1 hamsters with cardiomyopathy. The diagram shows the data ± SEM; * $P < 0.05$; ** $P < 0.001$ versus the untreated control group; other differences were not statistically significant (20).

15

Table 2. Weight data, heart and skeletal-muscle lesions and serum creatine kinase in hamsters with cardiomyopathy, after treatment with anipamil*

Group (number of animals)	Bodyweight gain (g) (initial weight 43 ± 1 g)	Heart weight (mg) Body weight (g)	Cardiac lesions Incidence (%)	Severity (Score 0–3)	Skeletal muscle lesions Incidence (%)	Severity (Score 0–3)	Serum CK (U/1)
Untreated (6)	26 ± 1	3.28 ± 0.09	100	2.03 ± 0.17	100	1.97 ± 0.23	28339 ± 5909
Anipamil (8)	30 ± 2	3.57 ± 0.10	0	0	100	1.80 ± 0.25	18295 ± 2435

x̄ ± SEM
* 3 mg/kg twice daily by subcutaneous injection

shift from the alpha-myosin isoform (V_1) to the beta-isoform (V_3) by treating the animals with gallopamil. The assessment was made by histochemical methods using labelled monoclonal antibodies (22). Figure 2 shows that the distribution pattern of the myosin forms in the normal heart were only slightly modified by 60 days' administration of gallopamil. However, despite the cardioprotective effect of gallopamil, it did not prevent the shift to the beta-myosin isoform in myopathic hearts. Evidently, the reduced contractility of the diseased heart is not directly related to the necrotizing process.

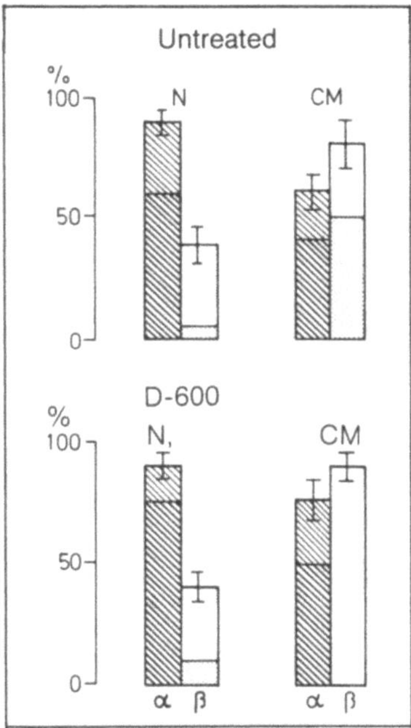

Figure 2. Effect of D 600 on the percentage distribution of myocardial cells labelled with fluorescent alpha-myosin antibodies and beta-myosin antibodies in normal (N) and myopathic (CM) mid-ventricular heart sections. Each bar represents the number of positive fibres established by point counting in four micrographs from 6 animals per group. The differences in hatching correspond to the degree of fluorescence.

Effect of long-term administration of gallopamil

1. Animal survival and time course of the cardiomyopathy

Three groups each of twenty 30-day-old hamsters with cardiomyopathy were used for this experiment. The first group of untreated animals served as the control. The other two groups were treated with 2 mg/kg gallopamil daily, the first group for 200 days and the second group for 330 days. The hearts were removed to assess the histological changes, to measure the Ca^{2+} and Mg^{2+} content in the homogenate and in isolated mitochondria, and to determine mitochondrial oxidative phosphorylation.

The survival rate of the treated animals, measured at 200 days, increased by 40%. After 300 days 73% of the hamsters treated with gallopamil were still alive as compared with 5% of the untreated control animals (Fig. 3).

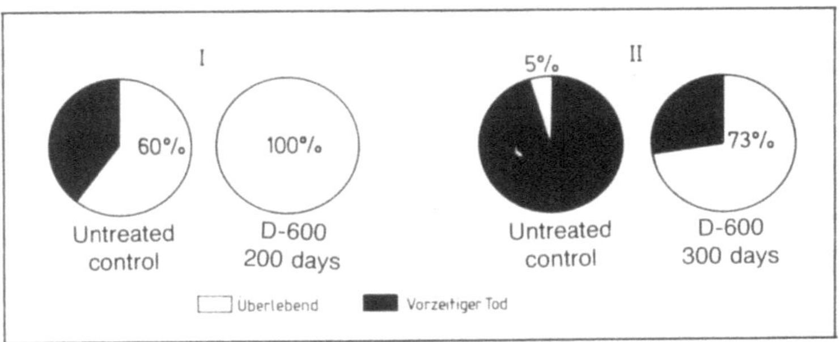

Figure 3. Life span of hamsters with polymyopathy, after long-term treatment with D 600

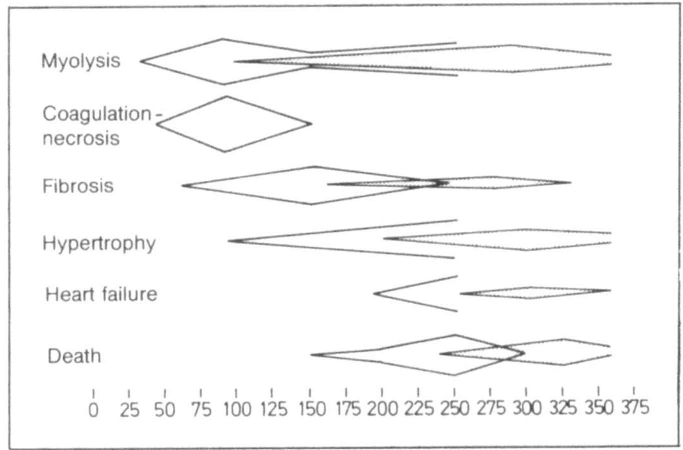

Figure 4. Diagram of the progression of myocardial changes in hamsters with hereditary cardiomyopathy under long-term treatment with gallopamil (shaded areas) (from 24)

Analysis of the pathological changes in the hearts (Fig. 4) showed that gallopamil successfully prevented the coagulation necrosis, but only retarded the myolysis. Fibrosis, hypertrophy and dilatation of the ventricles were less severe and progressed more slowly; only a few animals died with the typical signs of heart failure. The life span increased by 100 days.

2. Determination of calcium and magnesium

Figure 5 shows the calcium and magnesium content in heart homogenate and in the mitochondria. At the age of 200 days, in the treated animals the calcium levels in the homogenates were 20 times lower, and in the isolated mitochondria they were 3 times lower.

18

After 330 days the values were slightly higher, but they were still far below the control values for the untreated animals. The change in the Mg^{2+} content was less impressive and was only on the borderline of statistical significance.

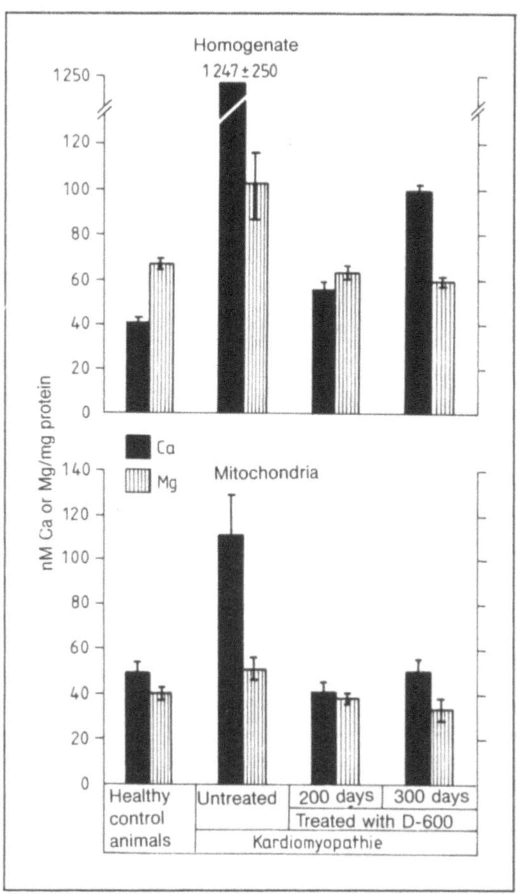

Figure 5. Effect of long-term gallopamil treatment on the Ca^{2+} and Mg^{2+} content of heart homogenates and heart mitochondria from hamsters with cardiomyopathy. The data are the means and standard deviations for two groups of six to eight animals given similar treatment (from 24)

3. Mitochondrial oxidative phosphorylation

As Fig. 6 shows, the mitochondrial Ca^{2+} loading resulted in a 40% reduction in the ratio of cell respiration with a significant reduction in the $ADP:O_2$ ratio as compared with the values for normal, healthy hamsters. Interestingly, these parameters remained virtually in the normal range after 200 days' gallopamil treatment. However, in the terminal stage of the disease, the effectiveness of gallopamil treatment was less obvious in that, despite relatively low Ca^{2+} loading of the mitochondria, the respiration control ratio had fallen to 5.5.

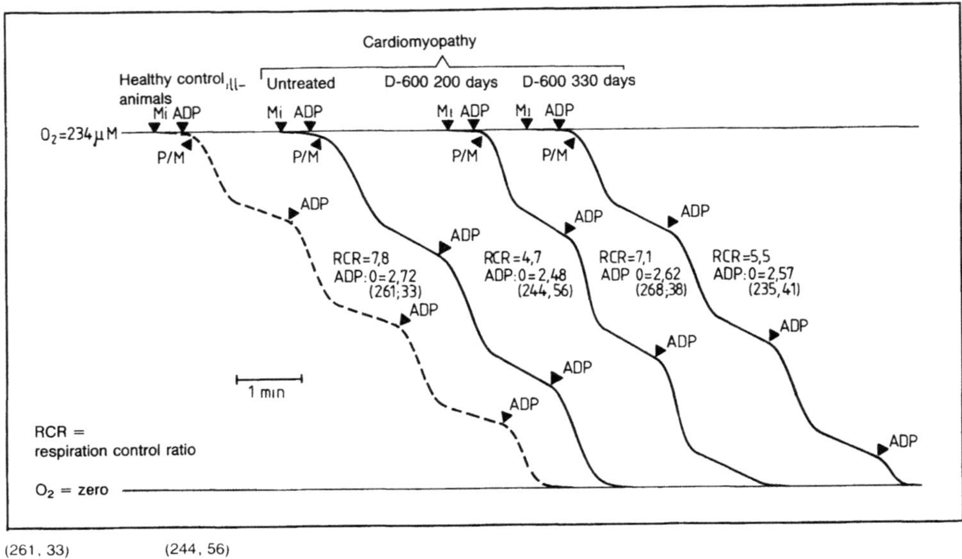

(261, 33)   (244, 56)

Figure 6. Polarographic measurements on isolated heart mitochondria from healthy control animals, untreated hamsters with cardiomyopathy and after treatment of the diseased animals with D 600 for 200 and 330 days. The determinations were carried out after stopping the treatment. Pyruvate and malate were used as substrates. The figures in parentheses show the oxygen uptake (µM/min/g protein) during stages III and IV.

Competition between gallopamil and other cardioactive drugs

The cardioprotective effect of isoprenaline (23) in cardiomyopathic hamsters prompted us to investigate the competitive therapeutic effects of adrenergic agonists and antagonists and of digoxin administered in combination with gallopamil. Table 3 shows the comparative effects of these cardio-active drugs given alone or in combination with gallopamil. The development of hypertrophy in myopathic hearts in response to isoprenaline was not dose-related and was virtually unaffected by gallopamil treatment. Similarly, there was no competition between the two drugs in preventing necrotic cardiac lesions. Methoxamine, an alpha$_1$-adrenoceptor stimulator, enhanced the necrotizing process; gallopamil abolished this stimulant effect. Propranolol, a beta-adrenoceptor blocker, reduced the necrotic changes in the heart, but the animals showed no response to the combined treatment with gallopamil, irrespective of the dosage selected. Metoprolol, a beta$_1$-adrenoceptor blocker, exhibited no preventive activity. When combined with gallopamil, in general only half the dose of each drug was needed. The preventive effect of gallopamil was still demonstrable. Treatment with digoxin did not antagonize the protective effect of gallopamil.

Summary

The fact that verapamil successfully prevented necrotic changes in the heart of hamsters with hereditary cardiomyopathy prompted us to investigate the therapeutic effects of other

20

Table 3. Effect of adrenergic agonists and antagonists and of digoxin given alone or combined with gallopamil in UM-X7.1 cardiomyopathic hamsters

Treatment (group)	Dose (mg/kg×d)	Heart weight (mg)* Body weight (g)		Necrotic cardiac lesions			
				Incidence %	Severity (Score 0–3)	Incidence %	Severity (Score 0–3)
		Control	Gallopamil**	Control		Gallopamil**	
Control	–	3.18 ± 0.03 (30)	3.44 ± 0.04 (24)	100	2.10 ± 0.13	10	0.18±0.05
Isoprenaline	3 sc	4.75 ± 0.15 (8)	4.29 ± 0.09 (8; p<0.05)	25	0.32 ± 0.12	0	0
	10 sc	4.57 ± 0.10 (8)	3.97 ± 0.07 (8; p<0.05)	50	0.66 ± 0.24	0	0
Methoxamine	3 sc	3.32 ± 0.09 (8)	3.49 ± 0.10 (8)	100	2.38 ± 0.33	0	0
Propranolol	20 ip	3.30 ± 0.11 (10)	ND*** (15)	70	1.45 ± 0.13		ND***
Metoprolol	20 ip	3.15 ± 0.08 (6)	3.27 ± 0.05 (10)	100	2.30 ± 0.18	10	1.5
Digoxin	2 sc	3.25 ± 0.08 (8)	3.53 ± 0.08 (10)	70	1.50 ± 0.35	0	0

$\bar{x}$ ± SEM; the number of animals is stated in parentheses;
 * ventricle alone;
 ** the gallopamil dose was gradually raised from 1 mg/kg×d in the first week to 2 mg/kg×d in the 3 ensuing weeks, except for the combined treatment with metoprolol — this group was only given half the dose (0.5–1 mg/kg×d);
 *** ND = no data because the animals died prematurely

calcium antagonists in this experimental model. The best results were obtained with two structural analogues, gallopamil and anipamil. Diltiazem and prenylamine also had a beneficial, but much less marked effect. However, neither nifedipine (or similar dihydropyridines, not included in this report) nor bepridil prevented the necrotic cardiac changes. Gallopamil treatment had no effect on the shift in heavy-chain (HC) myosins observed in animals with cardiomyopathy. Long-term treatment with gallopamil, up to 330 days, significantly slowed the progression of the cardiomyopathy by reducing the severity of the cardiac lesions, by lowering the calcium content of the myocardial cells and mitochondria and by improving mitochondrial respiratory function. After long-term administration the animals' life span was extended by almost 100 days and this was associated with a lower incidence of heart failure. Despite the lower calcium level in the mitochondria, there was a deterioration of oxidative phosphorylation in the terminal stage of the disease.

Acknowledgements

This research work was supported by a grant from the Medical Council of Canada and the Muscular Dystrophy Association of Canada. The authors would also like to thank the following companies for supplying the drugs we needed for these experiments: Astra Pharmaceutical Canada Ltd. (metoprolol), Ayerst Laboratories, Canada (propranolol),

Bayer AG, West Germany (nifedipine), Burroughs Welcome Inc., Canada (digoxin, methoxamine), Centre de Recherches Mauvernay, France (bepridil), Hoechst Canada Inc. (prenylamine), Knoll AG, West Germany (verapamil, gallopamil, anipamil) and Nordic Laboratories Inc., Canada (diltiazem). We are also grateful to Dr. J.-J. Léger of INSERM Montpellier, France, for providing the monoclonal antibodies for heavy-chain (HC) myosins.

References

1. Jasmin G, Eu HA (1979) Cardiomyopathy of hamster dystrophy. Ann NY Acad Sci 317:46–58
2. Jasmin G, Proschek I (1982) Hereditary polymyopathy and cardiomyopathy in the Syrian hamster. I. Progression of heart and skeletal muscle lesions in the UM-X7.1 line. Muscle & Nerve 5:20–25
3. Factor SM, Minase T, Cho S. Dominitz R, Sonnenblick EH (1982) Microvascular spasm in the cardiomyopathic Syrian hamsters: A preventable cause of local myocardial necrosis. Circulation 66:342–354
4. Berry B, Poulsen R, Yunge L, Bruneval P, Fitchell D, De Chastonay C, Gabbiani G, Huttner I (1983) Numerical densities of intramembrane partielles in the cardiac sarcolemma of normal and myopathic Syrian hamsters. J Mol Cell Cardiol 15:503–513
5. Wiegand V, Stroh E, Henniges A, Lossnitzer K, Kreuzer H (1983) Altered distribution of myosin isoenzymes in the cardiomyopathic Syrian hamsters (BIO 8.262). Basic Res Cardiol 78:665–670
6. Malhotra A, Karell M, Scheuer J (1985) Multiple cardiac contractile protein abnormalities in myopathic Syrian hamsters. J Mol Cell Cardiol 17:95–107
7. Makino N, Jasmin G, Beamish RE, Dhalla NS (1985) Sarcolemmal Na^+-Ca^{++} + exchange during the development of genetically determined cardiomyopathy. Biochem Biophys Res Comm 133:491–497
8. Sievers R, Wikman-Coffelt J, Parmley WW, Jasmin G (1986) Verapamil preserves adenine nucleotide pool in cardiomyopathic Syrian hamsters. Amer J Physiol H22–H28
9. Wagner JA, Reynolds IJ, Weissman HF, Dudek P, Weisfeld ML, Snyder SH (1986) Calcium antagonist receptors in cardiomyopathic hamster: Selective increase in heart, muscle, brain. Science 232:515–518
10. Jasmin G, Proschek L, Brisson G, Dhalla NS (1987) The hypothyroid state in cardiomyopathic hamsters. In: Dhalla NS, Singal PK, Beamish RE (eds.) Pathophysiology of heart disease. Martinus Nijhoff, Boston, in press
11. Fleckenstein A (1983) Calcium antagonism in heart and smooth muscle. John Wiley & Sons, New York, pp 153–164
12. Lindenmayer CE, Harigaya S, Bajusz E, Schwartz A (1970) Oxidative phosphorylation and calcium transport of mitochondria isolated from cardiomyopathic hamster hearts. J Mol Cell Cardiol 1:249–259
13. Wrogemann K, Nylen E (1978) Mitochondrial calcium overloading in cardiomyopathic hamsters. J Mol Cell Cardiol 10:185–195
14. Proschek L, Jasmin G (1982) Hereditary polymyopathy and cardiomyopathy in the Syrian hamster. II. Development of heart necrotic changes in relation to defective mitochondrial function. Muscle & Nerve 5:26–32
15. Lowry OH, Rosebrough NJ, Farr AL, Randall RJ (1951) Protein measurement with the folin phenol reagent. J Biol Chem 193:265–275
16. Jasmin G, Bajusz E (1973) Polymyopathie et cardiomyopathie héréditaire chez le hamster de Syrie. Inhibition sélective des lésions du myocarde. Ann Anat Pathol 18:49–66
17. Jasmin G, Bajusz E (1975) Prevention of myocardial degeneration in hamsters with hereditary cardiomyopathy. In: Fleckenstein A, Rona G (eds.) Recent Advances Pathophysiology and Morphology of Myocardial Cell Alteration. University Park Press, Baltimore, pp 219–229
18. Jasmin G, Solymoss B (1975) Prevention of hereditary cardiomyopathy in the hamster by Verapamil and other agents. Proc Soc Exp Biol Med 149:193–198

19. Jasmin G, Proschek L (1980) Prevention of myocardial degeneration in hamsters with hereditary cardiomyopathy. In: Fleckenstein A, Roskamm H (eds.) Calcium-Antagonismus. Springer, Berlin Heidelberg New York. pp 144–150
20. Jasmin G, Proschek L (1984) Comparative effects of Ca slow channel blockers on the hamster's hereditary cardiomyopathy. Symposium on Ca channel blocking agents. In: Spevelakis N, Caulfield JB (eds.) Calcium Antagonists. Mechanism of Action of Cardiac Muscle and Vascular Smooth Muscle. Martinus Nijhoff, Boston, pp 229–239
21. Jasmin G, Proschek L, Déchesne C (1986) The histochemistry of ventricular α- and β-myosin heavy chain (HC) in normal and cardiomyopathic hamsters treated with thyroxin (T$_4$). J Mol Cell Cardiol 18 (Suppl 1):233
22. Bouvagnet P, Léger J, Pons F, Déchesne C, Léger JJ (1982) Fiber types and myosin types in human atrial and ventricular myocardium. An anatomical description. Circ Res 55:794–804
23. Jasmin G, Proschek L (1983) The paradoxical effect of Isoproterenol on hamster hereditary polymyopathy. Muscle & Nerve 6:408–415
24. Jasmin G, Proschek L (1984) Calcium and myocardial cell injury. An appraisal in the cardiomyopathic hamster. Can J Physiol Pharmacol 62:891–898.

Author's address:

Prof. Dr. G. Jasmin
University of Montreal
Division of Medicine
Dept. of Pathology
Case postale 6128
Succursale "A"
Montreal, P. Q., H3C 3J7
Canada

Discussion

SPECCHIA

Which type of human cardiomyopathy is comparable to the hereditary cardiomyopathy of the hamster, the hypertrophic or congestive form? Have you found any differences in the build-up of calcium in the arterial wall in treated and untreated hamsters?

JASMIN

It is most a like human congestive cardiomyopathy. Hypertrophy does occur, but the main reason for the heart failure and profound oedema is dilatation of all four cavities of the heart. I have no definite information about the calcium level in the coronary wall. However, microcirculatory disorders may be responsible for the multifocal nature of the myocardial lesions.

STAUCH

Of course, using gallopamil to prevent necrosis in these cardiomyopathic hamsters is most interesting, but have there been any experiments in which calcium antagonists have been used to remove the calcium from these hearts?

JASMIN

At first we actually thought that calcium was responsible for the lesions. However, we now believe that calcium influx is promoted by a defective membrane transport. We cannot easily measure the amplitude of calcium movements in cardiac cell injury (ref. 24). Irreversibly damaged cells may well occur side by side with intact normal contractile cells. Using Langendorff's method to perfuse these myopathic hearts provides good evidence of preserving the nucleotides by verapamil; the calcium blocker clearly improves energy metabolism (see ref 8). It remains to be seen, however, whether removal of calcium is involved in this phenomenon.

MEINERTZ

Extrapolating the dosage you used in humans, what dose would have to be given to a patient to achieve a protective effect of this sort?

JASMIN

We used 2 mg/kg daily in our animals. In therapeutic trials in patients with muscular dystrophy we were concerned about arrhythmia; at that time a dose of 75 mg orally 3 times daily seemed recommendable. However, we would have to reconsider this dosage for better results.

Haemorheological effects of gallopamil in angina pectoris
– A controlled study

E. Ernst, A. Matrai †

Hemorheology Research Laboratory Department of Physical Medicine, University of Munich

Introduction

Under different experimental conditions, calcium antagonists alter (1, 2) or do not alter (3) parameters characterizing the flow properties of blood. Such changes could be of clinical relevance because they might increase perfusion in hypoxic tissues and thus improve the balance between oxygen supply and demand. Since experiments in vitro (4) indicated that gallopamil improves erythrocyte filterability and aggregation, we instituted a clinical trial with the aim of determining the effect of gallopamil on the flow properties of blood in patients suffering from angina pectoris.

Material and methods

Selection of patients

Twenty patients consented to take part in this study. The criterion for inclusion in the trial was clinical angina pectoris stages II–III. Criteria for exclusion were heart failure, hypotension, liver or kidney diseases, sick sinus syndrome, bradycardia (heart rate below 60/min) and AV or SA block.

Treatment schedule

During the first week of the trial the patients were given placebos. They were then treated with 50mg gallopamil (Procorum®) t.i.d. This phase was followed by another one-week placebo period. Throughout the trial the patients were allowed to take nitroglycerin p.r.n. Any other essential medications were continued unchanged.

Experimental methods

Blood was drawn, with minimal venous occlusion and without suction, into pre-heparinized (12.5 IU/ml) plastic tubes. The measurements were taken before treatment and thereafter at weekly intervals. The design of the study is shown in Fig. 1. The following variables were measured in triplicate within two hours of blood sampling:
– native blood viscosity at defined shear rates and 37 °C (Contraves LS30) (5);
– blood viscosity as above but at a haematocrit of 45% (6);
– haematocrit (microhaematocrit centrifuge);
– erythrocyte filterability (5 µm Nuclepore filters) (7);
– erythrocyte aggregation (Myrenne aggregometer) (8).

Design of the study

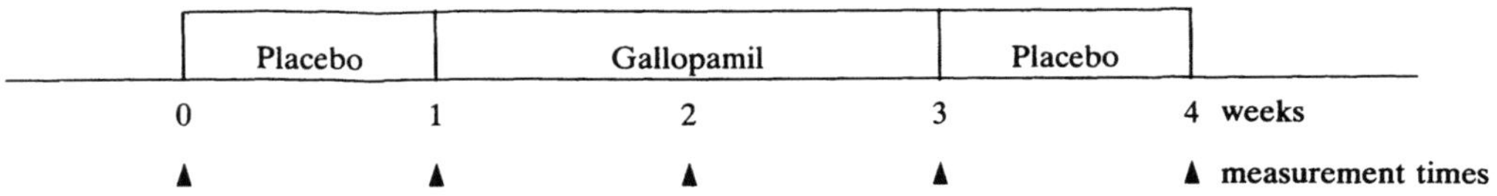

<table>
<tr><td></td><td>Placebo</td><td>Gallopamil</td><td>Placebo</td><td></td></tr>
<tr><td>0</td><td>1</td><td>2</td><td>3</td><td>4 weeks</td></tr>
<tr><td>▲</td><td>▲</td><td>▲</td><td>▲</td><td>▲ measurement times</td></tr>
</table>

Figure 1. After a one-week placebo phase, there was a two-week gallopamil phase followed by a one-week placebo phase. The measurements were made at weekly intervals. Throughout the study the patients were permitted to take nitroglycerin p.r.n.

Statistics

Student's t test and the non-parametric U test were used for the statistical comparisons. The null hypothesis was rejected if p was less than 0.05.

Results

The results are summarized in Table 1. The blood viscosities fell in the medication phase. The fall was reversible when gallopamil was stopped. There was a continuous fall of plasma viscosity, while erythrocyte filterability increased under the medication. The latter change reversed during the final week on placebo. Erythrocyte aggregation declined during the gallopamil phase and rose again thereafter.

Discussion

The results reported here reveal a significant reduction of blood viscosity in angina patients treated with gallopamil for two weeks. Most of the changes were reversible as soon as the drug was stopped. There were no significant changes during the initial placebo phase. Our findings appear to confirm those of other studies demonstrating that calcium antagonists improve the rheological properties of blood (1, 2). Results which indicate the contrary (3) may be explained by differences in the methods used and/or differences in the patient populations studied.

The flow properties of blood constitute the viscous component of peripheral resistance (9). Hence, haemorheological changes may modify blood flow and oxygen supply. From Poiseuille's law it would seem at first glance that the viscosity factor is irrelevant in the face of even minimal variations in vessel radius. Thus, while the autoregulation of vessel diameter is still intact, blood rheology is no more than a theoretical determinant of blood flow. However, if the vasomotor reserve is limited or exhausted (as occurs, for example, when hypoxia-induced dilatation is maximal) the rheological properties of blood become more relevant. Under these circumstances a reduction of blood viscosity, which was demonstrated in this study, may improve blood flow and the oxygen transport rate (10). It is therefore reasonable to postulate the rheological effects of gallopamil as being partly responsible for the anti-anginal action of the drug. However, generally speaking it is difficult to prove a causal relationship between pharmacological effects and clinical efficacy (11) and to do so would require a fundamentally different experimental approach.

26

Table 1. Haemorheological changes during the trial (means and standard deviations)

Parameter	A Baseline value	B After placebo for 1 week	C After one week of gallopamil	D After 2 weeks' gallopamil	E After 2 weeks' placebo
BV 0.7 s^{-1}	38.6 ± 5.3	37.6 ± 6.8*	35.2 ± 7.8	35.0 ± 6.2	38.5 ± 4.6°*
BV 94.5 s^{-1}	5.5 ± 0.4	5.3 ± 0.5	5.3 ± 0.5	5.3 ± 0.4	5.4 ± 0.4°*
BV (45) 0.7 s^{-1}	35.6 ± 5.4	35.0 ± 6.7°	33.1 ± 6.3	31.3 ± 6.0	38.3 ± 5.2°
BV (45) 94.5 s^{-1}	5.3 ± 0.4	5.2 ± 0.3°	5.1 ± 0.3	5.0 ± 0.3	5.3 ± 0.4°*
Haematocrit (%)	46.2 ± 2.1	46.1 ± 2.8	45.8 ± 2.3	46 7 ± 2.8	45.9 ± 1.9
Plasma- viscosity (mPa·s)	1.26 ± 0.06	1.28 ± 0.08°	1.26 ± 0.09	1.24 ± 0.06	1.25 ± 0.06
Erythrocyte aggregation (units)	11.5 ± 2.9	11.3 ± 3.0°*	8.2 ± 1.7	8.4 ± 1.2	12.6 ± 2.4°*
Erythrocyte filterability (units)	0.54 ± 0.12	0.54 ± 0.12°	0.60 ± 0.11	0.63 ± 1.1	0.51 ± 0.09°*

BV = viscosity of native blood; BV (45) = blood viscosity at a heamatocrit of 45%; * = significant difference versus C; ° = significant difference versus D

Summary

Preliminary studies showed that gallopamil like other calcium antagonists, alters the rheological properties of blood in vitro. An open clinical trial with 20 patients suffering from clinical angina pectoris stages II–III was therefore carried out to establish whether gallopamil (50 mg t.i.d.) modifies haemorheological parameters. Blood rheology was quantified by measuring blood viscosity, plasma viscosity, haematocrit, erythrocyte filterability and erythrocyte aggregation. After a one-week placebo phase there was a two-week gallopamil phase, followed by a second placebo phase. Gallopamil lowered blood and plasma viscosity and reduced erythrocyte aggregation. Erythrocyte filterability increased during the gallopamil phase. Most of the changes were reversible in the ensuing placebo phase. It is concluded that gallopamil increases the fluidity of blood. Further studies are needed to define whether these effects contribute to the anti-ischaemic action of gallopamil.

References

1. Walter D, Nicholson H, Roath S (1983) The acute effects of Nifedipine on red cell deformability in angina pectoris. Clin Hemorheol 3:294
2. Sowemino-Cocker SO, Kovacs JB, Kirby JDT, Turner P (1985) Effect of Verapamil on calcium induced rigidity and on filterability of red blood cells from healthy volunteers and patients with progressive systemic sclerosis. Brit J Clin Pharmacol 19:131

  3. Perret G, Garnier M, Modigliani E, Hanss M (1984) Lack of effect of nifedipine on erythrocyte filterability and on erythrocyte membrane lipids in healthy volunteers: A double blind cross-over study. Clin Hemorheol 4:401
  4. Ernst E, Matrai A (1986) Beeinflussung der Erythrozytenrheologie durch Gallopamil in vitro. In: Tillmann W, Ehrly AM (eds) Hämorheologie und Hämatologie. MPW, München, pp. 146–148
  5. Spinelli FR, Meier ChD (1974): Measurement of blood viscosity. Biorheology 11:301
  6. Matrai A, Whittington BBW, Ernst E (1979) Correction of blood viscosities to standardized hematocrit: a simple new method. Clin Hemorheol 5:622
  7. Dodds AJ, Flute P, Dormandy J et al. (1979) Haemorheological response to plasma exchange in Raynaud Syndrome. Brit Med J 2:1186
  8. Ernst E, Matrai A (1984) Messung des kolloidosmotischen Druckes. Labor Praxis Nov, p 8
  9. Chien S (1987) Physiological and pathophysiological significance of hemorheology. In: Chien S, Dormandy J, Ernst E, Matrai A (eds) Clinical Hemorheology. M. Nijhoff, The Hague, 1987
  10. Most AS, Ruocco NA, Gewirtz H (1986) Effect of reduction in blood viscosity on maximal myocardial oxygen delivery distal to a moderate stenosis. Circulation 74:1085–1092
  11. International Committee for Standardization in Haematology (1986) Guidelines for measurement of blood viscosity and erythrocyte deformability. Clin Hemorheol 6:439–453

Author's address:

P. D. Dr. med. E. Ernst
Hämorheologisches Forschungslabor
Klinik für physikalische Medizin
Universität München
Ziemssenstraße 1
D-8000 Munich 2
West Germany

Effect of gallopamil on local excitability, conduction and the index of arrhythmogenicity in the early phase of acute myocardial ischaemia

M. Budden, W. Meesmann

Department of Pathophysiology, Clinical Centre of the University (GHS) of Essen

During the first 30 minutes of acute LAD occlusion, ventricular arrhythmias and ventricular fibrillation occur with bimodal distribution. These characteristic, ischaemia-induced arrhythmic subphases Ia and Ib correlate with typical changes with time in local myocardial excitability thresholds and conduction times measured epicardially (at 6 electrode sites). Ia-arrhythmias develop during a rapid, pronounced and inhomogeneous rise in excitability thresholds and conduction times, whereas the Ib-arrhythmias are preceded by a spontaneous improvement in excitability and a speed-up in conduction.

In earlier experiments, from the changes in local diastolic excitability thresholds we developed an index of myocardial arrhythmogenicity in the early phase of acute myocardial ischaemia. In calculating this index, pathophysiologically important factors of arrhythmogenicity, namely the extent and rate of decrease in excitability and the evolving inhomogeneity, were weighted empirically. The resulting index curve is bimodal, with the index peaks coinciding with the occurrence of the Ia and Ib arrhythmias; in the arrhythmia-free interval the index values are low.

The experiments described below were performed on 15 anaesthetized dogs to investigate the effect of the calcium antagonist gallopamil on the excitability threshold, conduction time, the arrhythmogenicity index, arrhythmias in the early phase of ischaemia and on residual collateral perfusion (TM technique).

After two control occlusions with some arrhythmias, gallopamil was administered i.v. in a dose of 0.1 mg/kg body weight (25 µg/kg as a bolus; infusion of 2.5 µg/kg × min for 30 min, starting 20 minutes before the third occlusion). Coronary occlusion was repeated two and four hours after administration to monitor the effect of the calcium antagonist with time. Tracer microspheres were injected in the first few minutes of the second control occlusion and the first occlusion after gallopamil.

After gallopamil, the rise in the excitability thresholds and conduction times during occlusion was significantly delayed and reduced, and the partial re-decrease was retarded compared with the control occlusions. There were no ischaemia-induced arrhythmias and, correspondingly, the rise in the arrhythmogenicity index was delayed and less marked.

These effects of gallopamil were still evident two hours after administration. However, four hours after administering gallopamil time courses of excitability thresholds and conduction times were not significantly different from the courses during control occlusions and arrhythmias re-appeared. Thus, the antiarrhythmic effect of gallopamil in the early phase of acute myocardial ischaemia correlates with a delayed and reduced rise in the excitability threshold, conduction time and arrhythmogenicity index. The blood flow measurements made with the aid of tracer microspheres ruled out the possibility that these effects of gallopamil were due to a rise in residual collateral perfusion of the myocardium.

Author's address:

Dr. rer. nat. M. Budden
Abteilung für Pathophysiologie
Klinikum der Universität
Hufelandstraße 55
4300 Essen 1
West Germany

Discussion

STAUCH

My first question is, can you actually occlude a coronary artery as often as you like without altering the condition of the myocardium? Should there not have been a control study without gallopamil and another study in which the dogs were given gallopamil from the outset?
My second question is, what would have happened if gallopamil had been given only after coronary occlusion — did you try this? Is an effect still evident if there is still some residual flow?

BUDDEN

As regards your first question, we carried out repeated occlusions of suitable duration and found that the changes after the second and third occlusion were virtually the same. The major problem in carrying out a comparative study with a treated and untreated group would be that the residual collateral perfusion and area of ischaemia vary greatly from dog to dog. It would be necessary to use very large groups of animals. As to your second question, we did not administer gallopamil after coronary occlusion. However, studies have been carried out with verapamil. When verapamil was administered after acute coronary occlusion it had no discernible effect on the conduction times, but it did when it was administered before occlusion.

MEESMANN

As co-author I would like to add that an experiment in which 1) two to three initial ligations on the same animal with virtually the same baseline values elicit virtually the same changes, 2) administering the drug produces a characteristic and significant improvement in these changes, and 3) in the course of time with further ligations the values return to the baseline changes, will provide more reliable data than an experiment involving two different, treated groups comprising animals which differ in respect of, for example, collaterals and infarct size. In our studies each animal is actually its own control.

MÜLLER

Did your animals show pronounced reperfusion arrhythmias after occlusion and, if so, were these modified by gallopamil?

BUDDEN

For our studies we deliberately only considered small areas of ischaemia so as to minimize the possibility that the measurements would be interfered with by ventricular fibrillation.
Consequently, there were no, or only a few, isolated reperfusion arrhythmias. These were not modified by gallopamil.

30

Effects of gallopamil and nifedipine on ventricular arrhythmias, ventricular fibrillation, epicardial conduction delays and changes in the ventricular fibrillation threshold with time during myocardial ischaemia and reperfusion

W. Haverkamp, G. Hindricks, M. Kunert, J. Thale, Th. Behrenbeck and H. Gülker

Medical Department C, Münster University Hospital

Introduction

Malignant ventricular arrhythmias, especially ventricular fibrillation, which often occur within minutes after occlusion of a coronary vessel, are the commonest cause of sudden cardiac death (1–3). The ventricular arrhythmias which occur in animals after coronary occlusion performed once for 20–30 minutes close to the origin of the vessel show a phasic frequency distribution (4, 5). There is a build-up of the arrhythmias between the 2nd and 10th minute (phase Ia) and between the 15th and 20th minute (phase Ib). They are distinctly less severe in the interval between the two phases.

However, ventricular arrhythmias and ventricular fibrillation occur not only after occlusion of a coronary vessel but, depending on the duration of occlusion (6), they also occur when perfusion is re-established. If the areas of ischaemia are large enough (7, 8) in most cases ventricular fibrillation occurs within the first two minutes (6–13). Once sinus rhythm is re-established, between the 5th and 20th minute of the reperfusion phase (phase Id), there may be delayed, ventricular reperfusion arrhythmias which are very similar to an accelerated idioventricular rhythm (12, 13). Unlike phases Ia to Ic, in this phase of arrhythmia, ventricular fibrillation is extremely rare, even though there is high ectopic activity. It is not possible to estimate the contribution made by ventricular reperfusion arrhythmias to the pathogenesis of sudden cardiac death. Since the introduction of transluminal coronary angioplasty and coronary thrombolysis these arrhythmias have become more important from the practical, clinical point of view (14–17).

There are few published results on the anti-arrhythmic and antifibrillatory effect of gallopamil during acute myocardial ischaemia and reperfusion (18). Moreover, the data published on the effect of nifedipine are contradictory (19, 20 and other reports).

The aim of this study was

1. to investigate the effect of gallopamil versus nifedipine on ventricular arrhythmias, particularly ventricular fibrillation, during acute myocardial ischaemia and the ensuing early phase of reperfusion, and

2. to ascertain the underlying mechanisms of action by mapping the epicardial conduction delays and by measuring the ventricular fibrillation threshold.

Methods

General conditions for the study

The investigations were carried out with altogether 40 mongrel dogs under piritramide
(1 mg/kg x h)-nitrous oxide endotracheal anaesthesia ($N_2O/O_2 = 75/25$). Male and female
animals weighing from 20 to 30 kg were used.

All the animals were prepared as follows: after left lateral thoracotomy in the 5th intercostal
space and pericardiotomy, the descending ramus of the left coronary artery was exposed
close to its origin by blunt dissection, and snared with a silk thread. Tourniquet occlusions
were applied to induce acute myocardial ischaemia.

Electrophysiological investigations

The investigations were divided into two parts. In Part I we studied the effect of gallopamil
and nifedipine on the incidence of ventricular arrhythmias and ventricular fibrillation and
the effect of the two drugs on changes in epicardial conduction delays with time, during
myocardial ischaemia and reperfusion. In Part II, we analysed the effect of gallopamil and
nifedipine on the changes in the ventricular fibrillation threshold with time, during coronary
occlusion and reperfusion.

Ventricular arrhythmias and epicardial conduction delays (Part I)

The investigations were carried out on 28 dogs. In all 28 animals the descending ramus was
occluded for 20 minutes and then reperfused. Sixteen animals were used as the control. Ten
minutes before coronary occlusion, 6 other animals were given 0.125 mg/kg gallopamil i.v.
and another 6 animals were given 0.04 mg/kg nifedipine i.v. Animals which developed 2nd-
degree AV block under gallopamil were given atropine to restore 1:1 AV conduction.
Ventricular arrhythmias which occurred during the occlusion phase and reperfusion phase
were monitored continuously. If ventricular fibrillation occurred, the sinus rhythm was
restored within a few seconds by electrical defibrillation with 20 Ws.
The epicardial conduction times were determined with the aid of an epicardial multi-
electrode with 42 bipolar leads (Figure 1). The electrode was placed on the myocardium in
such a way that it would detect potentials from the non-ischaemic and from the ischaemic
myocardium. The location of the ischaemic myocardium was established from the epicardial
cyanosis which developed during a 5-minute test occlusion. The conduction times were
determined during supraventricular pacing at a rate of 160/min via a bipolar stimulation
catheter introduced into the coronary sinus. The measurements were taken continuously
twice before inducing myocardial ischaemia, every minute during myocardial ischaemia, in
the first 2 minutes after reperfusion and then in the 5th and 20th minutes. The epicardial
conduction time was regarded as the delay of the maximum deflection of the local potentials
in relation to the start of the R-wave upstroke in the ECG recorded simultaneously in lead
II. The conduction delay was calculated from the conduction times before and after
coronary occlusion and reperfusion. After the 20-minute reperfusion phase the vessel was
occluded again for 6 hours. We then determined the occluded perfusion bed of the
descending ramus, the area of myocardium exposed to ischaemia (determined by infusing 2
ml/kg methylene blue into the left atrium (21, 22)) and, after excising the heart, we
determined the infarct size by the triphenyl tetrazolium enzyme staining technique (23, 44).

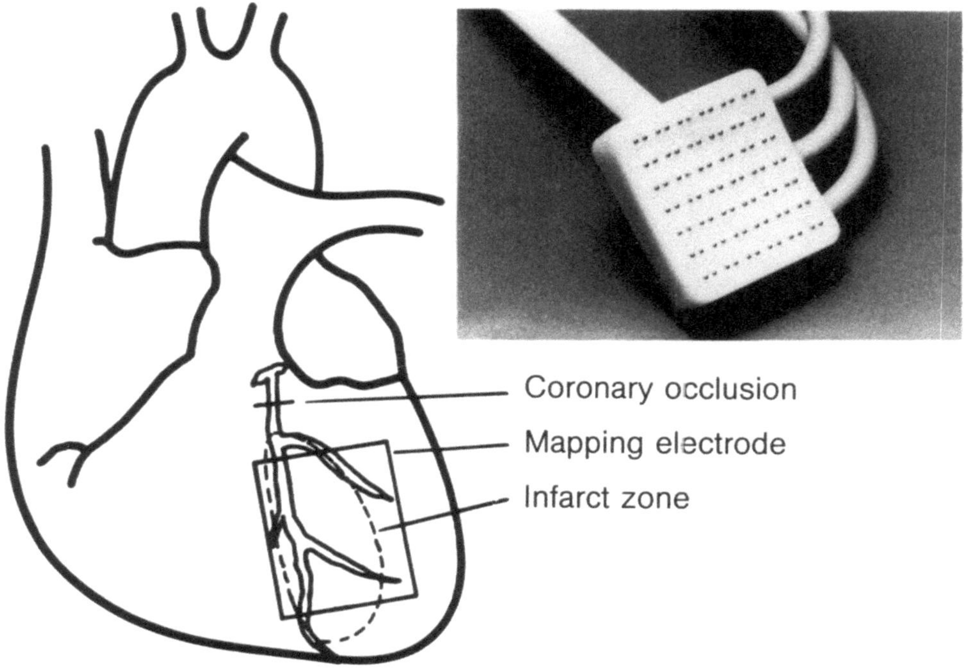

Figure 1. Position of the epicardial multi-electrode (3 × 4 cm, 42 bipolar leads) superimposed on the ischaemic zone. The gold-plated electrodes are 0.5 mm in diameter and the pairs of electrodes are arranged in 7 rows of 6 leads. The handle, which is 10 cm long, is used to position the electrode on the epicardium such that potentials can be recorded from ischaemic and non-ischaemic regions of the myocardium.

Determination of the ventricular fibrillation threshold (Part II)

In 12 dogs coronary occlusion lasting 20 minutes was carried out at 90-minute intervals. The first coronary occlusion was the control. Ten minutes before the second occlusion phase 6 animals were given gallopamil (0.1 mg/kg) and 6 animals were given nifedipine (0.04–0.08 mg/kg) i.v. To determine the ventricular fibrillation threshold, bipolar stimulation catheters were positioned in the apex of the right ventricle and in the anterolateral wall of the left ventricle in the region supplied by the descending ramus. Fibrillation was induced by microcomputer-controlled (25) electrical impulses triggered by the R wave, during the vulnerable phase of the cardiac cycle (13 single rectangular impulses, 2 ms duration, stimulus frequency 200 Hz) (Figure 2). The vulnerable phase was determined by "scanning" the relative refractory phase of the ventricle in 10-ms increments. That current which was just powerful enough to trigger ventricular fibrillation was defined as the ventricular fibrillation threshold. The sinus rhythm was restored within a few seconds by electrical defibrillation. In each case the fibrillation threshold was measured several times before coronary occlusion and 5 minutes after coronary ligation, by means of electrodes in the right ventricle. After 15 minutes it was measured within the ischaemic region in the left ventricle. The fibrillation

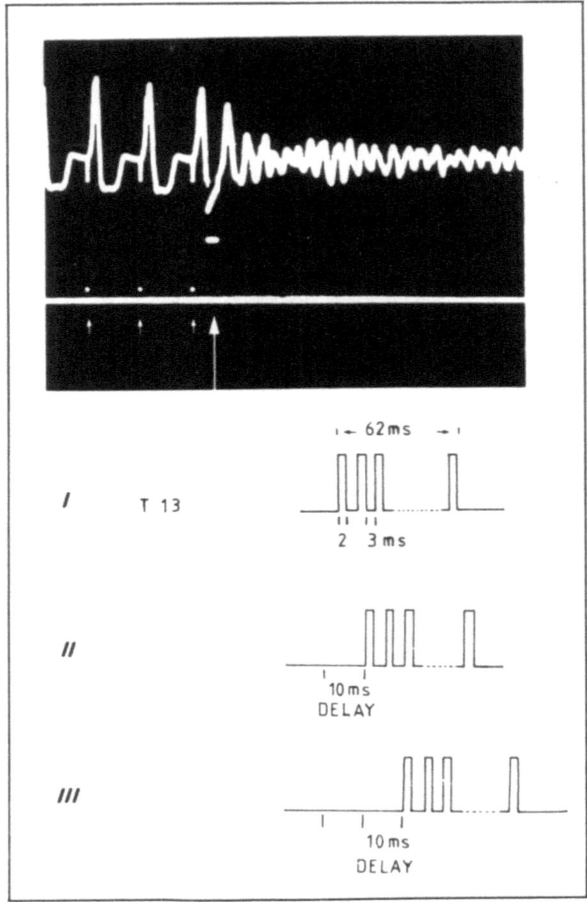

Figure 2. Determination of the ventricular fibrillation threshold: Top: Actual tracing (ECG, lead II; stimuli), Bottom: "Scanning" of the serial electrical impulses

threshold during the reperfusion phase (2 min, 5 min, 45 min and 60 min) was also measured via electrodes within the ischaemic region in the left ventricle. The sites and times of measurement were selected in the light of the characteristic changes which occur in the fibrillation threshold with time, after coronary occlusion and reperfusion (19, 26) (Figure 3): the fibrillation threshold measured by means of electrodes in the right ventricle outside the zone of ischaemia falls steeply in the first few minutes of ischaemia to a trough in the 5th minute. Even if ischaemia persists, the threshold values return to normal by the 20th minute. In contrast, the fibrillation threshold measured by means of electrodes in the ischaemic region of the left ventricle remains virtually constant in the first few minutes after coronary occlusion and does not fall to a trough until phase Ib. After reperfusion the fibrillation threshold of the right ventricle briefly falls steeply, but then rises again to the control values in the ensuing minutes. The ensuing rise of the fibrillation threshold in the ischaemic region is clearly delayed; it takes some 60 minutes for the threshold to rise again to the control level.

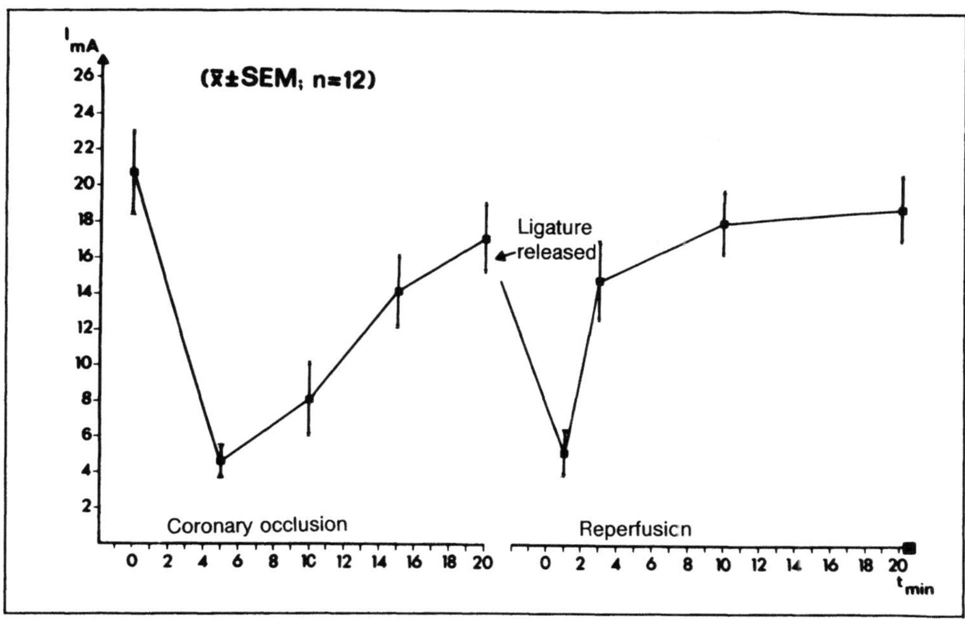

Figure 3. Changes in the ventricular fibrillation threshold with time, after acute coronary occlusion and after reperfusion (I = current; x̄ ± SEM)
a) Measured by means of electrodes outside the zone of ischaemia in the right ventricle;

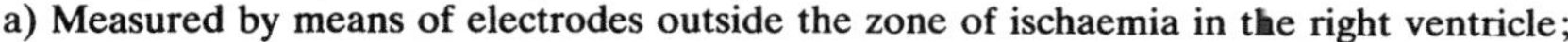

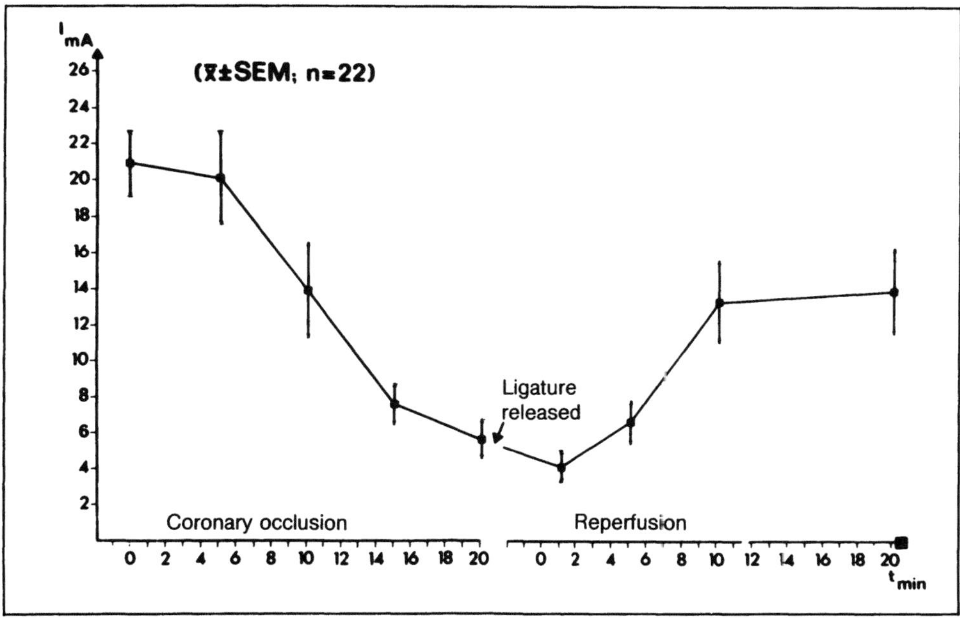

b) Measured by means of electrodes within the zone of ischaemia in the left ventricle

Statistics

The results are stated as means, with standard deviations. The statistical analysis for Part I was carried out with the aid of the Mann-Whitney-Wilcoxon test and for Part II by means of the unpaired Student's t test.

Results

Effect of gallopamil and nifedipine on the incidence of ventricular arrhythmias and ventricular fibrillation during acute myocardial ischaemia

The results are shown in Figure 4. In the control group ventricular arrhythmias and ventricular fibrillation showed a biphasic frequency distribution with arrhythmia peaks in

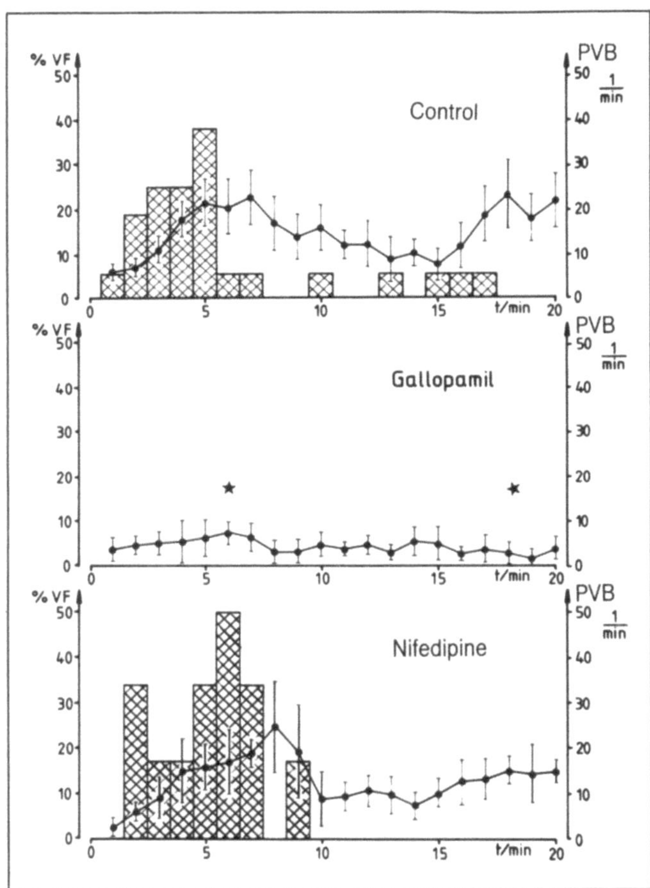

Figure 4. Effect of gallopamil and nifedipine on the incidence of ventricular arrhythmias (●—●) and of ventricular fibrillation ▩ (the diagram shows the percentage frequency of fibrillation events per minute) after acute coronary occlusion

36

the 7th and 18th minute. Recurrent ventricular fibrillation occurred in 8 of the 16 control
animals (50%) in phase 1a between the 2nd and 10th minute and in 3 of 16 animals (19%) in
phase 1b between the 13th and 17th minute. After gallopamil the incidence of premature
ventricular beats, with a peak of 7.7 ± 2.4 in the 6th minute was significantly lower than in
the control group. None of the animals pretreated with gallopamil showed ventricular
fibrillation.

In contrast, nifedipine had no effect on the severity or incidence of ventricular arrhythmias
following coronary occlusion. 50% of the animals showed recurrent ventricular fibrillation.

*Effect of gallopamil and nifedipine on epicardial conduction delays during acute myocardial
ischaemia.*

The results are shown in Figure 5. In the control group, in the first few minutes after
coronary occlusion there were pronounced changes in the local electrogram derived from
the ischaemic region, with a reduction in amplitude, fragmentation and delayed onset of the
local potentials. The delay in epicardial conduction in the ischaemic region peaked in the 5th
minute at an average of 38.0 ± 10 ms. Thereafter the conduction delays partially reversed to
10–15 ms between the 10th and 20th minute. In non-ischaemic areas of the myocardium
there were no significant changes in conduction during the phase of ischaemia.

After gallopamil there was a clear-cut reduction in the peak of the epicardial conduction
delays. The peak delay, 18.4 ± 1.4 ms, reached in the 6th minute, was significantly lower
than in the control group. On the other hand, pretreating the animals with nifedipine did not
have any effect on the peak height of conduction delays in the ischaemic region. There were

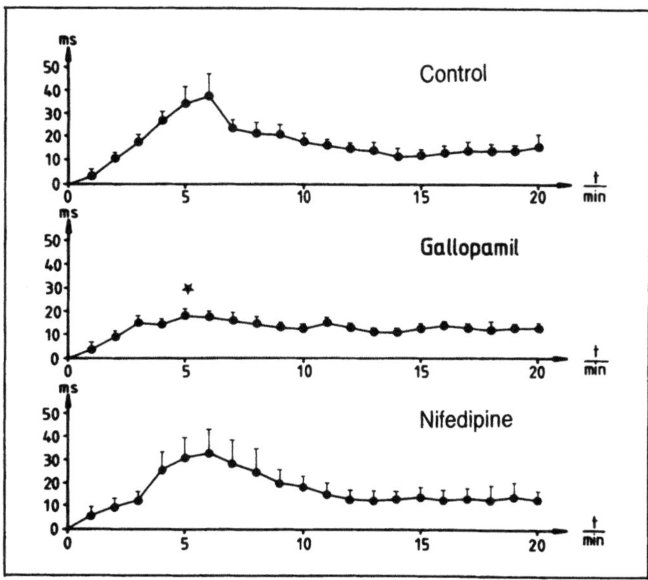

Figure 5. Effect of gallopamil and nifedipine on epicardial conduction delays in the ischaemic region
after acute coronary occlusion (x̄ ± SEM; * = p<0.05)

no significant differences between the three groups as regards conduction delays between the 10th and 20th minute.

Effect of gallopamil and nifedipine on the ventricular fibrillation threshold during acute myocardial ischaemia

The results are shown in Figure 6. Neither gallopamil nor nifedipine had a significant effect on the ventricular fibrillation threshold prior to coronary occlusion. Under control condition the fibrillation threshold measured in the right ventricle 5 minutes after coronary occlusion

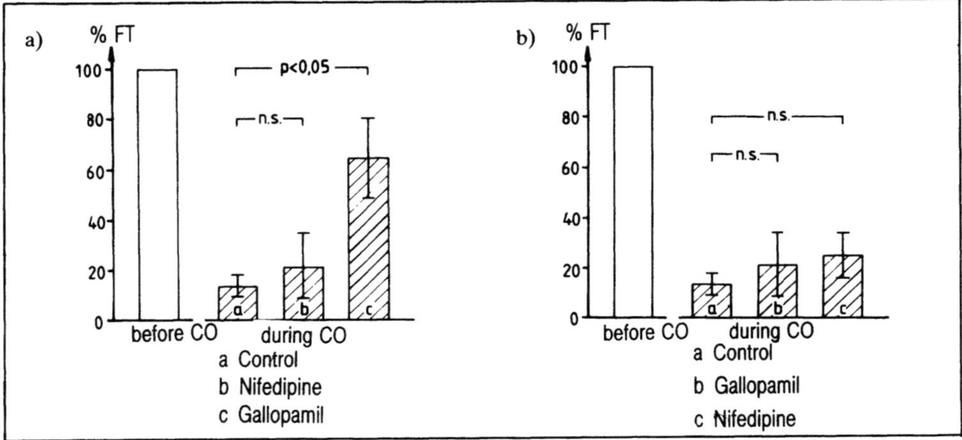

Figure 6. Effect of gallopamil and nifedipine on the lowering of the fibrillation threshold (FT)
a) Electrodes positioned outside the zone of ischaemia in the right ventricle; 5 min after acute coronary occlusion (CO); b) Electrodes positioned within the zone of ischaemia in the left ventricle; 15 min after acute coronary occlusion

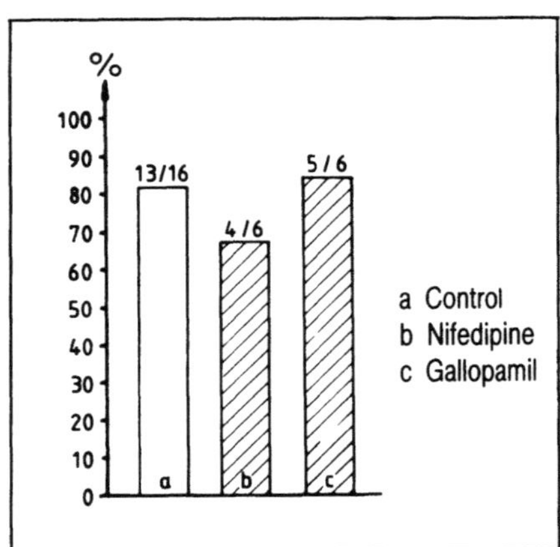

Figure 7. Effect of gallopamil and nifedipine on the incidence of initial reperfusion ventricular fibrillation after releasing the coronary ligature

fell by 85%, from 25.6 ± 3.1 mA to 3.8 ± 2.9 mA (p<0.001), in the gallopamil group and by 87%, from 20.0 ± 2.0 mA to 2.5 ± 1.5 mA (p<0.001), in the nifedipine group. After pretreatment with gallopamil coronary occlusion only reduced the fibrillation threshold by 36%, from 18.7 ± 3.7 mA to 12.0 ± 3.2 mA (p<0.01 versus the control occlusion). In contrast, nifedipine did not inhibit the decrease in the fibrillation threshold, which fell by 91%, from 17.0 ± 1.0 mA to 1.5 ± 0.5 mA (n.s. versus the control occlusion).

Under control conditions the ventricular fibrillation threshold measured within the ischaemic region 15 minutes after coronary occlusion fell by 79%, from 22.9 ± 2.8 mA to 4.9 ± 2.1 mA, in the gallopamil group and by 74%, from 17.0 ± 1.0 mA to 4.5 ± 2.0 mA, in the nifedipine group. The changes were statistically significant (p<0.001) in both groups. After gallopamil the fibrillation threshold fell by 75%, from 21.2 ± 3.1 mA to 5.2 ± 2.1 mA (p<0.001), and after nifedipine it fell by 79%, from 17.0 ± 3.5 mA to 3.6 ± 2.5 mA (p<0.001). The differences in the fibrillation thresholds were not statistically significant.

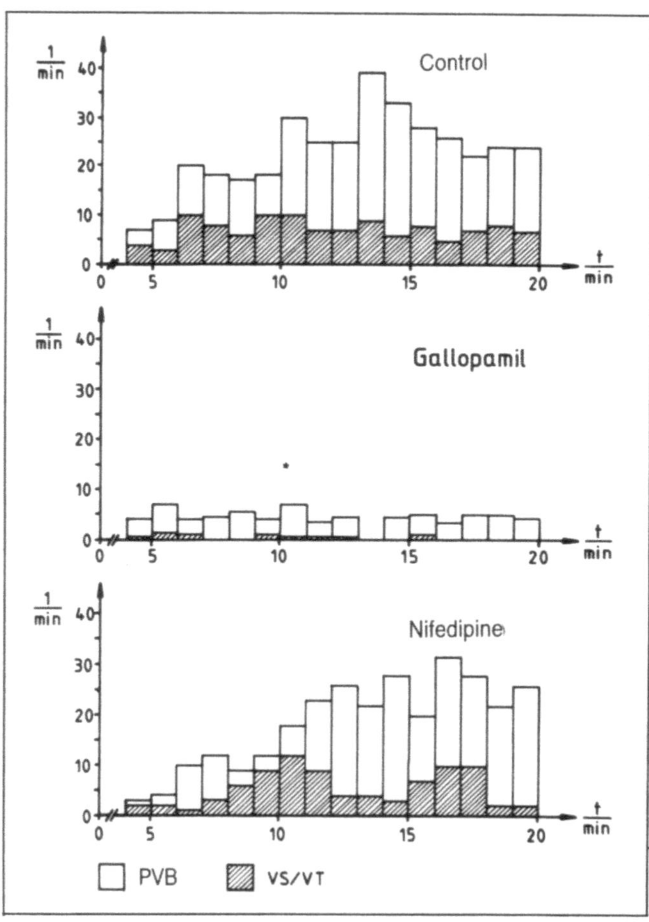

Figure 8. Effect of gallopamil and nifedipine on the delayed arrhythmias after reperfusion (PVB = premature ventricular beats, VS = ventricular salvoes, VT = ventricular tachycardia; * = p < 0.05)

Effect of gallopamil and nifedipine on the incidence of ventricular arrhythmias after reperfusion

Under control conditions 13 of 16 animals (81%) developed initial ventricular fibrillation within 3 minutes of the blood flow being restored (Figure 7). After pretreatment with gallopamil reperfusion ventricular fibrillation occurred in 4 of 6 animals (67%) and after nifedipine it occurred in 5 of 6 animals (86%). The differences were not statistically significant.
Eight of 16 animals (50%) in the control group showed delayed reperfusion arrhythmias (Figure 8). Gallopamil suppressed these arrhythmias virtually completely, whereas pretreating the animals with nifedipine did not significantly affect the incidence of delayed reperfusion arrhythmias.

Effect of gallopamil and nifedipine on epicardial conduction delays after reperfusion

The results are shown in Figure 9. The restoration of perfusion at the end of the occlusion phase caused a sudden and inhomogeneous reversal of the epicardial conduction delays in the ischaemic region, with restitution of the amplitude and less fragmentation of the local

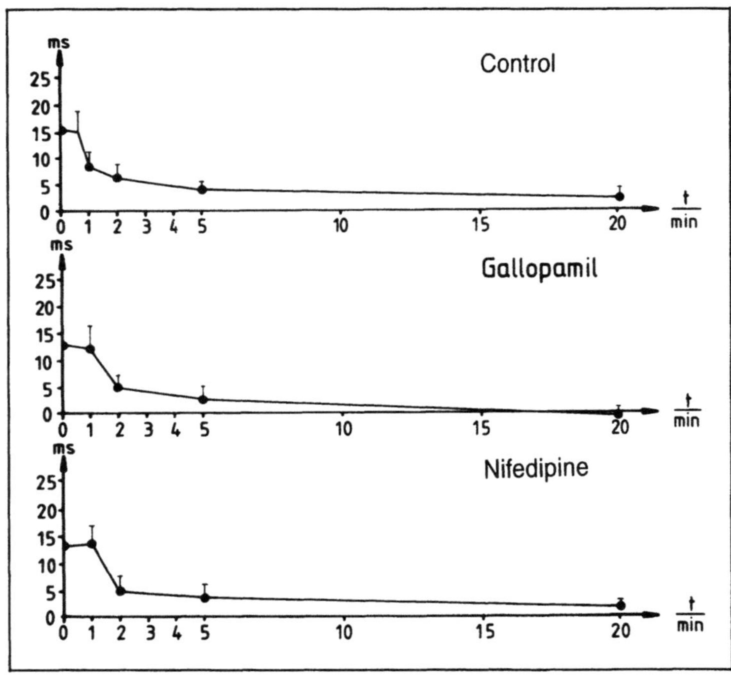

Figure 9. Effect of gallopamil and nifedipine on epicardial conduction delays in the ischaemic region after reperfusion ($\bar{x}$ ± SEM)

potentials. Just 5 minutes after releasing the ligation, epicardial conduction in the ischaemic region had almost completely returned to normal both under control conditions and after gallopamil and nifedipine. There were no statistically significant differences in conduction delays.

Effect of gallopamil and nifedipine on changes in the fibrillation threshold with time, after reperfusion

The results are shown in Figure 10. Under control conditions, immediately after reperfusion the fibrillation threshold measured within the ischaemic region was 2.9 ± 1.6 mA in the gallopamil group and 1.0 ± 0.5 mA in the nifedipine group. There were no significant changes in the fibrillation threshold after treatment with gallopamil or nifedipine. Gallopamil and nifedipine significantly hastened the rise in the fibrillation threshold during the reperfusion phase. Under control conditions it took 60 minutes for the values to return to the baseline. After pretreatment with gallopamil the values returned to the baseline after only 15 minutes, whereas under nifedipine it was 30 minutes before the fibrillation threshold had returned to the control values. The difference in the rise of the fibrillation threshold in the two groups was statistically significant ($p < 0.05$) 15 minutes after the restoration of perfusion.

Effect of gallopamil and nifedipine on infarct size

Under control conditions the area of myocardium exposed to ischaemia was $40.5 \pm 3.4\%$ of the left ventricle and the area was not statistically significantly different in the animals pretreated with gallopamil or nifedipine ($38.8 \pm 2.3\%$ and $39.8 \pm 2.9\%$ respectively) (Figure 11). Gallopamil reduced the infarct size in terms of the left ventricle significantly, by 41% ($14.5 \pm 1.6\%$ compared with $24.5 \pm 2.8\%$ in the control group, $p < 0.05$). Pretreating the animals with nifedipine had no significant effect on infarct size ($23.1 \pm 2.3\%$ of the left ventricle, n.s. versus the control group).

Discussion

Effect of gallopamil and nifedipine on ventricular arrhythmias and ventricular fibrillation during myocardial ischaemia

Unlike nifedipine, in the study reported here gallopamil exhibited pronounced anti-arrhythmic and antifibrillatory effects after coronary occlusion. Although it was as long ago as the late 1960s that Fleckenstein et al. (27) characterized gallopamil as a highly specific calcium antagonist, hitherto there has only been one study on the effect of gallopamil on ischaemia-induced ventricular arrhythmias. Müller and Beckmann (18) showed in rats that, administered 3 minutes after occluding the left coronary artery, (+)-gallopamil significantly reduced the incidence of ventricular arrhythmias and ventricular fibrillation between the 5th and 10th minute after coronary ligation. Our findings confirmed these initial results, which were of limited general value because they were obtained in rats which generally do not exhibit constant arrhythmias associated with ventricular fibrillation. We obtained comparable results when using Verapamil (19, 34) consistent with published findings (28–33). Since then,

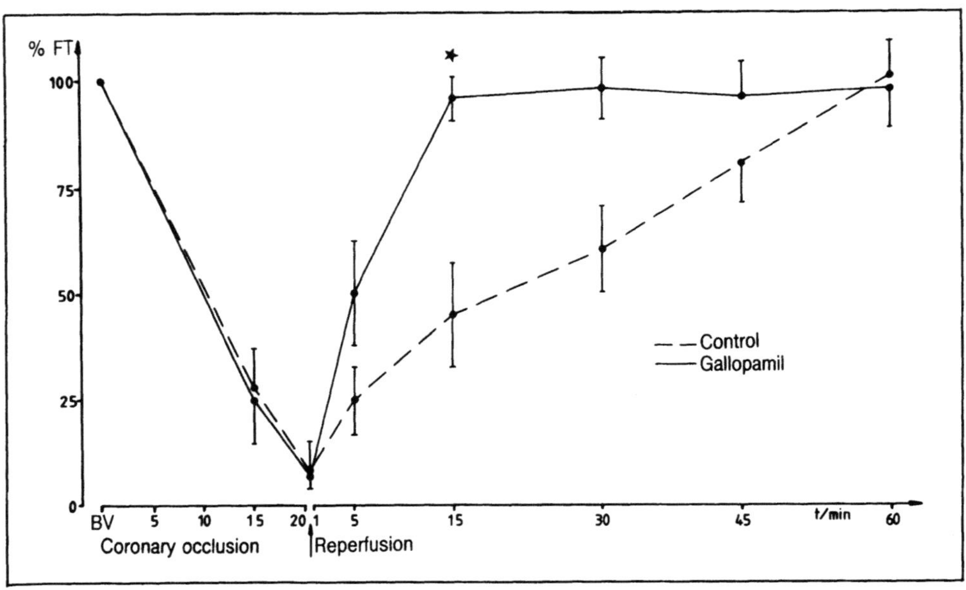

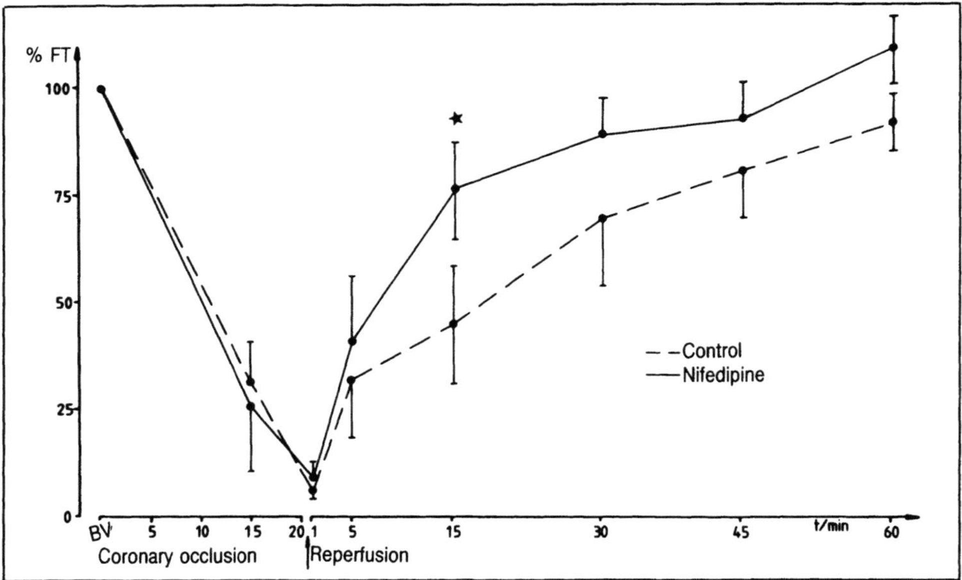

Figure 10. Effect of gallopamil and nifedipine on the rise in the fibrillation threshold after reperfusion (electrodes positioned within the zone of ischaemia in the left ventricle); BV = baseline
a) Gallopamil * = p<0.01;   b) Nifedipine * = p<0.05

42

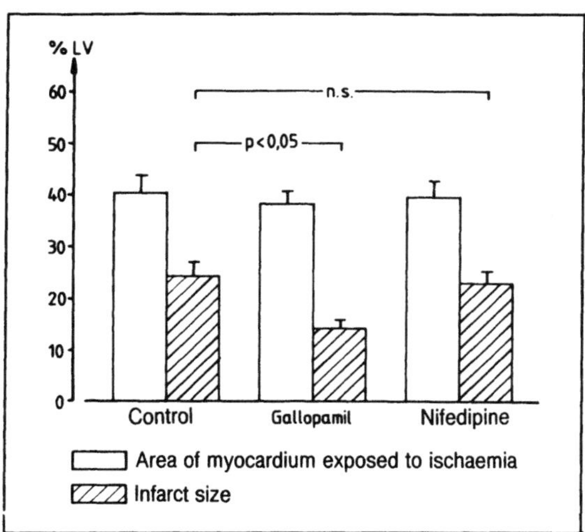

Figure 11. Area of myocardium exposed to ischaemia and infarct size in the control group and after pretreatment with gallopamil and with nifedipine (the data are expressed in terms of the mass of the left ventricle)

tiapamil, another phenylalkylamine, has also been shown to have significant anti-arrhythmic and antifibrillatory effects (35–37).

In contrast, studies on nifedipine have produced inconsistent and to some extent contradictory results. Promising results with nifedipine were obtained mainly in rats (38, 39), whereas the results of studies by Henry (40) and Verrier and Lown (41) in dogs, like our results, and the data obtained by Verdouw et al. (42) in pigs, did not reveal any evidence that nifedipine has anti-arrhythmic or antifibrillatory effects after coronary occlusion.

Effect of gallopamil and nifedipine on epicardial conduction delays and changes in the ventricular fibrillation threshold with time, after coronary occlusion

The pronounced anti-arrhythmic and antifibrillatory effects of gallopamil in phase Ia were associated with a significant reduction in the lowering of the fibrillation threshold measured in the non-ischaemic myocardium. It has also been reported that other phenylalkylamines inhibit the lowering of the fibrillation threshold during this phase of arrhythmia (19, 30, 31, 36, 37, 43). An explanation for the effect of gallopamil in reducing cardiac vulnerability at this time may be that it reduces the disparity in conduction between non-ischaemic and ischaemic regions of the myocardium and within ischaemic areas by reducing maximum epicardial conduction delays in the ischaemic region. The fact that there was no alteration of conduction delays under nifedipine indicates that this drug does not modify the lowering of the right ventricular fibrillation threshold or the incidence of ventricular fibrillation.

One possible reason for the reduction of epicardial conduction delays and of the lowering of the fibrillation threshold in phase Ia under gallopamil is that this drug slows the rise in the extracellular potassium concentration in the ischaemic region. Meesmann et al. (44) demonstrated this effect with gallopamil, but not with nifedipine. Slowing the rise in the extracellular potassium concentration reduces the fall in the resting membrane potential of ischaemic myocardium cells and thus improves depressed fast response potentials in this phase of arrhythmia.

Other factors which may be responsible for slowing conduction during myocardial ischaemia are hypoxia (45–47) and acidosis (45, 47–50). Gallopamil reduces the hypoxia-induced depletion of energy-rich phosphate compounds and glycogen in the myocardium (51). It reduces the enzyme loss under low-flow conditions and ensuing normal perfusion (51). It has been reported that nifedipine exhibits cardioprotective effects (52, 53), but recent comparative studies have shown that the effects of phenylalkylamines are significantly more marked than those of dihydropyridines (54, 55). This hypothesis is corroborated by the study reported here. Gallopamil significantly reduced infarct size, by on average 41%, whereas nifedipine did not significantly affect the extent of myocardial necrosis. A possible explanation for these differences is that gallopamil causes a more marked reduction of calcium influx, which increases under conditions of ischaemia. The effect of phenylalkylamines such as gallopamil and verapamil, and of the benzothiazepine derivative diltiazem, on the slow inward current of calcium is markedly rate-dependent (56–60), whereas this is much less pronounced with dihydropyridines (59, 61). Also, gallopamil and verapamil markedly delay the recovery from the inactivation of calcium-dependent action potentials (58, 60), whereas the delaying effect of dihydropyridines is minimal (59, 61).

Haemodynamic effects do not appear to be of any relevance as regards the different electrophysiological effects we observed. Gallopamil does afford a fairly marked reduction in cardiac oxygen demand, and it reduces the blood pressure and, unlike nifedipine, the heart rate. However, these effects were largely nullified because the measurements of epicardial conduction delays and ventricular fibrillation threshold were taken during constant supraventricular or ventricular pacing.

The pronounced anti-arrhythmic and antifibrillatory effects of gallopamil in phase Ib following coronary occlusion did not coincide with any effect on epicardial conduction delays or on the lowering of the fibrillation threshold within the ischaemic region. The effect of gallopamil in inhibiting ventricular fibrillation during this phase of arrhythmia is best explained by the pronounced anti-arrhythmic action, thus being an indirect effect.

Effect of gallopamil and nifedipine on ventricular arrhythmias, epicardial conduction delays and changes in the fibrillation threshold with time, after reperfusion

In the study reported here, neither gallopamil nor nifedipine prevented early reperfusion ventricular fibrillation or the heterogeneous reversal of conduction delays and the initial fall in the fibrillation threshold after the restoration of perfusion. The effect of gallopamil on early reperfusion ventricular fibrillation had never previously been investigated. However, the published results for verapamil (19, 31, 33, 62, 64), tiapamil (37) and nifedipine (19, 63, 64) also indicated that in the main these drugs have no effects. Discrepancies in the published results are mainly due to lack of standardization of the experimental model (13, 62). It is also conceivable that calcium antagonists such as gallopamil reduce reperfusion fibrillation when there are relatively small areas of the myocardium exposed to ischaemia, since in the study reported here gallopamil significantly hastened the restoration of electrical stability later on during the reperfusion phase.

Cardioprotective properties also explain this effect of the drug. The significance of increased calcium influx into the myocardial cells, particularly during reperfusion, has been alluded to repeatedly in the literature (65–68). This probably also explains the marked suppression of the delayed reperfusion arrhythmias, the underlying cause of which is thought to be abnormal automaticity of subendocardial Purkinje fibres damaged by ischaemia or reperfusion (69, 70). However, neither gallopamil nor nifedipine is effective in short-term i.v. treatment for "late" reperfusion arrhythmias (unpublished investigations).

Nifedipine did in fact hasten the rise of the fibrillation threshold following reperfusion and thus it did afford some degree of cardioprotection, but its effects were significantly less pronounced than those of gallopamil and evidently did not suffice to suppress the delayed reperfusion arrhythmias.

Summary

The effect of gallopamil and nifedipine on ventricular arrhythmias, ventricular fibrillation, epicardial conduction delays and the change in the ventricular fibrillation threshold with time, following acute coronary occlusion and ensuing reperfusion, was studied in altogether 40 anaesthetized dogs. Gallopamil caused a clear-cut reduction in the incidence of spontaneous arrhythmias and ventricular fibrillation and, at the same time, it significantly reduced peak conduction delays and the lowering of the fibrillation threshold in phase Ia. Nifedipine exhibited none of these effects. There were no effects on the epicardial conduction delays or the lowering of the fibrillation threshold in phase Ib.

Neither gallopamil nor nifedipine reduced the incidence of initial ventricular fibrillation after reperfusion. However, both drugs, but particularly gallopamil, accelerated the rise in the fibrillation threshold in the ischaemic region. Unlike nifedipine, gallopamil also significantly reduced delayed reperfusion arrhythmias.

The differences in the anti-arrhythmic and antifibrillatory effects of gallopamil and nifedipine during acute myocardial ischaemia and after reperfusion can be explained by differences in their bioelectrical pharmacological properties and in the degree of cardio-protection.

References

1. Goldstein S, Lanids JR, Leighton R (1981) Characteristics of the resuscitated out-of-hospital cardiac arrest victims with coronary heart disease. Circulation 64:977–982
2. Myerburg RJ, Conde CA, Sung RJ (1980) Clinical electrophysiologic and hemodynamic profile of patients resuscitated from prehospital cardiac arrest. Am J Med 68:658–572
3. Iseri LT, Humphrey SB, Siner EJ (1978) Prehospital bradyasystolic cardiac arrest. Ann intern Med 88:741–748
4. Kaplinsky E, Ogawa S, Balke CW, Dreifus LS (1979) Two periods of early ventricular arrhythmia in the canine acute myocardial infarction model. Circulation 60:397–403
5. Meesmann W, Gülker H, Krämer B, Stephan K, Menken U, Wiegand V (1979) Ventrikuläre Arrhythmien und Vulnerabilität des Herzens in der Frühphase nach akutem experimentellem Koronarverschluß und nach Reperfusion – mögliche Mechanismen. In: Antoni H, Bender F, Gerlach E, Schlepper M (eds) Herzrhythmusstörungen. Schattauer, Stuttgart, pp. 27–43
6. Balke CW, Kaplinsky E, Michelson EL, Naito M, Dreifus LS (1981) Reperfusion tachyarrhythmias: correlation with antecedent coronary artery occlusion tachyarrhythmias and duration of myocardial ischemia. Am Heart J 101:449–456

7. Sheehan FH, Epstein SE (1983) Determinants of arrhythmic death during coronary artery reperfusion: effect of perfusion bed size. Am Heart J 105:911–914

8. Austin M, Wenger TL, Harrell FE, Luzzi FA, Strauss HC (1982) Effect of myocardium at risk on outcome after coronary occlusion and release. Am J Physiol 243:H340–364

9. Axelrod PJ, Verrier RL, Lown B (1974) Vulnerability to ventricular fibrillation during acute coronary arterial occlusion and release. Am J Cardiol 36:776–782

10. Battle WE, Naimi S, Avitall B, Brilla AH, Banas JS, Bete JM, Levine JH (1974) Distinctive time course of ventricular vulnerability to fibrillation during and after release of coronary ligation. Am J Cardiol 34:42–47

11. Cox SL, Thomas MD, Boineau JP (1977) The electrophysiological time course of acute myocardial ischemia and the effects of early coronary artery reperfusion. Circulation 48:971–983

12. Kaplinsky E, Ogawa S, Michelson EL, Dreifus LS (1981) Instantaneous and delayed ventricular arrhythmias after reperfusion of acutely ischemic myocardium: evidence for multiple mechanisms. Circulation 63:333–340

13. Thale J, Gülker H, Haverkamp W, Hindricks G, Bender F (1986) Pharmakologische Beeinflussung von Reperfusionsarrhythmien. In: Brisse B, Bender F (eds) Autonome Innervation des Herzens. Myokardiale Hypoxie. Steinkopff, Darmstadt, pp. 225–246

14. Goldberg S, Greenspan AJ, Urban PL, Muza B, Berger B, Walinsky P, Marokko PR (1983) Reperfusion arrhythmia: a marker of restoration of antegrade flow during intracoronary thrombolysis for acute myocardial infarction. Am Heart J 105:26–32

15. Mathey DG, Kuck K-H, Tilsner V, Krebber H-J, Bleifeld W (1981) Nonsurgical coronary artery recanalization in acute transmural myocardial infarction. Circulation 63:489–497

16. Westveer DC, Stewart J, Hauser AM, Gangadharan V, Ramos RG, Kanelas C, Gordeon S, Timmis GC (1983) The significance of reperfusion arrhythmias with thrombolytic coronary recanalization. Circulation 68 (Suppl III):410

17. Timmis GC, Ramos RG, Gangadharan V, Gordeon S (1985) Determinants of reperfusion arrhythmias in a randomized trial of streptokinase vs angioplasty for acute myocardial infarction. Circulation 72 (Suppl III):219

18. Müller B, Beckmann K (1982) Effects of the optical isomers of D 600 on cardiovascular parameters and on arrhythmias caused by aconitine and coronary artery ligation in anesthetized rats. J Cardiovasc Pharmacol 4:615–621

19. Gülker H, Thale J, Brisse B, Bender F (1984) Vergleichende Untersuchungen zur antiarrhythmischen und antifibrillatorischen Wirksamkeit von Verapamil und Nifedipin nach akutem Koronarverschluß und nach Reperfusion. Z Kardiol 73:515–524

20. Crome R, Hearse DJ, Manning AS (1986) Ischaemia and reperfusion-induced arrhythmias. Beneficial effects of nifedipine. In: Lichtlen PR (Ed) 6th international Adalat symposium. New therapy of ischaemic heart disease and hypertension. Excerpta Medica, Amsterdam, pp 100–107

21. Darsee JA, Kloner RA (1980) The no reflow phenomenon: a time-limiting factor for reperfusion after coronary occlusion? Am J Cardiol 46:800–806

22. Lo HM, Kloner RA, Braunwald E (1985) Effect of intracoronary verapamil on infarct size in the ischemic, reperfused canine heart: Critical importance of the timing of treatment. Am J Cardiol 56:672–677

23. Lie JT, Pairolero PC, Holley KE, Titus JL (1975) Macroscopic enzyme-mapping verification of large, homogeneous, experimental myocardial infarcts of predictable size and location in dogs. J Thorac Cardiovasc Surg 69:599–605

24. Fishbein MC, Meerbaum S, Rit J, Lando U, Kanmatsuse K, Mercier JC, Corday E, Ganz W (1981) Early phase acute myocardial infarct size quantification: validation of the triphenyl tetrazolium chloride tissue enzyme staining technique. Am Heart J 101:593–600

25. Heuer H, Gülker H, Bender F (1981) Mikrocomputergesteuerte 3-Kanal-Stimulationseinrichtung zur Analyse der atrialen und ventrikulären Vulnerabilität des Herzens. Biomed Techn 26:130–135

26. Gülker H, Thale J, Bender F (1983) Different time course of the ventricular fibrillation threshold following acute coronary artery occlusion and release in ischemic and non-ischemic areas of the heart. Pace (Suppl II):34

27. Fleckenstein A (1983) Calcium antagonism in heart and smooth muscle. Experimental facts and therapeutic prospects. John Wiley & Sons, New York

28. Kaumann AJ, Aramendia P (1968) Prevention of ventricular fibrillation induced by coronary ligation. J Pharmacol 164:326–332

29. Elharrar V, Gaum WE, Zipes DP (1977) Effect of drugs on conduction delay and incidence of ventricular arrhythmias induced by acute coronary occlusion in dogs. Am J Cardiol 39:544–549

30. Fondacaro JD, Han J, Yoon MS (1979) Effects of verapamil on ventricular rhythm during acute coronary occlusion. Am Heart J 96:81–86

31. Brooks WW, Verrier RL, Lown B (1980) Protective effect of verapamil on vulnerability to ventricular fibrillation during myocardial ischemia and reperfusion. Cardiovasc Res 14:295–302

32. Schwartz PJ, Vandi E, Zaza A (1981) The prevention of cardiac arrhythmias associated with myocardial ischemia and dependent upon increases in sympathetic activity. In: Zanchetti A, Krikler (eds) Calcium antagonism in cardiovascular therapy. Experience with verapamil. Excerpta Medica, Amsterdam, pp. 314–325

33. Pelleg A, Pardo Y, Belhassen B, Shargordsky B, Chagnac A, Laniado S (1985) Effects of verapamil and bepridil on occlusion and reperfusion arrhythmias in the canine heart. Cardiology 72:185–201

34. Haverkamp W, Thale J, Gülker H, Hindricks G, Niedermeyer J, Bender F (1985) Effects of different calcium antagonists on ventricular arrhythmias and epicardial conduction delay during acute coronary occlusion and reperfusion. Naunyn-Schmiedeberg's Arch Pharmacol 332 (Suppl):R45

35. Saini R, Antonaccio M (1982) Antiarrhythmic, antifibrillatory activities and reduction of infarct size after the calcium antagonist Ro 11–1781 (tiapamil) in anaesthetized dogs. J Pharmacol Exp Ther 221:29–36

36. Thandroyen F, Higginson L, Opie L (1982) Protective effect of a calcium channel antagonist agent (CCAA), tiapamil (Ro-11-1781) against ventricular fibrillation during acute myocardial ischemia and reperfusion. Circulation 66 (Suppl II):140

37. Raeder EA, Verrier RL, Lown B (1986) Protective effect of tiapamil against ventricular fibrillation during coronary artery occlusion. Am Heart J 111:878–882

38. Fagbemi O, Parratt JR (1981) Calcium antagonists prevent early postinfarction ventricular fibrillation. Eur J Pharmacol 75:179–185

39. Parratt JR, Coker SJ (1983) Cardioprotection with calcium antagonists by suppression of early ischaemia and reperfusion-induced arrhythmias. Eur Heart J 4 (Suppl C):49–54

40. Henry PD (1982) Comparative pharmacology of calcium antagonists: nifedipine, verapamil and diltiazem. Am J Cardiol 46:107–1058

41. Verrier RL, Lown B (1981) Contrasting effects of verapamil and nifedipine on vulnerability to ventricular fibrillation in the normal and ischemic heart. In: Zanchetti A, Krikler DM (eds) Calcium antagonism in cardiovascular therapy. Experience with verapamil. Excerpta Medica, Amsterdam, pp. 326–337

42. Verdouw PD, Wolffenbuttel BHR, Ten Cate FJ (1983) Nifedipine with and without propranolol in the treatment of myocardial ischemia: effect on ventricular arrhythmias and recovery of regional wall function. Eur Heart J 4 (Suppl C):101–108

43. Thandroyen FT (1982) Protective action of calcium channel antagonist agents against ventricular fibrillation in the isolated perfused rat heart. J Moll Cell Cardiol 14:21–32

44. Vogt B, Budden M, Kirchengast M, Zhang KM, Martin C, Meesmann W (1987) Zeitverlauf der extracellulären myokardialen Kalium-Aktivität während akuter Myokardischämie und der Einfluß von Gallopamil bei Hunden und Schweinen. In this book, p. 52

45. Morena H, Janse ML, Durrer D (1980) Comparison of the effects of regional ischemia, hypoxia, hyperkalemia and acidosis on intracellular and extracellular potentials and metabolism in the isolated porcine heart. Circ Res 46:634–646

46. Futura T, Kodama I, Shimuzu T, Toyama J, Yamada K (1983) Effects of hypoxia on the electrical activity of canine cardiac Purkinje fibers. Jpn Heart J 24:417–425

47. Kodama I, Wilde A, Janse MJ, Durrer D (1984) Combined effects of hypoxia, hyperkalemia and acidosis on membrane potential and excitability of guinea-pig ventricular muscle. J Moll Cell Cardiol 16:247–259

48. Marrannes R, deHemptinne, Leusen I (1979) Influence of lactate and other organic ions on conduction velocity in mammalian heart fibers depressed by "metabolic" acidosis. J Mol Cell Cardiol 11:800–814

49. DeMello WC (1980) Influence of intracellular injection of H^+ on the electrical coupling in cardiac Purkinje fibers. Cell Biol Int Rep 4:51–58

50. Kagiyama Y, Hill JL, Gettes LS (1982) Interaction of acidosis and increased extracellular potassium on action potential characteristics and conduction in guinea pig ventricular muscle. Circ Res 51:614–623

51. Raschak M, Gries J, Bühler V, Maurer R (1983) Untersuchungen zur kardialen und vasalen Wirksamkeit von Gallopamil. In: Kaltenbach M, Hopf R (eds) Gallopamil. Pharmakologisches und klinisches Wirkungsprofil eines Kalziumantagonisten. Springer, Berlin Heidelberg New York, pp. 75–82
52. Nayler WG, Ferrari R, Williams A (1980) Protective effect of pretreatment with verapamil, nifedipine and propranolol on mitochondrial function in the ischemic and reperfused myocardium. Am J Cardiol 46:242–248
53. Nayler WG, Dillon JS, Panagiotopoulos S, Sturrock WJ (1986) Dihydropyridines and the ischaemic myocardium. In: Lichtlen PR (ed) 6th inernational Adalat symposium. New therapy of ischaemic heart disease and hypertension. Excerpta Medica, Amsterdam, pp. 386–399
54. Ym R, Patterson RE, Markle D, McGuire D, Goldstein SR, Speir EH, Greene R, Aamodt R, Epstein SE (1983) Contrasting effect of verapamil and nifedipine on pH of ischemic myocardium during fixed coronary occlusion. JACC 1:677
55. Rosenberger LB, Jacobs LW, Stanton HC (1984) Evaluation of cardiac anoxia and ischemia models in the rat heart using calcium antagonists. Life Sci 34:1379–1387
56. Ehara T, Kaufmann R (1978) The voltage- and time-dependent effects of (-)-verapamil on the slow inward current in isolated cat ventricular myocardium. J Pharmacol Exp Ther 207:49–55
57. Kohlhardt M, Mnich Z (1978) Studies on the inhibitory effect of verapamil on the slow inward current in mammalian ventricular myocardium. J Moll Cell Cardiol 10:267–272
58. McDonald TF, Pelzer D, Trautwein W (1980) On the mechanism of slow calcium channel block in heart. Pflügers Arch 385:175–179
59. Lee KS, Tsien RW (1983) Mechanism of calcium channel blockade by verapamil, D 600, diltiazem and nitrendipine in single dialysed heart cells. Nature 302:790–794
60. Pelzer D, Trautwein W, McDonald TF (1982) Calcium channel block and recovery from block in mammalian ventricular muscle treated with organic channel inhibitors. Pflügers Arch 394:97–105
61. Sanguetti MC, Kass RC (1984) Voltage-dependent block of calcium channel current in the calf cardiac Purkinje fiber by dihydropyridine calcium channel antagonists. Circ res:336–348
62. Naito M, Michelson EL, Kmetzi JJ, Kaplinsky E, Dreifus LS (1981) Failure of antiarrhythmic drugs to prevent experimental reperfusion ventricular fibrillation. Circulation 63:70–79
63. Sheehan FH, Epstein SE (1982) Effects of calcium channel blocking agents on reperfusion arrhythmias. Am Heart J 103:973–977
64. Ribeiro LGT, Brandon TA, Bebauche TL, Maroko PR, Miller RR (1981) Antiarrhythmic and hemodynamic effects of calcium channel blocking agents during coronary artery reperfusion. Comparative effects of verapamil and nifedipine. Am J Cardiol 48:49–74
65. Shen AC, Jennings RB (1972) Kinetics of calcium accumulation in acute myocardial ischemic injury. Am J Pathol 67:441–452
66. Poole-Wilson PA, Harding DP, Bourdillon PDV, Tones MA (1984) Calcium out of control. J Moll Cell Cardiol 16:175–187
67. Cheung JY, Bonventre JV, Malis CD, Leaf A (1986) Calcium and ischemic injury. N Eng J Med 314:1670–1676
68. Ferrari R, Ceconi C, Curello S, Cargnoni A, Agnoletti G, Boffa GM, Visiolo O (1986) Intracellular effects of myocardial ischaemia and reperfusion: role of calcium and oxygen. Eur Heart J (Suppl C):3–12
69. Friedman PL, Stewart JR, Wit AL (1973) Spontaneous and induced cardiac arrhythmias in subendocardial Purkinje fibers surviving extensive myocardial infarction in dogs. Circ Res 33:612–626
70. Lazzara R, El-Sherif N, Scherlag BJ (1973) Electrophysiological properties of canine Purkinje cells in one-day-old myocardial infarction. Circ Res 33:722–734

Author's address:

Dr. med. W. Haverkamp
Medizinische Universitätsklinik
Abt. Innere Medizin C
Albert-Schweitzer-Str. 33
D–4400 Münster
West Germany

Discussion

MEINERTZ

It was reported previously that gallopamil does not affect collateral flow, but now we hear that it reduces infarct size. How else can you explain this, or do you regard this as a secondary phenomenon, that is to say the infarcts might be smaller because the animals have fewer arrhythmias?

HAVERKAMP

In the dog, after coronary occlusion for about six hours the infarct extends to almost 90% of the potential area of infarction. The infarct progresses from endocardium to epicardium. I believe that here gallopamil has a direct cardioprotective effect by reducing calcium influx into the cells. The importance of increased calcium influx, particularly during the acute phase and in later phases of myocardial ischaemia and after reperfusion has been pointed out many times.
However, we largely nullified any effects on haemodynamic parameters such as a reduction of blood pressure or heart rate during acute myocardial ischaemia by measuring the electrophysiological parameters during constant supraventricular or ventricular pacing.

MEESMANN

I would like to go back to the question asked by Dr. Meinertz. Should we not look very critically at your statement that you found a 41% reduction in infarct size after 6 hours' ligation? I mean that we must look more critically at the time factor. You yourself alluded to the development of infarction in the dog. The spread and development of the infarct with time certainly depends on collateral flow and other factors which affect this progression. Is it not more likely that the reduction in infarct size which you found was only apparent and was in fact due to delayed development of the infarct? We know from other studies, from numerous clinical discussions and from the Viennese cardiologists, that a genuine response, that is to say a reduction in infarct size, cannot be proven for at least 24 hours. I therefore believe that what you observed was probably the effect of delayed spread of the infarction rather than a genuine reduction in infarct size.

HAVERKAMP

Time is, of course, an important factor in determining infarct size, and so basically I agree with you. We did not examine the effect of gallopamil on infarct size after, say, 12, 24 and 48 hours. However, our results show that there are differences between nifedipine and gallopamil.

MEESMANN

Good, so we are not dealing with a phenomenon of infarct size, but rather with factors which affect the time it takes for the infarct to develop.

HAVERKAMP

In the final analysis I believe that the effect of calcium antagonists on infarct size is not yet fully understood. We have to consider whether a medication was given before or after coronary occlusion and here the published results are very different, so further research is needed to settle this question.

MEESMANN

Have you ever observed any effect on the arrhythmias or on ventricular fibrillation when the drug is administered after ligation?

HAVERKAMP

Unfortunately we have never administered gallopamil or nifedipine after coronary occlusion. There is published evidence that giving verapamil to dogs after coronary occlusion increases the epicardial conduction delay. These results were published a few years ago in Circulation, but unfortunately only as an abstract. Since then, as far as I am aware there have been no published studies on this topic. However, it seems to me unlikely that concentrations high enough to exert anti-arrhythmic and antifibrillatory effects could be achieved in the myocardium by such a method.

FROM THE AUDITORIUM

A question for Dr. Bender. Calcium antagonists are very often prescribed prophylactically for patients with coronary insufficiency. Are there any differences between nifedipine and gallopamil in this respect or is there any clinical evidence that their effects differ?

BENDER

Dr. Fischer-Hansen in Copenhagen has designed a broadly based epidemiological study with patients at risk following a recent myocardial infarction. The study, which is still in progress, shows that verapamil, used prophylactically, reduces cardiac death following myocardial infarction. This is the only large study I am aware of and it is nearly finished. I do not know of any comparative studies with other calcium antagonists, and of course this would be very problematic.

PFENNIGSDORF

Dr. Bussmann, who is with Kaltenbach's team in Frankfurt, has investigated recent myocardial infarction patients. They were given an infusion of verapamil; I believe the dose was 0.1 mg/kg over 24 hours. There was a definite reduction in infarct size here.

HEUSCH

I would like to re-emphasize the point made by Dr. Meesmann. I believe that we must distinguish between a rather vaguely defined cardioprotective effect, or in other words a reduction of acute heart death as a result of, for example, the anti-arrhythmic effects of calcium antagonists, and a reduction in the size of myocardial infarction. I would like to underline your comment that it might simply have been a matter of delayed development of the infarct. Two years ago the American Heart Association set up a commission, headed by the pathologist Keith Reimer, which last year published a comprehensive study in Circulation Research. It was found that any reduction of infarct size cannot actually be assessed until there has been coronary occlusion for at least 24 hours with at least one week's reperfusion. This study also showed that of the 30 or so drugs which had proved effective in Kloner and Braunwald's experiments, in which the occlusion time had been too short (about 4 or 6 hours), verapamil was the only drug which had possibly produced reproducible, although not statistically significant, improvements under those conditions.

HAVERKAMP

To my knowledge, in this study the drugs were administered shortly after, and a few hours after, coronary occlusion. So this is not directly comparable. However, basically, I agree with you too. Once again may I emphasize the differences in cardioprotection. I showed the incidence of phase-Id arrhythmias, that is arrhythmias which occur some time after reperfusion and which, in morphological terms, are due to an accelerated idioventricular rhythm. Pretreatment with gallopamil virtually abolished these cardiac arrhythmias. However, if gallopamil is administered in the early necrotic stage of myocardial infarction, the calcium antagonist has no anti-arrhythmic effect. This is evidence of pronounced cardioprotective effects and in this respect dihydropyridines differ from phenylalkylamines such as gallopamil.

Dr. Heusch, I agree with you, but not with your use of the word "vague" for the definition of coronary protection. This phrase has been used very precisely here. It is the incidence of ventricular fibrillation and the incidence of ventricular arrhythmias in a defined, reproducible, fixed period of myocardial ischaemia. When clinicians use this term, they do not always mean the same thing; there you are right.

Time courses of extracellular myocardial potassium activity during acute myocardial ischaemia and the effect of gallopamil in dogs and pigs [*]

B. Vogt, M. Budden, M. Kirchengast*, K. M. Zhang, C. Martin, W. Meesmann

Department of Pathophysiology, Clinical Centre of the University of Essen (GHS) and
* Knoll AG, Biological Research and Development, Ludwigshafen

Introduction

The previous papers described in detail the two distinct phases of ventricular arrhythmias occurring during the first 30 minutes of acute coronary occlusion. This phenomenon is observed in both dogs and pigs and we have every reason to believe that it is equally relevant in humans. This early phase of arrhythmias following acute occlusion of the left anterior descending coronary artery (LAD) is illustrated by the results from 65 dogs shown in Fig. 1. Ventricular fibrillation and ventricular arrhythmias show a bimodal distribution with, typically, two separate arrhythmic subphases, designated Ia and Ib (15). Simultaneously, the

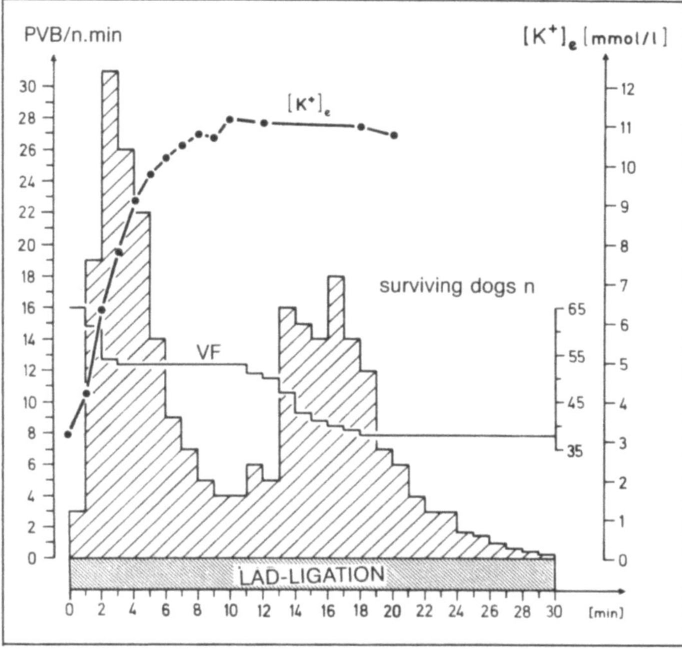

Fig 1. Extracellular myocardial K^+ activity ($[K^+]_e$), arrhythmias (PVB) and ventricular fibrillation (VF) during acute coronary occlusion in dogs. The PVB and VF data were obtained from 65 dogs, the $[K^+]_e$ data from 12 other dogs.

extracellular myocardial potassium activity ($[K^+]_e$) measured epicardially within the ischaemic area rises rapidly in the first few minutes, reaching a plateau during phase Ia and remaining at this plateau throughout phase Ib (8, 9, 17). The rapid increase in $[K^+]_e$ during acute myocardial ischaemia correlates with marked inhomogeneous electrophysiological changes which are invariably associated with the occurrence of early arrhythmias (3, 10). We now know that some calcium antagonists reduce the incidence of ischaemia-induced arrhythmias or abolish them completely. This was originally demonstrated by Kaumann and Aramendia in 1968 (11) and has also been clearly demonstrated by previous papers. Direct blockade of the slow channel, but also haemodynamic, metabolic and direct effects of calcium antagonists on cell function have been postulated as possible mechanisms. Published results (1, 7, 12, 13, 14, 16) and our own research (2, 4, 5) indicate that calcium antagonists reduce the ischaemia-induced release of potassium in the myocardium.

This paper is a report on experiments to investigate the ischaemia-induced changes in $[K^+]_e$ after gallopamil and nifedipine. They were carried out on dogs in the Department of Pathophysiology at the Clinical Centre, Essen, and on pigs in the laboratories of Knoll AG, Ludwigshafen.

Methods

General experimental conditions

The dogs, weighing 25–41 kg, were anaesthetized with morphine-urethane-chloralose and the pigs, weighing 19–29 kg, were anaesthetized with Stresnil-Hypnodil and nitrous oxide. All animals were ventilated mechanically and if necessary the respiratory parameters were adjusted in order to maintain normal blood gas values. ECG (lead II), aortic pressure, and left ventricular pressure with the derived parameter $(dp/dt)_{max}$ were recorded continuously. In the dogs, the heart rate was kept constant by atrial pacing in order to eliminate the effects of varying heart rates on the measurements.

Measurement of extracellular myocardial K^+ activity

$[K^+]_e$ was measured epicardially with an ion-selective multi-electrode sutured to the area subsequently to be rendered ischaemic. This multiple electrode consisted of 8 individual electrodes and a central calibration channel. All electrodes were covered with a direct-contact PVC-valinomycin membrane. A calomel electrode with an electrolyte bridge as the transmission medium was used as the common reference for the potassium electrodes. This was positioned as near to the multi-electrode as possible in order to minimize the effect of DC potentials (17).

Short-term myocardial ischaemia was induced by occluding the distal bifurcation of the LAD or, in the pigs, also by ligation of two adjacent lateral branches of the LAD. Before drug administration, control ligation with $[K^+]_e$ measurement was performed once (in pigs) or twice (in dogs) so that each animal served as its own control. The reperfusion time between each ligation was always at least 45 minutes. The ischaemia-induced change in $[K^+]_e$ was readily reproducible in repeated, short-term coronary occlusions. This is shown in Fig. 2 illustrating the mean time courses of the $[K^+]_e$ obtained from 6 pigs during three successive short-term ligations of the LAD.

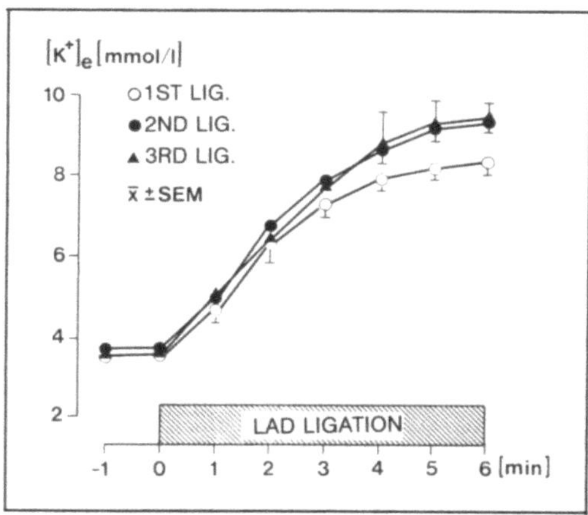

Fig. 2. Extracellular myocardial K$^+$ activity ([K$^+$]$_e$) during repeated coronary occlusions in pigs (n = 6)

The [K$^+$]$_e$ values during the second ligation (shaded circles) were slightly higher than during the first ligation (open circles), but the values remained virtually constant during subsequent ligations. Similar results have been found by other authors for pigs (6) and by us for the canine heart. In the studies on dogs, there was also a good correlation between the K$^+$ activities measured epicardially before ligation (gallopamil group: 3.62–3.90 mmol/l; nifedipine group: 3.26–3.44 mmol/l) and the K$^+$ activities in arterial blood sampled at the same time (gallopamil group: 3.70–3.81 mmol/l; nifedipine group: 3.22–3.69 mmol/l).

Dosages and mode of administration of the drugs

After the second control occlusion, each dog (n=11) was given a total dose of gallopamil of 0.1 mg/kg i.v. (bolus of 25 µg/kg followed by a 30-minute infusion of 2.5 µg/kg·min), starting 20 minutes before the third ligation. The pigs (n=6) were given 0.02 mg/kg gallopamil i.v. in 2 minutes, starting 10 minutes before the next ligation. This dose was limited by the marked fall in blood pressure and the excessive loss of contractility which would occur at higher doses.

The effect of nifedipine on the ischaemia-induced increase in [K$^+$]$_e$ was studied in 6 other dogs and 6 other pigs. Unlike gallopamil, nifedipine has no antiarrhythmic or antifibrillatory effect in the early phase of ischaemia (see paper by Haverkamp et al.). Here again, the dosages administered to dogs and pigs were different. This is explained by the different effects of the initial reflex sympathetic stimulation and peripheral dilation. The dogs were given 0.01 mg/kg nifedipine i.v. within 5 minutes and the pigs 0.05 mg/kg i.v. within 2 minutes. In each case the LAD was acutely ligated 10 minutes later.

Evaluation of the results and statistical analysis

During each occlusion [K$^+$]$_e$ was measured via 6 electrodes. We calculated Δ[K$^+$]$_e$ for each electrode, i.e. the difference between the baseline value and each value obtained during ischaemia, and then used these data to calculate the mean for the 6 electrodes. The data thus

55

obtained for $\Delta[K^+]_e$ during each ligation were then averaged for the whole group. In the dogs, the changes in $\Delta[K^+]_e$ during the ligations after drug administration were compared with the corresponding baseline profiles obtained during the second control occlusion. All data are expressed as $\bar{x} \pm$ SEM. The t test for paired samples was used for the statistical calculations.

Results

Effect of gallopamil on the ischaemia-induced rise in extracellular myocardial K^+ activity

Figure 3 shows the typical time courses of $\Delta[K^+]_e$ established in 11 dogs and 6 pigs during acute LAD occlusion for 9 and 6 minutes respectively, in each case before and after treatment with gallopamil. In both groups, the ischaemia-induced changes in $[K^+]_e$ were significantly different for the control occlusion and the LAD ligation after gallopamil.

The degree of the ischaemia-induced extracellular K^+ accumulation is characterized by the mean rate of rise and the level of the plateau reached by $\Delta[K^+]_e$. Both parameters were reduced significantly by gallopamil. Comparison of these characteristic parameters of changes in $[K^+]_e$ during acute coronary occlusion before and after gallopamil in dogs and pigs shows that the gallopamil-induced reduction of both the mean rate of rise and of the $[K^+]_e$ plateau was virtually the same (Table 1). Blood flow measurements with radiotracer

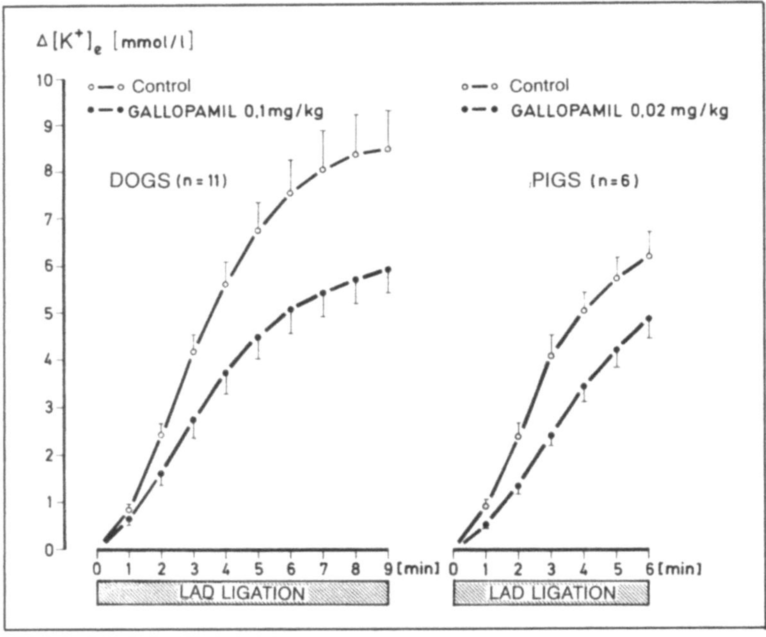

Figure 3. Effect of gallopamil on the ischaemia-induced rise in extracellular myocardial K^+ activity $(\Delta[K^+]_e)$ in dogs and pigs

microspheres in dogs (5) verified that gallopamil has no effect on collateral blood flow in the ischaemic myocardium. Thus, gallopamil does not reduce the ischaemia-induced rise in $[K^+]_e$ by increasing the residual collateral perfusion.

Table 1. Mean rise and plateau values of extracellular myocardial K^+ activity ($\Delta[K^+]_e$) during acute coronary occlusion before and after gallopamil in dogs (0.1 mg/kg) and pigs (0.02 mg/kg)

$\Delta[K^+]_e$	Dogs (n = 11)		Pigs (n = 6)	
	Control	Gallopamil	Control	Gallopamil
Mean rise	1.18	0.82*	1.04	0.81*
[mmol/l · min]	±0.12	±0.10	±0.09	±0.07
Plateau	8.39	5.88*	6.21	4.88*
[mmol/l]	±0.84	±0.51	±0.52	±0.42

$\bar{x} \pm$ SEM   * p < 0,05

Haemodynamic effects of gallopamil

The baseline haemodynamic data for both groups of animals before the coronary occlusions, in each case without and after administration of gallopamil, are given in Table 2. The heart rate of the dogs was fairly high and constant due to pacing, but in the pigs it also hardly changed. In both groups the arterial blood pressure fell significantly as a result of the peripheral dilator action of gallopamil. Concomitantly, a clear-cut negative inotropic effect was observed, which was significant in the pigs.

Table 2. Effect of gallopamil on haemodynamics in dogs (0.1 mg/kg) and pigs (0.02 mg/kg). Baseline values before the control occlusion and before coronary ligation under gallopamil

Haemodynamics	Dogs (n = 11)		Pigs (n = 6)	
	Control	Gallopamil	Control	Gallopamil
Heart rate	135	135	104	101
(beats/min)	±5	±5	±10	±10
AOP syst.	109	97*	93	87*
[mm Hg]	±2	±4	±4	±4
AOP diast.	64	51*	55	50
[mm Hg]	±3	±3	±4	±4
LV $(dp/dt)_{max}$	1855	1500	2600	1700*
[mm Hg/s]	±144	±141	±210	±180

$\bar{x} \pm$ SEM   * p < 0.05

Effect of nifedipine on the ischaemia-induced rise in extracellular myocardial K^+ activity

At the dosage used, nifedipine did not on average modify the ischaemia-induced rise in $[K^+]_e$ with time (Fig. 4). In the dogs, both the rate of rise and the $\Delta[K^+]_e$ plateau reached were virtually unchanged. Nor did nifedipine significantly alter the time course of the ischaemia-induced release of K^+ in the pigs. The slight difference in the curves before and after the relatively high dose of nifedipine was no longer observed when the customary dosage of 0.01 mg/kg was applied. This was ascertained by a supplementary study carried out in the Knoll laboratories.

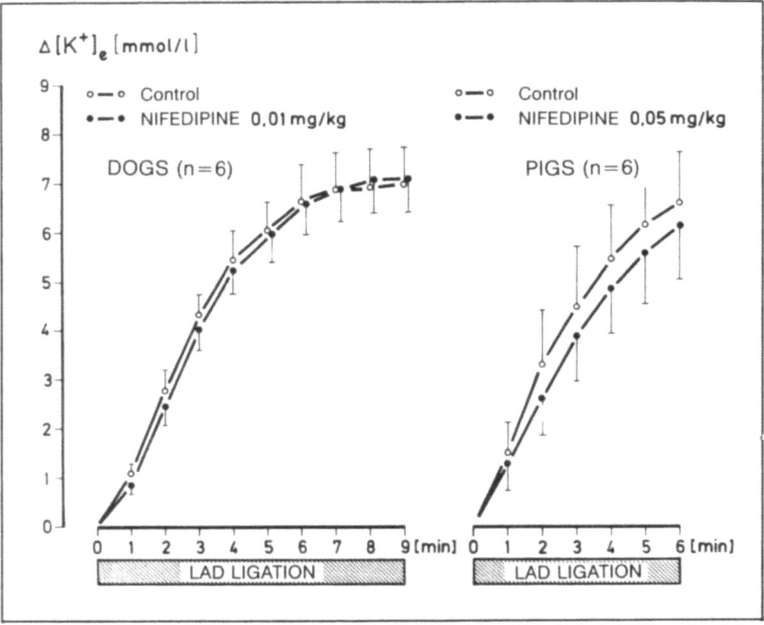

Figure 4. Effect of nifedipine on the ischaemia-induced rise in extracellular myocardial K^+ activity ($\Delta[K^+]_e$) in dogs and pigs

Haemodynamic effects of nifedipine

The haemodynamic effects of nifedipine, administered to dogs and pigs shortly before the ensuing ligations, are shown in Table 3. Here, the reflex sympathetic stimulation was still evident from the pronounced rise in $LV(dp/dt)_{max}$ in both species and the marked increase in heart rate in the pigs. The peripheral dilation resulted in a significant fall in blood pressure, which was even more evident in the pigs, in which control values were low and the dosage of nifedipine was higher.

Table 3. Effect of nifedipine on haemodynamics in dogs (0.01 mg/kg) and pigs (0.05 mg/kg). Baseline values before the control occlusion and before coronary ligation under nifedipine

Haemodynamics	Dogs (n = 6)		Pigs (n = 6)	
	Control	Nifedipine	Control	Nifedipine
Heart rate	160	162	90	120*
(beats/min)	± 0	± 2	± 9	± 8
AOP syst.	108	106	83	75*
[mm Hg]	± 3	± 6	± 3	± 5
AOP diast.	73	65*	46	37*
[mm Hg]	± 2	± 3	± 2	± 3
LV $(dp/dt)_{max}$	2133	2508	2480	2730
[mm Hg/s]	± 307	± 551	± 280	± 370

$\bar{x} \pm$ SEM $* \, p < 0.05$

Discussion

Nayler et al. (16) have already shown that, where the entire heart is hypoxic, verapamil reduces the loss of K^+ from the myocardium and Lefer et al. (13) have demonstrated that verapamil reduces K^+ loss from myocardial tissue. However, it was the use of epicardial (9, 17) or intramyocardial (8) ion-selective K^+ electrodes which first provided accurate data on the extent of the changes in $[K^+]_e$ and thus furnished information about the exact time at which they start and how they develop during acute myocardial ischaemia.

Our investigations prove that, in dogs and pigs, gallopamil significantly reduces both the rate of rise of $[K^+]_e$ and the height of the plateau. This correlates, particularly in the phase Ia, with the effect of gallopamil in delaying and reducing ischaemia-induced electrophysiological inhomogeneities (3). All this corresponds well with experimental evidence of the antiarrhythmic and antifibrillatory effects of gallopamil in the early phase of ischaemia. In contrast, at the doses used nifedipine has no effect upon $[K^+]_e$ and this is consistent with the lack of any experimental or clinical evidence of antiarrhythmic or antifibrillatory effects in early myocardial ischaemia.

These differences between gallopamil and nifedipine as regards their effects on $[K^+]_e$ and the incidence of arrhythmias would appear to suggest that the effect of gallopamil in reducing the ischaemia-induced release of K^+ is directly responsible for its antiarrhythmic activity. However, we do not believe that it is yet possible to decide to what extent the ischaemia-induced increase in $[K^+]_e$ is responsible for causing the arrhythmias, or whether it is a conditioning factor, merely a precondition for arrhythmias. In either case, however, $[K^+]_e$ might be used as an indicator of the antiarrhythmic efficacy of a drug.

References

1. Blake K, Clusin WT (1986) Effects of diltiazem on ischemic myocardial depolarization and extracellular K^+ accumulation. European J Pharmacol 127:261–265
2. Budden M, Kirchengast M, Zhang KM, Römer B, Meesmann W (1984) Reduced increase of extracellular myocardial potassium activity during acute coronary occlusion in dogs as an effect of the calcium-antagonist gallopamil (D 600). Pflügers Archiv European J Physiol 400 (Suppl):R 5
3. Budden M, Kichengast M, Neumann M, Meesmann W (1984) Einfluß des Ca^{2+}-Antagonisten Gallopamil (D 600) auf den Zeitverlauf der Dispersion (D) der Erregbarkeiten (E) und Erregungsleitungszeiten (ELZ) nach LAD-Ligatur (L) bei Hunden. Z Kardiol 73 (Suppl):49
4. Budden M, Waldhelm M, Meesmann W (1986) Extrazelluläre myokardiale K^+-Aktivität während akuter Ischämie vor und nach Applikation des neuen Calciumantagonisten Anipamil. Z Kardiol 75 (Suppl):73
5. Budden M, Kirchengast M, Zhang KM, Meesmann W (1987) Effects of the calcium antagonist gallopamil on the increase of myocardial extracellular potassium activity during LAD occlusion in dogs. Basic Res Cardiol 82:279–289
6. Fleet WF, Johnson TA, Graebner CA, Gettes LS (1985) Effect of serial brief ischemic episodes on extracellular K^+, pH, and activation in the pig. Circulation 72:922–932
7. Fleet WF, Johnson TA, Graebner CA, Engle CL, Gettes LS (1986) Effects of verapamil on ischemia-induced changes in extracellular K^+, pH, and local activation in the pig. Circulation 73:837–846
8. Hill JL, Gettes LS (1980) Effect of acute coronary artery occlusion on local myocardial extracellular K^+ activity in swine. Circulation 61:768–778
9. Hirche HJ, Franz C, Bös L, Bissig R, Lang R, Schramm M (1980) Myocardial extracellular K^+ and H^+ increase and noradrenaline release as possible cause of early arrhythmias following acute coronary artery occlusion in pigs. J Mol Cell Cardiol 12:579–593
10. Horacek T, Neumann M, von Mutius S, Budden M, Meesmann W (1984) Nonhomogenous electrophysiological changes and the bimodal distribution of early ventricular arrhythmias during acute coronary artery occlusion. Basic Res Cardiol 79:649–667
11. Kaumann AJ, Aramendia P (1968) Prevention of ventricular fibrillation induced by coronary ligation. J Pharmacol Exp Ther 164:326–332
12. Kirchengast M, Raschack M (1986) Effects of anipamil upon epicardial ischaemic ST-elevation and K^+-liberation in pig hearts. Naunyn-Schmiedeberg's Arch Pharmacol 332 (Suppl):R 45
13. Lefer AM, Polansky EW, Bianchi CP, Narayan S (1979) Influence of verapamil on cellular integrity and electrolyte concentrations of ischemic myocardial tissue in the cat. Basic Res Cardiol 74:555–567
14. Lopez JF, Orchard RC (1985) Effects of verapamil on the extracellular K^+ rise during myocardial ischaemia in dogs. Cardiovasc Res 19:363–369
15. Meesmann W, Wiegand V, Menken U, Komhard W, Rehwald U (1978) Early mortality due to ventricular fibrillation, and the vulnerability of the heart following acute experimental coronary occlusion: possible mechanisms and pharmacological prophylaxis. In: Bauer RD, Busse R (eds) The arterial system. Springer Berlin Heidelberg New York. pp 275–284
16. Nayler WG, Grau A, Slade A (1976) A protective effect of verapamil on hypoxic heart muscle. Cardiovasc Res 10:650–662
17. Wiegand V, Güggi M, Meesmann W, Kessler M, Greitschus F (1979) Extracellular potassium activity changes in the canine myocardium after acute coronary occlusion and the influence of beta-blockade. Cardiovasc Res 13:297–302

Author's address:

Dipl.-Biol. B. Vogt
Abteilung für Pathophysiologie
Klinikum der Universität
Hufelandstraße 55
D-4300 Essen 1
West Germany

Discussion

MEINERTZ

That is most interesting. Have you ever carried out measurements with an electrode in the coronary sinus or determined potassium in blood samples, in other words have you checked to see whether these changes can also be detected in the coronary sinus? The reason I ask is that it might then be possible to use this technique in humans, for example during PTCA, in order to determine the degree of ischaemia from the release of potassium.

VOGT

No, we have not measured potassium in the coronary sinus. We chose to determine potassium epicardially because this is the only way to obtain usable data. The coronary sinus also receives blood from non-ischaemic areas of the myocardium.

KIRCHENGAST

At the European Congress of Cardiology in 1984 Mr. Poole-Wilson reported his results, which have since been published, from patients undergoing PTCA. During ischaemia potassium rose by about 0.6 mM/l – within 2 minutes, I believe.

MEINERTZ

That is why I believe it might be interesting to measure potassium in the coronary sinus.

MEESMANN

There are fundamental objections to this. If I remember rightly, and Mr. Bender should probably know more about this, the first attempts to demonstrate that potassium in the coronary sinus rises during myocardial ischaemia were reported a long time ago by Hauss' group from Münster. This surprised us, even at the time. If potassium really is liberated from the ischaemic myocardium, then in the coronary sinus it would only be possible to detect a minute fraction of the amount released by the cells during ischaemia. During reperfusion, the potassium would be diluted enormously by the initially excessive influx of blood. In my opinion such investigations designed to evaluate the potassium released are simply not relevant. Secondly, as regards the actual electrophysiological effects, we must assume even with our measurements, that in the central ischaemic region where we are measuring with the six surface electrodes, the mean value we obtain is appreciably lower than the real potassium activity at the outer cell membrane. This is why the potassium values we find are also distinctly lower than those used by Cranefield in his three-compartment model of potassium depolarization of cells to demonstrate the slow-response action potentials with noradrenaline.

BENDER

Mr. Meesmann, we too were surprised by these results from Hauss, but they were not ours.

MEESMANN

I do beg your pardon, but I did not say "yours".

TRITTHART

I have a question concerning the rise in potassium and the changes in conduction in the centre of the hypoxic region, which have also been alluded to in other papers. A rise of potassium to 10 mM would at best increase the velocity of conduction, and could not in itself cause a delay in conduction. What may we actually assume? If I understand correctly, the inhomogeneities in conduction appear long after the start of the potassium plateau phase. So, I would like to ask whether this means that this plateau actually implies quasi-constant conditions, or is there something else which evades measurement going on here, something which in the final analysis is the key determinant of the other conduction disorders? Is there any evidence for this? Or, how do you see it?

VOGT

It is difficult to explain the practically constant plateau, and why there is such a plateau, which neither rises nor falls. One might envisage that potassium continues to diffuse out of the cells, but there is still residual collateral perfusion, at least in the dogs, which removes some of the potassium from the ischaemic myocardium and this results in a plateau. However, I do not know whether that is the case.

MEESMANN

I should like to add something to that. I think that what we are measuring is largely correct, but our interpretation of the results must not necessarily be appropriate. We calculate a mean from the data obtained from the six electrodes. These means, averaged over all the animals, are used for our computations and are used to plot the curves shown. However, if the six separate values from each electrode in the centre of the ischaemic zone are plotted as a histogram, we find a marked scatter of the values, sometimes even in the initial phase of ischaemia, which then persists in the plateau phase as well. The values do not approximate with time. In extreme cases the differences may be as much as several mM/l. The scatter is reproducible with repeated occlusions. We know of no convincing explanation for this variation, but this rather stimulates the discussion. In my opinion this sometimes fairly marked scatter of the virtually constant values during the plateau phase suggests that the potassium plateau does not represent an equilibrium between constantly rising and falling potassium activities in the extracellular space.
To answer your actual question I would repeat what we ourselves realized in the course of many discussions: We are taking our measurements, as it were, a long way from the surface of the cell. Therefore, when measuring epicardially we have to consider a substantial diminution in potassium activity and this loss would be even greater if we were to measure potassium in the coronary sinus. In this context I believe that our data are only a relative indication of the changes in the actual extracellular activities outside the cell membrane, and that the absolute values are undoubtedly higher. It is also conceivable that the rate of changes in potassium at the outer membrane is steeper. The early arrhythmias do in fact occur while potassium is still rising.

FLEISCHMANN

As a clinician may I ask once again what is the basis of this cardioprotective effect? If it is so pronounced, will it be used in heart surgery, for example? Can Mr. Tritthart give us some idea about what is to be understood from this effect of gallopamil?

TRITTHART

I cannot give a definite answer to that. There are a number of claims. Perhaps you know that there is a potassium channel which is normally closed, but which opens if there is a deficiency of ATP under hypoxic conditions. This channel is considered to be partly responsible for the excessive loss of potassium. The protective effect of calcium antagonists invariably involves membrane functions which are energy-dependent. In other words any cell which can save energy by reducing its force of contraction, which consumes large amounts of energy, also has more energy available for its membrane function. One would anticipate, and this has been shown long ago, that the break down in ATP would happen more slowly and to a lesser degree.
It is also likely that, in the presence of calcium antagonists, more of the ATP fraction near the membrane can be maintained for longer. This could also be the basis of a specific protective effect. I summarized the cascades which occur during hypoxia. With the intervention of phospholipases, this can induce leaks in the membrane, that is to say major membrane defects amounting to irreversible damage. However, long before that, the operation of the sodium-potassium pump is the key to the survival of a cell and determines how long it can maintain its homoeostasis. However, if nifedipine and verapamil or gallopamil only exerted their effect via energy metabolism or on ATP fraction near the membrane, then they would have much the same effects. At the moment I have no other explanation as to why this is not the case. Perhaps the outflow of potassium might be due not only to inhibition of the pump, but also to additional channels. I only say "might be". As yet, no one knows. But this certainly needs further investigation.

MEESMANN

So, we have no satisfactory answer as to how the calcium antagonists actually exert their cardioprotective effect, or indeed about the different effects of different calcium antagonists.

HOLZGREVE

The last three papers have certainly provided us with some very convincing data and to some extent have distinguished gallopamil/verapamil from nifedipine. But I would like to hear a little more about the difference between these drugs and other classes of compounds which have exhibited similar anti-arrhythmic properties and cardioprotective effects in the acute infarction model in that they reduced infarct size. I am thinking mainly of the alpha-blockers, the combined alpha- and beta-blocker labetalol, and of course of the beta-blockers. Have you looked into this? In other words, I would like to have some comment on published evidence that other drugs have similar effects.

VOGT

Beta-blockers were studied some time ago at the Essen Institute. Beta-blockade merely delayed the rise in extracellular potassium activity in acute myocardial ischaemia. However, the same plateau was still reached in phase Ia, albeit a little later. Without medication, extracellular potassium activity showed virtually the same response to regional myocardial chemical sympathectomy, a procedure which eliminates sympathetic effects within the ischaemic area. The ischaemia-induced rise in potassium is then also slowed and reaches the plateau with a delay of about 2 minutes. The other calcium antagonists which have been studied include verapamil, diltiazem and anipamil. The effects of these drugs on extracellular potassium activity are similar to those of gallopamil. We have not tested alpha-adrenoceptor blockers, and I know of no published results obtained by this method with these drugs.

New aspects on the pathophysiology of coronary heart disease

G. Heusch[1], B. D. Guth[2]

[1] Abteilung für Pathophysiologie, Univ. Essen, FRG, and
[2] Division of Cardiology, Univ. of California, San Diego, USA

Introduction

Myocardial ischemia is the underlying pathological process for all clinical events which are referred to as coronary heart disease. Angina pectoris and myocardial infarction are the classic manifestations of myocardial ischemia. In many cases heart failure is also caused by chronic recurrent ischemia and the replacement of irreversibly injured cardiomyocytes by scar tissue (1). The initiation of malignant arrhythmias, sometimes leading to sudden cardiac death, may also be the result of myocardial ischemia.

Myocardial ischemia may be defined as hypoperfusion of the myocardium. Thus, the term myocardial ischemia is largely synonymous with the term coronary insufficiency coined by Hermann Rein and Franz Büchner.

Three essential mechanisms of myocardial ischemia can be distinguished:

1. thrombotic coronary occlusion, which may be primarily due to activation of the plasmatic cascade or to platelet aggregation
2. coronary vasoconstriction, which may primarily affect the large epicardial coronary arteries – as true spasm or as critical narrowing of a pre-existing stenosis – or predominantly affect the coronary resistance vessels – α-adrenergic coronary constriction plays a major role here
3. an increase in myocardial demand with an inadequate increase in coronary supply – the importance of this mechanism will be questioned in this paper.

These three causes of myocardial ischemia can only be distinguished schematically, but not in the pathophysiology and clinical course. Therefore, the present manuscript will emphasize the dynamic nature of myocardial ischemia, i.e., the interaction of the previously distinguished factors and the temporal and spatial dynamics of myocardial ischemia.

Coagulation and myocardial ischemia

The basic underlying substrate of all mechanisms contributing to the initiation of myocardial ischemia is a functional or morphologically demonstrable damage of the coronary vascular wall. An endothelial lesion appears to be the first step in the development of coronary vascular damage (2). There is evidence that hemodynamic factors determine the formation and localization of the primary endothelial lesion. Whereas endothelial cells line up in the direction of laminar flow, they change their orientation in the presence of turbulences (3). The predilective sites of atherosclerotic lesions in the coronary vascular system coincide with the sites of strong turbulence in coronary blood flow (4, 5). The classic risk factors for coronary artery disease are not important determinants of the site of coronary atherosclerosis (6), but hyperlipidemia is involved in the development of an endothelial lesion (7).

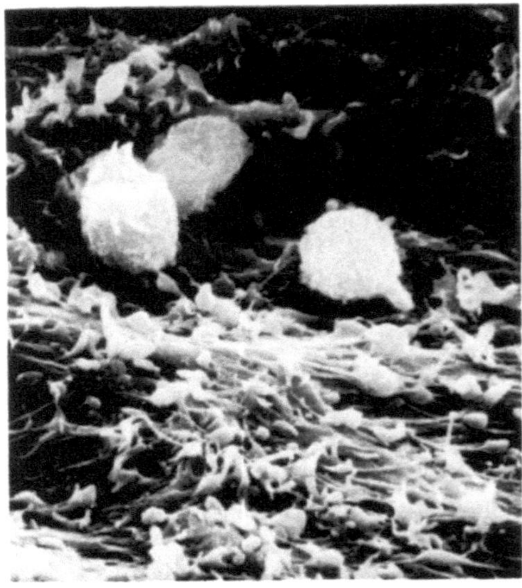

Fig. 1. Scanning electron microscopy of an endothelial lesion covered with platelets and leukocytes. From (9) by permission of the Am. Heart Assoc.

A further step in the development of vascular damage is based on the interaction of the endothelial lesion with coagulation (8, 9) (Fig. 1). Platelets and leukocytes adhere to the endothelial lesion. The plasmatic factor VIII (or v. Willebrand factor) is essentially involved in the platelet adhesion and activation (10). This is supported by the observation that pigs with a genetic deficiency of factor VIII, i.e., v. Willebrand's disease, are resistant against spontaneous and cholesterol-induced atherosclerosis (11, 12). During activation of aggregated platelets, factors are released which may contribute to further damage of the vascular wall: a platelet-derived growth factor stimulates the proliferation of vascular smooth muscle cells (13), and the platelet factor 4 is chemotactic (14) and could also be involved in the proliferation of vascular smooth muscle cells in the intima. Furthermore, hyperlipidemia enhances platelet reactivity (15).

The plasmatic and platelet-related coagulation phenomena are involved in the early phase of coronary vascular wall damage. Advanced atherosclerosis, however, predisposes for local coagulation due to increased turbulence; the importance of turbulence for the development of coronary atherosclerosis was demonstrated above. There is also increased shear stress in stenotic segments (16) which may further add to the vascular wall damage and finally, in concert with other hemodynamic factors such as sudden changes in blood pressure or coronary constriction, induce rupture of an atheroma (17, 18, 19) (Fig. 2).

Platelets aggregate on the ruptured plaque and a red thrombus may be formed (20) which may be organized and further narrow the coronary artery or even acutely occlude the vessel. Coronary thromboses leading to fatal myocardial infarction are nearly always the result of plaque rupture (20). Not only the plasmatic coagulation resulting from plaque rupture, but also the enhanced platelet aggregation in stenotic segments can decrease coronary blood flow critically (21, 22, 23) (Fig. 3). In animal studies an often cyclical reduction of coronary blood flow with a progressive decrease followed by a rapid increase in coronary blood flow has been demonstrated. Aspirin prevents platelet aggregation and the resulting cyclical fluctuations of coronary blood flow. Platelet aggregates may not only mechanically occlude

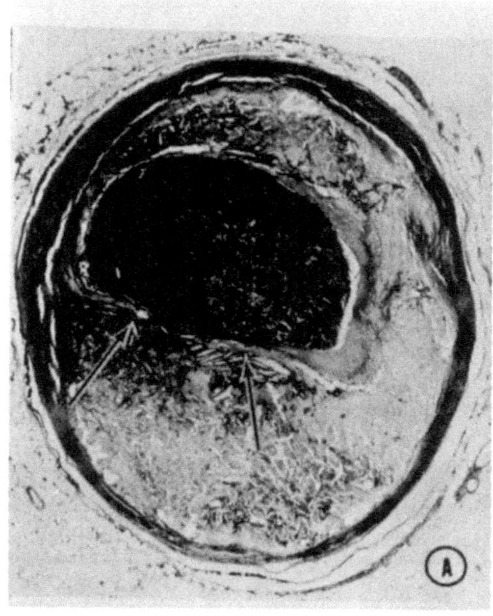

Fig. 2. Cross-section of a coronary artery occluded by a thrombus which originates from an ulcerated atheroma. From (17) by permission of the C. V. Mosby Comp.

the coronary vascular lumen, but also release coronary constrictor substances such as serotonin and thromboxane A2 (24) which may aggravate the reduction in coronary blood flow.

In summary, plasmatic and platelet-related factors play a key role even in the early phase of the development of coronary vascular wall damage. In turn, a preexisting stenosis enhances both the plasmatic and platelet-related coagulation. Platelet aggregates and/or thrombi on pre-existing stenoses may acutely reduce coronary blood flow and initiate acute myocardial ischemia. The release of coronary constrictor substances may also be involved in the initiation of myocardial ischemia. Thus, the initiation of myocardial ischemia may be caused by a complex interaction between the mechanical obstruction of the stenotic segment, plasmatic and platelet-related coagulation and coronary vasoconstriction.

In patients with unstable angina pectoris, enhanced platelet activity is found within the first few hours after the onset of clinical symptoms (23). In the first few hours of an acute myocardial infarction, coronary angiography reveals a thrombotic occlusion in the majority of patients (25); the incidence of occlusion decreases thereafter, probably as a result of spontaneous lysis and recanalization. In recent years, invasive-intracoronary thrombolysis (26) or intravenous thrombolysis with streptokinase (27) have been used successfully in the treatment of acute myocardial ischemia. In the future, thrombolysis with a tissue plasminogen activating factor (28) appears promising.

Coronary constriction and myocardial ischemia

For clarity, the constriction of epicardial coronary arteries will be distinguished from the constriction of coronary resistance vessels.

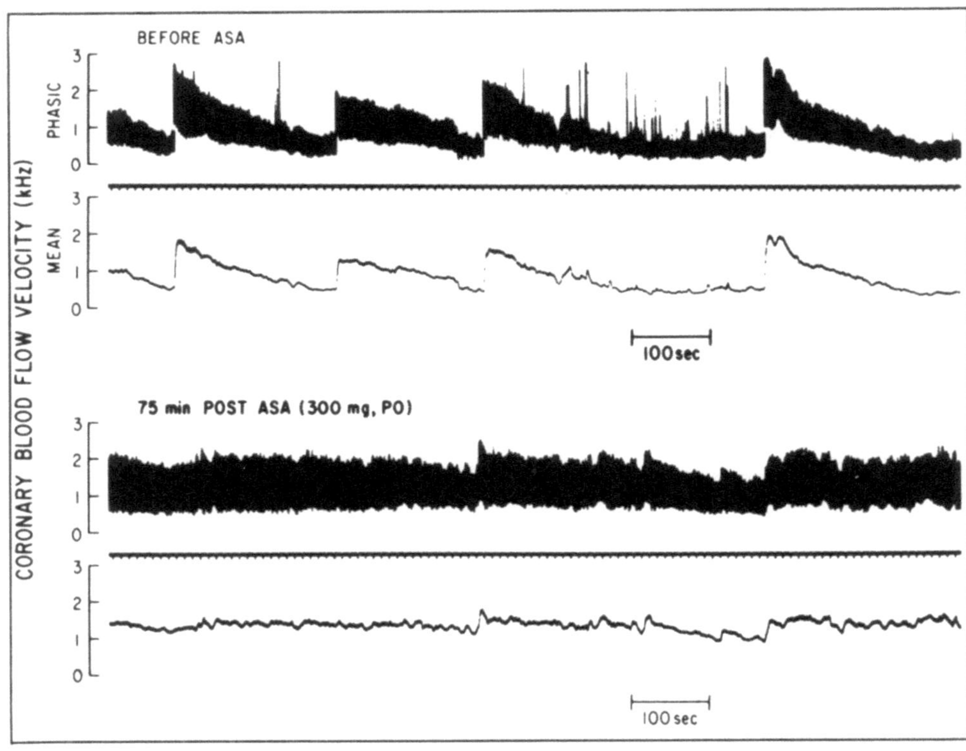

Fig. 3. Original tracing demonstrating cyclical fluctuations of coronary blood flow in a dog with severe coronary stenosis. Aspirin prevents these cyclical flow fluctuations (22)

Epicardial coronary constriction

A critical reduction of coronary blood flow at the site of epicardial coronary arteries underlies a range of pathophysiological processes from spasm to dynamic coronary stenosis, and finally to changes in the hemodynamic severity of a fixed coronary stenosis. These pathophysiological processes differ in the quantitative contribution of active coronary vasoconstriction and fixed mechanical coronary occlusion to the initiation of myocardial ischemia. However, a common underlying feature is again a functional or morphologically demonstrable damage of the local vascular wall.

The hemodynamic severity of a coronary stenosis may change even if the stenosis is morphologically fixed. Apart from the angles of entry and exit which determine the extent of turbulences at the transition from the normal to the stenotic vascular segments, the intraluminal pressure determines the actual cross-sectional area of the stenotic segment. The relation between coronary blood flow and perfusion pressure is nonlinear and only an apparent coronary resistance can be calculated from the actual ratio of perfusion pressure to coronary blood flow (30) Nevertheless, changes in intraluminal perfusion pressure may change the hemodynamic severity of a coronary stenosis. In the presence of a fixed severe coronary stenosis, an acute dilation of the poststenotic coronary vascular bed with a resulting decrease in poststenotic perfusion pressure can markedly decrease coronary blood

68

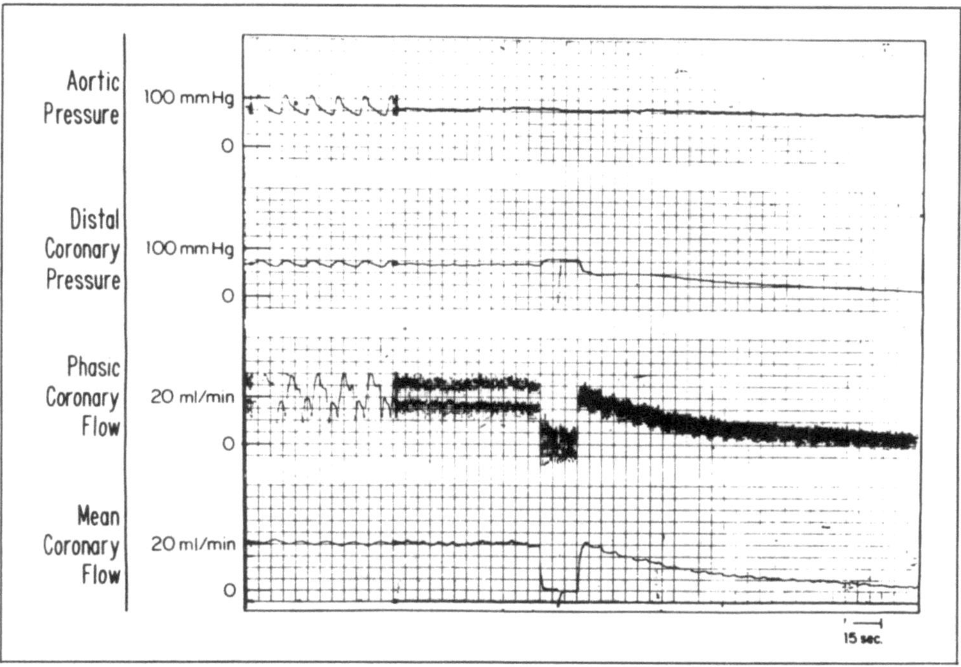

Fig. 4. A brief complete occlusion of a critically stenotic coronary artery induces a dilation of the poststenotic vascular bed. Poststenotic perfusion pressure therefore decreases after release of the occlusion. Despite an unchanged aortic pressure, the resistance of the stenotic segment markedly increases and coronary blood flow drops (31)

flow (31) (Fig. 4). The increase in the hemodynamic severity of the stenosis is real and is not pretended by the calculation of stenosis resistance according to Ohm's law, since rather than the observed increase in stenosis resistance with decreasing coronary blood flow, a decrease in stenosis resistance should result from the nonlinear pressure-flow relation. An increase in the hemodynamic severity of a fixed coronary stenosis as the result of poststenotic coronary dilation and a consequent drop in poststenotic coronary perfusion pressure has been demonstrated in experiments after transient coronary occlusion (31), with intracoronary contrast medium (31), in tachycardia during atrial pacing (32) and exercise (33). Conversely, the hemodynamic severity of a stenosis is decreased when coronary perfusion pressure increases (34).

Changes in the hemodynamic severity of a coronary stenosis are much more marked if the stenotic segment includes not only an atherosclerotic segment, but also a segment which retains vasomotion. Histological examination often reveals a vascular segment with an eccentric atherosclerosis and intact vascular smooth muscle cells (35). There may be a dynamic coronary stenosis (30, 36) when active coronary vasoconstriction is superimposed on the pre-existing atherosclerosis, and acute myocardial ischemia may be initiated. Acute ischemic myocardial dysfunction may be induced by isometric exercise in patients with a compensated coronary stenosis at rest (37). Myocardial ischemia is induced by the reflex constriction of the stenotic segment (Fig. 5) and not by the increase in myocardial

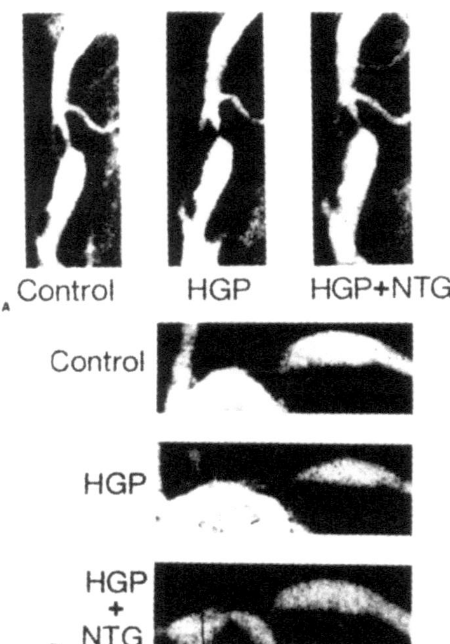

Fig. 5. Coronary arteriography demonstrates a constriction of a significant coronary stenosis during reflex sympathetic activation by isometric exercise (handgrip HGP); dilation of the stenotic segment by nitroglycerin (NTG) (37)

performance; nitroglycerin prevents the constriction of a stenotic vascular segment and, despite unchanged increases in myocardial performance, also myocardial ischemia (37). The calcium antagonist diltiazem also prevents the reflex coronary constriction of a significant coronary stenosis and the resulting myocardial ischemia (38). Brown et al. attribute the reflex constriction of the stenotic vascular segment to the activation of α-adrenoceptors.

Potentially there are only gradual differences between the previously discussed dynamic coronary stenosis and coronary spasm. In fact, critical coronary constriction as well as spasm occur preferentially in the immediate vicinity of organic lesions (39). With respect to this observation, McAlpin developed the theory that a critical coronary occlusion is merely the geometric result of normal vasoconstriction in a stenotic vascular segment (Fig. 6). A given decrease in the external radius of a vascular segment having a pre-existing luminal reduction results in a proportionally larger decrease in the internal radius (40). In contrast to this purely geometric theory of coronary spasm, studies by Serruys et al. (41) emphasize the unpredictable vasomotion of a stenotic epicardial coronary segment. During a provocation test with methergine, the angiographically determined luminal reduction of the stenotic segment matched the luminal reduction predicted from the vasoconstriction of normal segments by geometric assumptions in only a minority of cases.

At present, the causes of local hypercontractility of the coronary vascular wall remain speculative. However, a few interesting observations in this context will be discussed: α_1-adrenoceptor mediated constriction of epicardial coronary arteries can be induced by sympathetic activation. However, the reduction in vessel caliber is not sufficient to cause a measurable reduction in coronary blood flow (42). The provocation of coronary spasm by ergonovine is considered a classic challenge for the diagnosis of spastic angina pectoris (43, 44). The provocation of coronary spasm appears to be related to a serotonergic action of ergonovine, whereas the α-adrenergic action appears to be of minor importance (45).

70

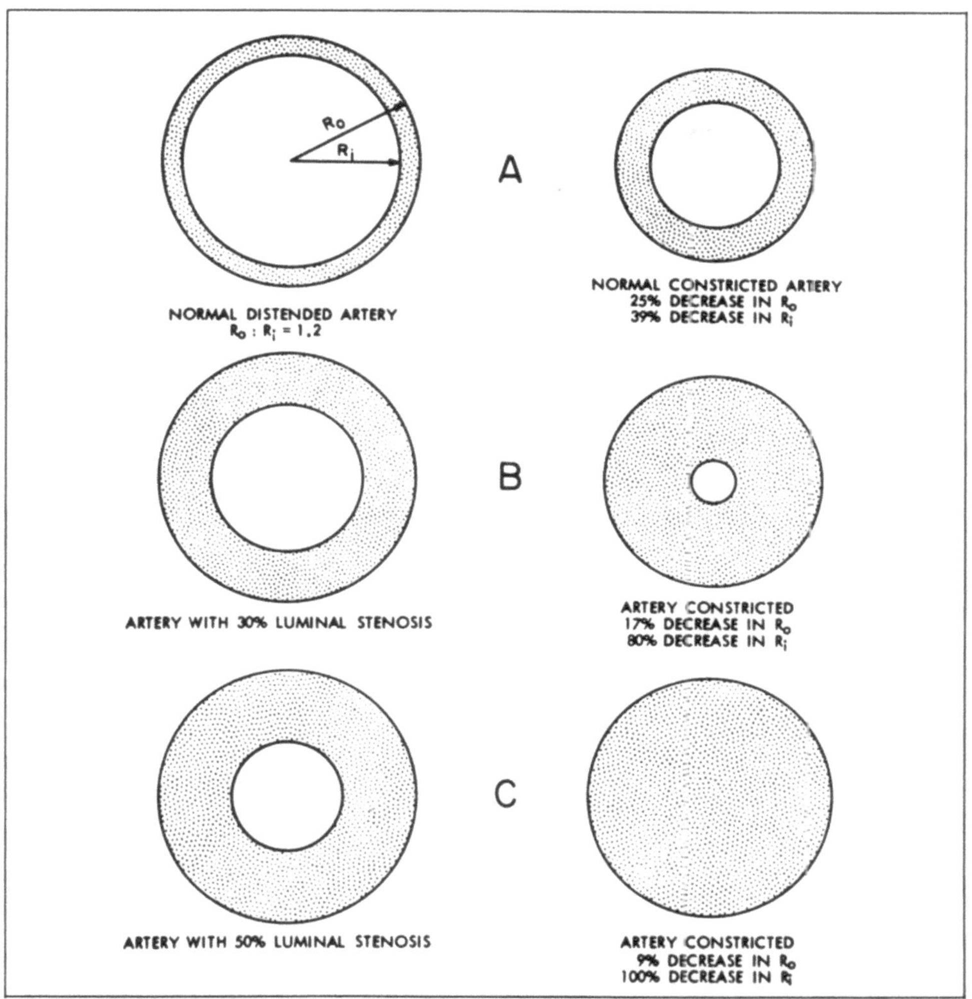

Fig. 6. Geometric theory of coronary spasm. The same decrease in external diameter induces a progressive decrease in internal diameter with increasing severity of coronary stenosis (40)

With the development of cholesterol-induced atherosclerosis, the constrictor effects of serotonin in large arterial segments are enhanced (46, 47). Histamine has also been implicated in the initiation of coronary spasm (48).

The predisposition of epicardial coronary arteries to local hypercontractility by endothelial damage appears as a particularly attractive hypothesis. The endothelium can release relaxant factors (49, 50). After experimental endothelial damage an enhanced vasoconstriction of large femoral arteries during α_1-adrenoceptor activation was found (51). In canine epicardial coronary arteries the acetylcholine-induced vasodilation is reversed to constriction after removal of the endothelium (52). In this context, the interaction between the

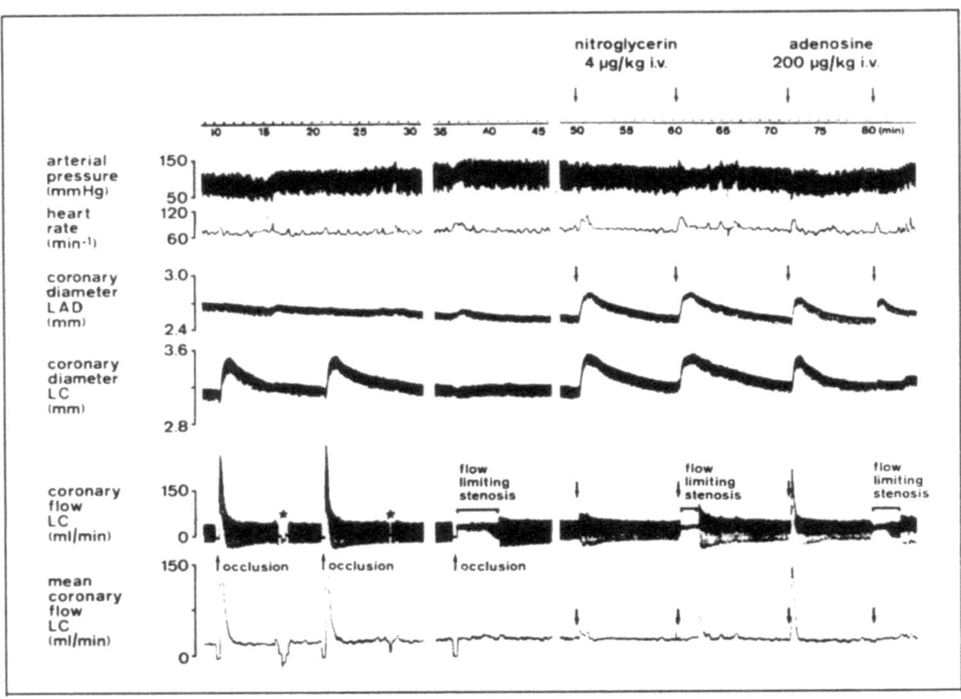

Fig. 7. Dilation of coronary resistance vessels by transient coronary occlusion or adenosine induces, with some delay, also a dilation of epicardial coronary arteries which is prevented by limitation of the increase in coronary blood flow with a stenosis. Nitroglycerin, in contrast, induces a flow-independent dilation of epicardial coronary arteries (41)

coronary microcirculation and the diameter of epicardial coronary arteries (Fig. 7) which was first described by Holtz et al. (53, 54) and shortly thereafter by Hintze and Vatner (55), appears to be particularly important. An increase in coronary blood flow induced by postocclusive reactive hyperemia or by adenosine also induces with some delay an increase in the diameter of epicardial coronary arteries. Holtz proposes the hypothesis that a dilation of coronary arterioles increases coronary blood flow and induces increased shear stress at the luminal surface of the endothelium which, in turn, releases a vasodilator factor. Prostanoids have been excluded as potential mediators of this endothelium-mediated dilation of epicardial coronary arteries, since the inhibition of cyclooxygenase by indomethacin or diclofenac does not change these responses. According to this hypothesis, the increased frequency of episodes of vasospastic angina pectoris in the night and early morning hours can be explained by the reduction in myocardial function and metabolism, and a respective attenuation of flow-dependent, endothelium-mediated coronary dilation at that time. In contrast to stress-induced myocardial ischemia in which there is a primary increase in myocardial oxygen demand, a primary reduction in myocardial demand is supposed to be initiating myocardial ischemia at rest. However, it must be cautioned that the experimentally observed changes in the diameter of epicardial coronary arteries in all previously mentioned studies have been so small that they could only contribute to a reduction in coronary blood flow when extrapolated to pre-existing critical coronary stenoses. However,

72

experimental proof for this is still lacking. Also, although there is experimental evidence for
enhanced α-adrenergic or serotonergic epicardial coronary constriction, a respective clinical
therapy of vasospastic angina pectoris has not been proven successful (56, 57, 58).

In summary, coronary blood flow can be critically reduced at the level of epicardial coronary
arteries. While the hemodynamic severity of a fixed stenosis may change, epicardial
vasoconstriction predominates in a dynamic stenosis with an eccentric atherosclerosis and a
normal wall segment and, particularly, in coronary spasm. Despite many interesting
experimental observations, the causes of local hypercontractility in epicardial coronary
arteries and, thus finally the cause of vasospastic angina pectoris, are still unclear.

Constriction of the coronary resistance vessels

The classic view of the pathogenesis of myocardial ischemia assumes that coronary
resistance vessels are maximally dilated during myocardial ischemia and do not respond to
constrictor stimuli. The mechanisms which contribute to the compensatory dilation of
coronary resistance vessels distal to stenoses and during myocardial ischemia are essentially
unclear. Adenosine, a purported key mediator in this process, has been demonstrated in
recent studies as not being an important mediator of the compensatory poststenotic
coronary dilation, since inactivation of endogenously released adenosine by deaminase does
not change poststenotic coronary resistance (59). Recent studies indicate that the idea of
maximal coronary dilation during myocardial ischemia is not correct. Even after maximal
pharmacological coronary dilation with exogenous adenosine (60) and in the presence of
coronary stenoses (61), coronary vessels remain responsive to the α-adrenergic constrictor
effects of the sympathetic transmitter norepinephrine. Under resting conditions, hypoper-
fused coronary arteries retain a vasoconstrictor tone, whereas the pharmacological
attenuation of that tone improves myocardial perfusion (62, 63, 64, 65).

Our own studies focussed on the importance of α-adrenergic coronary constrictor
mechanisms in the initiation of myocardial ischemia. In compensation for a proximal
coronary stenosis, the dilator reserve of the poststenotic coronary vascular bed is partially
recruited. While the recruitment of coronary dilator reserve may preserve poststenotic
myocardial blood flow and contractile function at rest, it also reduces the potential for
increases in coronary blood flow during acute stress. Thus, electrical stimulation of cardiac
sympathetic nerves induces a marked dilation of intact coronary arteries. In the presence of
a moderate coronary stenosis, however, this dilation is much less marked (Fig. 8). In the
presence of a severe coronary stenosis which actually exhausts poststenotic coronary dilator
reserve, electrical stimulation of cardiac sympathetic nerves can even induce coronary
vasoconstriction. This poststenotic coronary constriction, in turn, induces poststenotic
myocardial ischemia as evidenced by contractile dysfunction, net lactate production and
malignant arrhythmias (66). The sympathetically induced poststenotic constriction is
mediated by vascular α2-adrenoceptors. The nonselective α-antagonist phentolamine, or the
selective α2-antagonist rauwolscine can prevent the sympathetically induced poststenotic
coronary constriction. The calcium antagonist nifedipine has also been shown to functionally
antagonize the α2 – adrenoceptor – mediated vasoconstriction (67). Poststenotic coronary
constriction and myocardial ischemia can also be induced by reflex sympathetic activation,
subsequent to carotid occlusion and pain (68, 69). Furthermore, there is a positive feed-back
between myocardial ischemia, once initiated, and the activity of cardiac sympathetic nerves

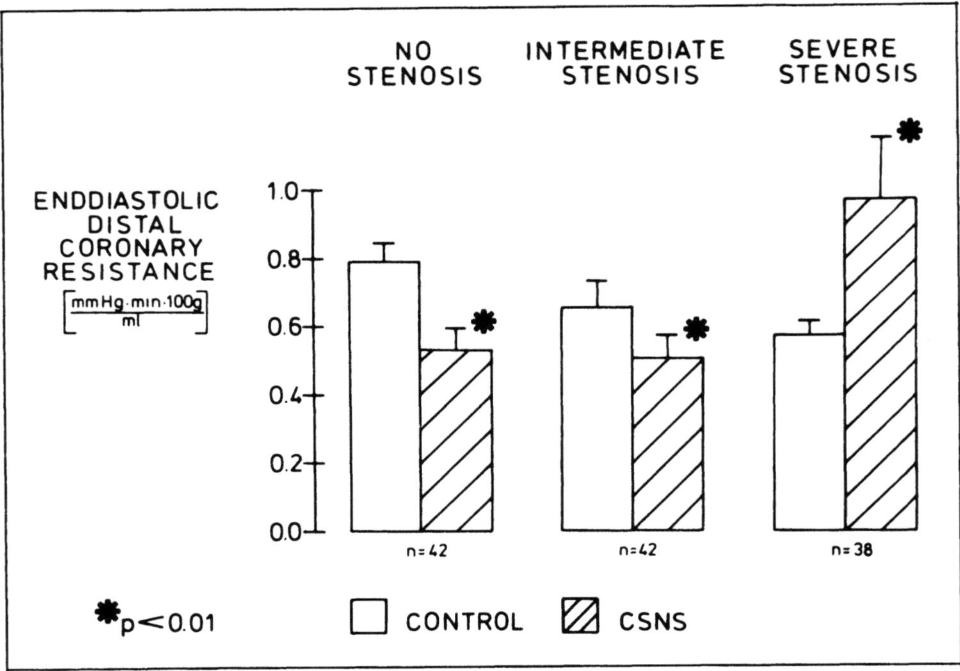

Fig. 8. Electrical stimulation of cardiac sympathetic nerves (CSNS) induces a marked decrease in coronary resistance of intact coronary arteries. With a compensatory decrease in poststenotic resistance distal to an intermediate stenosis at rest, the sympathetically induced decrease in resistance is attenuated. Distal to a severe coronary stenosis, cardiac sympathetic nerve stimulation even increases coronary resistance. (From (66) by permission of the Am. Heart Assoc.) (66)

which may lead to a progressive aggravation of myocardial ischemia (70). This vicious cycle can be interrupted not only by α_2-blockade or nifedipine, but also by segmental epidural anesthesia of cardiac sympathetic nerves with procaine and central nervous inhibition of sympathetic activity with clonidine (71). Significant α_2-adrenoceptor mediated poststenotic coronary constriction is not only induced by electrical and reflex sympathetic activation in anesthetized dogs, but also during treadmill exercise in conscious dogs (72). Intracoronary infusion of the selective α_2-antagonist idazoxan improves poststenotic regional myocardial blood flow and function during continued treadmill exercise. Nifedipine also attenuates poststenotic coronary constriction and reduces exercise-induced myocardial ischemia (73).

A significant increase in coronary resistance is also induced in patients with coronary heart disease by reflex sympathetic activation during the cold pressor test (74, 75, 76, 77). In two recent clinical trials the therapeutic effectiveness of intracoronary α-blockade with the nonselective α-antagonist phentolamine was demonstrated (78, 79) (Fig. 9).

In summary, coronary resistance vessels are not maximally dilated during myocardial ischemia but retain significant constrictor tone. Sympathetic activation in experimental animals or in patients can induce poststenotic α-adrenoceptor-mediated coronary constriction which, in turn, may precipitate or aggravate myocardial ischemia. These results from experimental and clinical studies being in good agreement, there appears to be a sound pathophysiological basis for the therapeutic use of coronary dilators, in particular calcium antagonists, which

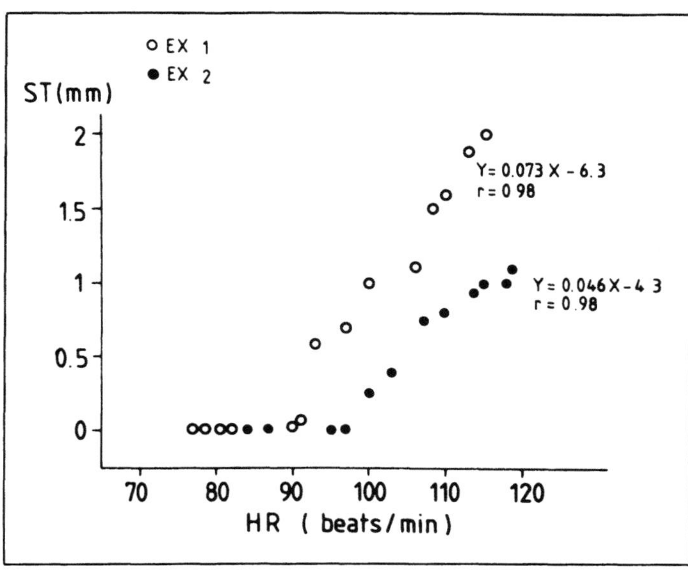

Fig. 9. With a comparable tachycardia, the exercise-induced ST-depression is markedly reduced by the α-antagonist phentolamine. O = control, ● = phentolamine (78)

can functionally prevent the α-adrenoceptor mediated coronary constriction (67, 73, 80). The dynamic component of coronary vasoconstriction, either predominantly of the epicardial coronary arteries or of the resistance vessels, cannot be overestimated as a key factor for the initiation of acute myocardial ischemia. This dynamic component may be responsible for the often marked variation in the susceptibility of patients to angina pectoris during daily life, despite an unchanged coronary morphology (81).

Increase in myocardial oxygen demand and myocardial ischemia

Hermann Rein and Franz Büchner postulated that a discrepancy between myocardial oxygen demand and supply was the underlying cause of myocardial ischemia. This hypothesis has often been interpreted to mean that after exhaustion of coronary dilator reserve distal to a severe coronary stenosis such that coronary blood flow can no longer be increased, myocardial ischemia can be induced by increases in poststenotic myocardial oxygen demand. This interpretation is overly simplistic since neither the regional nature of myocardial ischemia, and thus the problem of myocardial blood flow distribution, nor the time course of the interaction between regional myocardial function as an indicator of oxygen demand, on the one hand, and regional blood flow as an indicator of oxygen supply on the other hand are accounted for. The regional nature of myocardial ischemia requires to respect the interactions between the ischemic area and the adjacent nonischemic area (Fig. 10). Myocardial blood flow to a poststenotic area depends on two sources, i.e. coronary arterial inflow through the stenotic vessel (F_2) and collateral blood flow originating from adjacent non or less stenotic coronary arteries (F_1). During physical or mental stress,

75

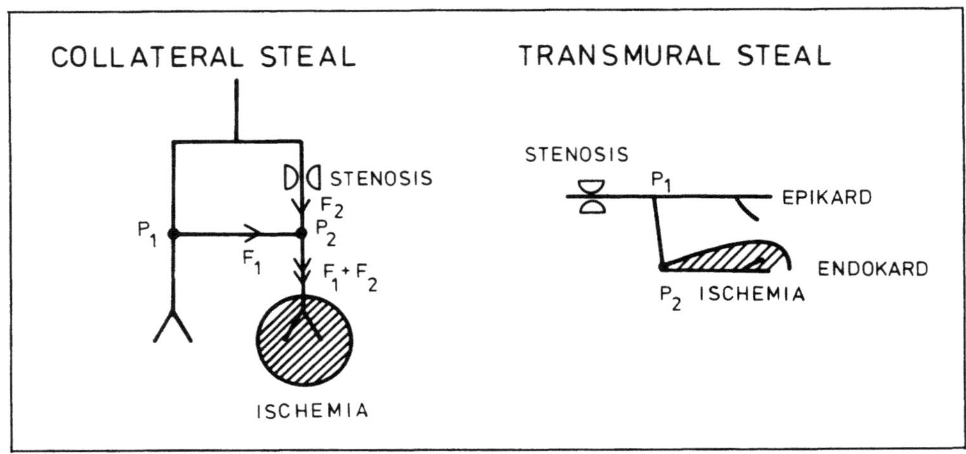

Fig. 10. Schematic diagram of collateral steal and transmural steal. Detailed discussion in the text.

the function of the nonischemic myocardium is increased, and the increased metabolic demand is adequately met by an increase in coronary blood flow after dilation of the terminal coronary vascular bed. The dilation of the nonischemic terminal vascular bed reduces the driving pressure for collateral blood flow $(P_1–P_2)$ thereby reducing blood flow to the ischemic region, a phenomenon referred to as collateral steal (82). Collateral steal is not only the result of metabolic dilation in nonischemic myocardium, but also of enhanced extravascular coronary compression within the ischemic myocardium. Both factors contribute to the reduction in the driving pressure for collateral flow (83). In essence, myocardial ischemia is caused by an actual reduction of myocardial blood flow in the ischemic region.

This applies not only to laterally adjacent areas, but also to the transmural distribution of blood flow within an area supplied by the stenotic coronary artery. The dilation of subepicardial coronary vessels in concert with the greater mechanical compression of subendocardial coronary vessels by left ventricular pressure, induces a redistribution of blood flow from the subendocardium to the subepicardium i.e. a transmural steal (84). Such a transmural redistribution of regional myocardial blood flow during myocardial ischemia can be observed experimentally during treadmill exercise in dogs having a chronic single vessel coronary stenosis which is compensated at rest (Fig. 11). A transmural steal phenomenon can be considered as the cause of the predominantly subendocardial myocardial ischemia during angina pectoris and nontransmural myocardial infarction. With respect to the importance of increased myocardial demand for the initiation of myocardial ischemia, it must be emphasized that an increase in oxygen demand of the nonischemic, laterally or transmurally adjacent myocardium induces a redistribution of blood flow, thus causing a reduction in absolute blood flow in the ischemic myocardial region and precipitating myocardial ischemia.

A detailed analysis of the time course of exercise-induced myocardial ischemia also emphasizes the importance of absolute regional myocardial blood flow. An increase in regional function and thus in the regional oxygen demand of the poststenotic myocardium occurs only during the first few seconds of acute treadmill exercise. During the subsequent steady state response which is achieved within a few minutes, regional function and regional oxygen demand are reduced (Fig. 12). During exercise in dogs with single vessel coronary stenosis (85, 86), there exists a close linear relationship between regional contractile function

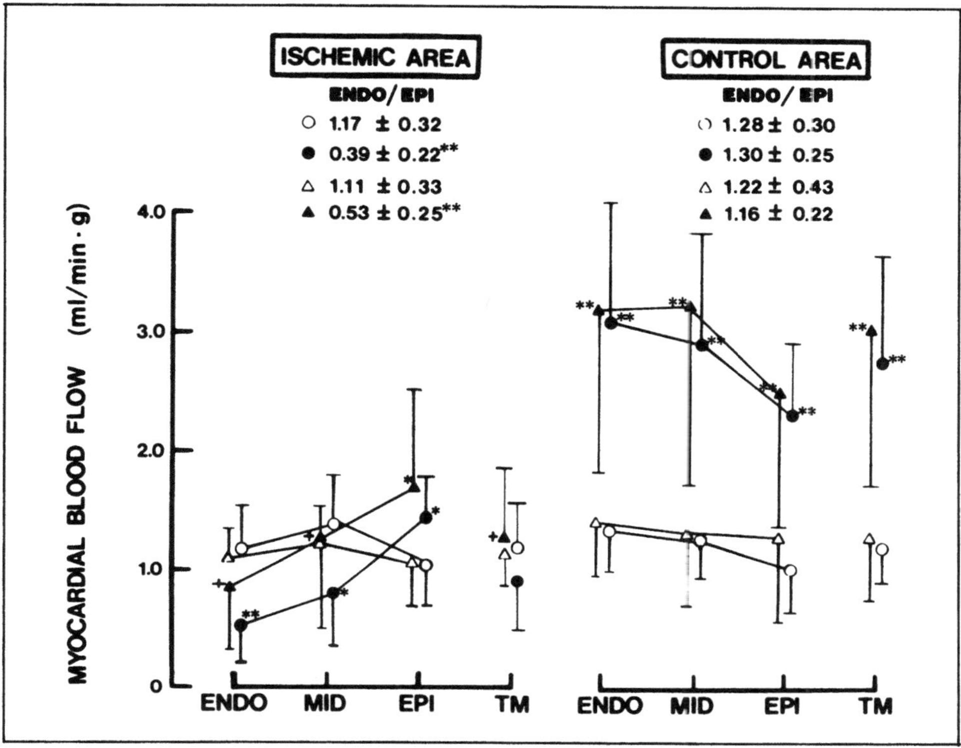

Fig. 11. Transmural distribution of regional myocardial blood flow in an ischemic and a nonischemic area. At rest (O) the distribution of blood flow in the ischemic and nonischemic area is not different. During exercise (●) blood flow in the nonischemic area is increased in all transmural layers. In contrast, in the ischemic area, a transmural gradient with a decrease in subendocardial and an increase in subepicardial blood flow develops. Nifedipine does not change blood flow at rest (△), but attenuates the decrease in perfusion of the subendocardium and midmyocardium during exercise (▲). (73)

and regional myocardial blood flow in the steady state (Fig. 13). Furthermore, when regional myocardial blood flow is normalized to account for changes in heart rate by calculating blood flow per beat, the flow-function relationships at rest and during exercise become superimposable (85). These data suggest that a state of "relative" ischemia with a discrepancy between enhanced function and oxygen demand on the one hand and a limited blood flow and oxygen supply on the other hand, exists only transiently at the onset of exercise-induced ischemia. In the steady state, however, there is "absolute" ischemia with a proportional reduction in regional function and blood flow, in particular blood flow per beat (85, 87). Thus, the degree of regional contractile dysfunction during myocardial ischemia appears to be determined by the absolute amount of regional myocardial blood flow reduction (85). According to this hypothesis, during ischemia the cause-effect relationship between myocardial function and blood flow is reversed: under normal conditions an increase in myocardial contractile function induces an increase in myocardial blood flow through metabolic coronary dilation; in contrast, during ischemia absolute myocardial blood flow determines the actual contractile function.

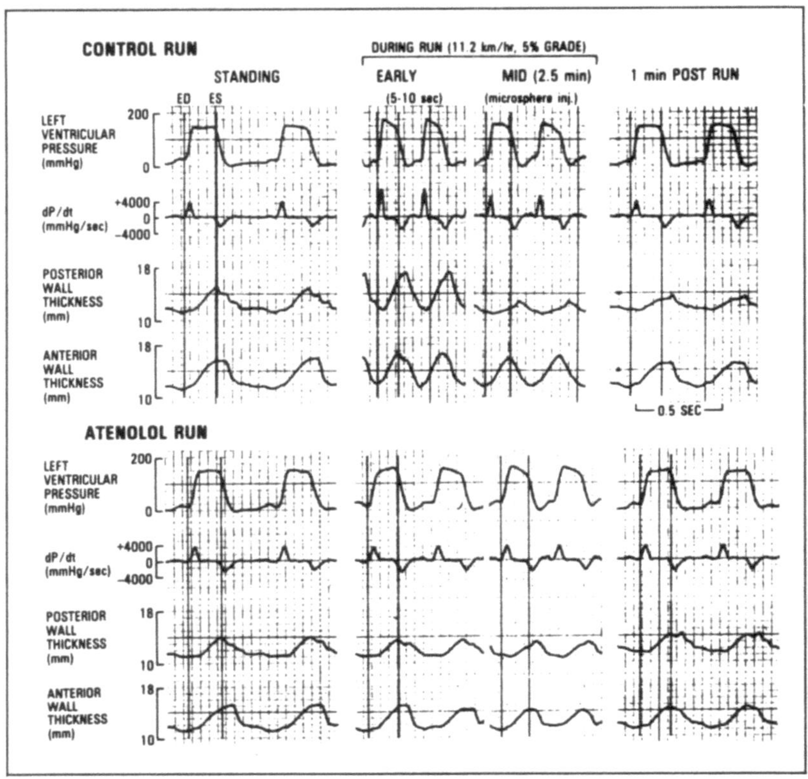

Fig. 12. Original tracing demonstrating the hemodynamic responses to treadmill exercise in a dog with chronic coronary stenosis. Regional myocardial function is only increased for seconds, but in the steady state there is marked ischemic regional myocardial dysfunction. After β-blockade with atenolol, ischemic myocardial dysfunction is less marked (88)

The previously outlined phenomena in the spatial and temporal development of myocardial ischemia are, of course, also important for therapeutic interventions. Thus, the attenuation of exercise-induced myocardial ischemia by β-blockade with atenolol cannot be attributed to a reduction in demand of the ischemic region. It results rather from a reduction in the demand of the nonischemic regions which induces a redistribution of blood flow to the ischemic region, thereby permitting increased contractile function matched to the increase in perfusion (88) (Fig. 12). The attenuation of the exercise-induced tachycardia is particularly important for the anti-ischemic action of atenolol since prevention of the negative chronotropic action of atenolol by atrial pacing prevents the increases in regional myocardial blood flow and function. Thus, the prolongation of diastolic duration and the concomitant improvement of regional myocardial blood flow are of greater importance for reducing ischemia than the negative inotropic actions of atenolol, which are not anti-ischemic per se (89). Consequently, a specific bradycardic agent without negative inotropic effect markedly attenuated exercise-induced myocardial ischemia in dogs with chronic coronary stenosis (90). The calcium antagonists verapamil (91) and diltiazem (87), or a combination of calcium antagonists with β-blockers (92, 93) not only exert negative chronotropic actions but in

78

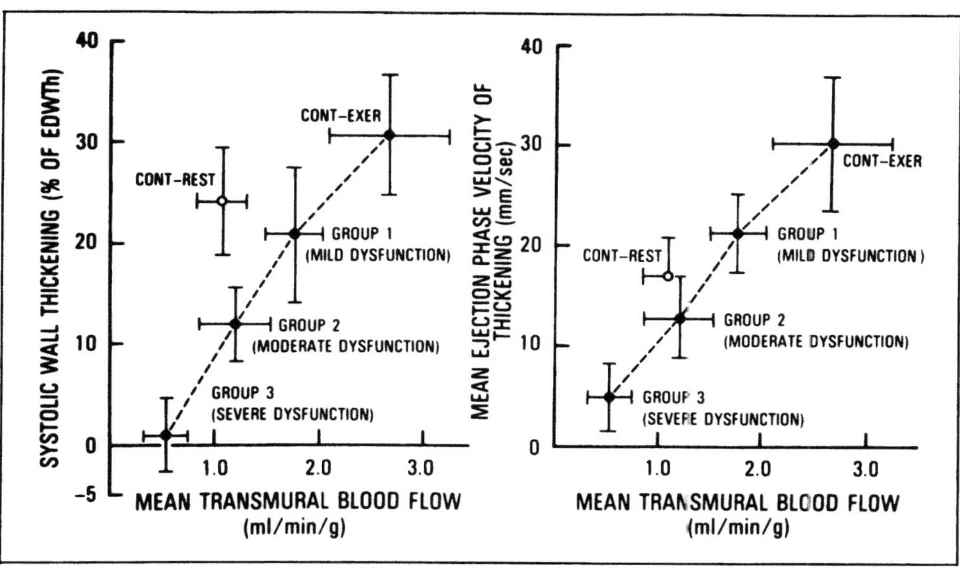

Fig. 13. Linear relationship between regional myocardial blood flow and function during several degrees of exercise-induced myocardial ischemia (85)

addition a coronary dilator effect, thus preventing exercise-induced coronary constriction (see above).

These studies demonstrate that apart from a transient phase lasting only a few seconds, in the ischemic region the discrepancy between regional myocardial function and oxygen demand on the one hand and regional myocardial blood flow and oxygen supply on the other hand is minimized by the contractile dysfunction. The amount of absolute myocardial blood flow to the ischemic region determines the actual level of myocardial function. Whether this determination of ischemic myocardial function by the actual myocardial blood flow is an active adaptation of function to the reduced perfusion in terms of a "downregulation" (94, 95) or whether the impairment in regional myocardial function is merely a consequence of the loss of energy-rich phosphates remains to be investigated. In the future, the combination of NMR-spectroscopy with analyses of regional myocardial blood flow and function may help to clarify this issue (96). In conclusion, it must be emphasized that the concept of Hermann Rein and Franz Büchner, i.e. a discrepancy of oxygen demand and supply as the underlying mechanism of myocardial ischemia, is not entirely refuted by the fact that there is little discrepancy between regional myocardial blood flow and function during steady state ischemia. It appears necessary to distinguish the demand for contractile function from the demand for the structural integrity of myocardial cells. Thus there might be a discrepancy between demand and supply at the cellular level, but not at the hemodynamic level. This hypothesis is supported by the regular post-mortem finding of disseminated myocardial necroses in patients with angina pectoris. It may also be argued that the obvious close linear relationship between regional myocardial function and blood flow when normalized per beat does not simply reflect the relationship of demand and supply. Flow per beat may already reflect a supply-demand ratio and the actual contractile function may be the result of this supply-demand balance. Nevertheless, at any given heart rate, absolute blood flow and function are adequately matched.

Finally, the dynamic nature of myocardial ischemia is again emphasized, i.e. the dynamic interaction of coagulation, coronary vasomotion and myocardial demand in the initiation of myocardial ischemia as well as the dynamic local and temporal development of myocardial ischemia. A rational therapy of myocardial ischemia and its secondary complications must be based on these dynamic pathophysiological interactions. Thus, the ultimate goal must be an improvement of absolute blood flow to the ischemic myocardium.

References

1. Roskamm H (1977) Die Coronarerkrankungen. In: Reindell H, Roskamm H (Hrsg.) Herzkrankheiten. Springer, Berlin Heidelberg New York, S. 529–617
2. Fuster V, Steele PM, Chesebro JH (1985) Role of platelets and thrombosis in coronary atherosclerotic disease and sudden death. J Am Coll Cardiol 5:175B–184B
3. Bürrig K, Hort W (1987) Werdegang der Koronarsklerose. Antrag des Sonderforschungsbereichs 242 Koronare Herzkrankheit der Universität Düsseldorf
4. Wesolowski SA, Fries CC, Sabini AM, Sawyer PN (1965) The significance of turbulence in hemic systems and in the distribution of the atherosclerotic lesion. Surgery 57:155–161
5. Nauth HF, Hort W, Hubinger R (1979) Untersuchungen über die Lokalisation sklerotischer Veränderungen in den Koronararterien und ihren großen epikardialen Ästen. Z Kardiol 68:832–838
6. Hort W, Moosdorf R, Kalbfleisch H, Köhler F, Milzner-Schwarz U, Frenzel H (1977) Postmortale Untersuchungen über Lokalisation und Form der stärksten Stenosen in den Koronararterien und ihre Beziehung zu den Risikofaktoren. Z Kardiol 66:333–340
7. Ross R, Harker L (1976) Hyperlipidemia and atherosclerosis. Science 193:1094–1100
8. Jorgensen L, Packham MA, Rowsell HC, Mustard JF (1972) Deposition of formed elements of blood on the intima and signs of intimal injury in the aorta of rabbit, pig, and man. Lab Invest 27:341–350
9. Nichols TC, Bellinger DA, Johnson TA, Lamb MA, Griggs TR (1986) von Willebrand's disease prevents occlusive thrombosis in stenosed and injured porcine coronary arteries. Circ Res 59:15–26
10. Meyer D, Baumgartner HR (1983) Role of von Willebrand factor in platelet adhesion of the subendothelium. Brit J Haemat 54:1–19
11. Fuster V, Bowie EJW, Lewis JC, Fass DN, Owen CA, Brown AL (1978) Resistance to arteriosclerosis in pigs with von Willebrand's disease. J Clin Invest 61:722-730
12. Fuster V, Fass DN, Kaye MP, Josa MP, Zinsmeister AR, Bowie EJW (1982) Arteriosclerosis in normal and von Willebrand pigs. Circ Res 51:587–594
13. Ross R, Glomset J, Kariya B, Harker L (1974) A platelet-dependent serum factor that stimulates the proliferation of arterial smooth muscle cells in vitro. Proc Nat Acad Sci USA 71:1207–1210
14. Deuel TF, Senior RM, Chang D, Griffin GL, Heinrikson RL, Kaiser ET (1981) Platelet factor 4 is chemotactic for neutrophils and monocytes. Proc Nat Acad Sci USA 78:4584–4587
15. Carvalho ACA, Colman RW, Lees RS (1974) Platelet function in hyperlipoproteinemia. N Engl J Med 290:434–438
16. Fry DL (1968) Acute vascular endothelial changes associated with increased blood velocity gradients. Circ Res 22:165–197
17. Ridolfi RL, Hutchins GM (1977) The relationship between coronary artery lesion and myocardial infarcts: Ulceration of atheroscletoric plaques precipitating coronary thrombosis. Am Heart J 93:468–486
18. Hellstrom HR (1979) Evidence in favor of the vasospastic cause of coronary artery thrombosis. Am Heart J 97:449–452
19. Gertz SD, Uretsky G, Wajnberg RS, Navot N, Gotsman MS (1981) Endothelial cell damage and thrombus formation after partial arterial constriction: Relevance of the role of coronary artery spasm in the pathogenesis of myocardial infarction. Circulation 63:476–487
20. Hort W (1974) Kreislauforgane. In: Eder M, Gedigk P (Hrsg.) Lehrbuch der Allgemeinen Pathologie und der Pathologischen Anatomie. Springer, Berlin Heidelberg New York, pp. 291–334
21. Folts JD, Crowell EB, Rowe GG (1976) Platelet aggregation in partially obstructed vessels and its elimination with aspirin. Circulation 54:365–370

22. Gallagher KP, Osakada G, Kemper WS, Ross J Jr (1985) Cyclical coronary flow reductions in conscious dogs equipped with ameroid constrictors to produce severe coronary narrowing. Basic Res Cardiol 80:100–106

23. Sobel M, Salzmann EW, Davies GC, Handin RI, Sweeney J, Ploetz J, Kurland G (1981) Circulating platelet products in unstable angina pectoris. Circulation 63:300–306

24. Needleman P, Kulkarni PS, Raz A (1977) Coronary tone modulation: formation and actions of prostaglandins, endoperoxides, and thromboxanes, Science 194:409–412

25. DeWood MA, Spores J, Notske R, Mouser LT, Burroughs R, Golden MS, Lang HT (1980) Prevalence of total occlusion during early hours of transmural myocardial infarction. New Engl J Med 303:897–902

26. Rentrop P, Blanke H, Karsch KR, Kaiser H, Köstering H, Leitz K (1981) Selective intracoronary thrombolysis in acute myocardial infarction and unstable angina pectoris. Circulation 63:307–317

27. Schröder R (1984) Intravenous short-term infusion of streptokinase in acute myocardial infarction. Int J Cardiol 5:631–637

28. Sobel BE, Geltman EM, Tiefenbrunn AJ, Jaffe AS, Spadaro JJ, Ter-Pogossian MM, Collen D, Ludbrook PA (1984) Improvement of regional myocardial metabolism after coronary thrombolysis induced with tissue-type plasminogen activator or streptokinase. Circulation 69:983–990

29. Mates R, Gupta RL, Bell AC, Klocke FJ (1978) Fluid dynamics of coronary artery stenosis. Circ Res 42:152–162

30. Gould KL (1980) Dynamic coronary stenosis. Am J Cardiol 45:286–292

31. Schwartz JS, Carlyle PF, Cohn JN (1979) Effect of dilation of the distal coronary bed on flow and resistance in severely stenotic coronary arteries in the dog. Am J Cardiol 43:219–224

32. Heusch G, Yoshimoto N, Müller-Ruchholtz ER (1982) Effects of heart rate on hemodynamic severity of coronary artery stenosis in the dog. Basic Res Cardiol 77:562–573

33. Schwartz JS, Tockman B, Cohn JN, Bache RJ (1982) Exercise-induced decrease in flow through stenotic coronary arteries in the dog. Am J Cardiol 50:1409–1413

34. Schwartz, JS, Carlyle PF, Cohn JN (1980) Effects of coronary arterial pressure on coronary stenosis resistance. Circulation 61:70–76

35. Freudenberg H, Lichtlen PR (1981) Das normale Wandsegment bei Koronarstenosen – eine postmortale Studie. Z Kardiol 70:863–869

36. Rafflenbeul W, Lichtlen PR (1982) Zum Konzept der dynamischen Koronarstenose. Z Kardiol 71:439–444

37. Brown BG, Lee AB, Bolson EL, Dodge HT (1984) Reflex constriction of significant coronary stenosis as a mechanism contributing to ischemic left ventricular dysfunction during isometric exercise. Circulation 70:18–24

38. Hossack KF, Brown BG, Stewart DK, Dodge HT (1984) Diltiazem-induced blockade of sympathetically mediated constriction of normal and diseased coronary arteries: lack of epicardial coronary dilatory effect in humans. Circulation 70:465–471

39. MacAlpin RN (1980) Relation of coronary arterial spasm to sites of organic stenosis. Am J Cardiol 46:143–153

40. MacAlpin RN (1980) Contribution of dynamic vascular wall thickening to luminal narrowing during coronary arterial constriction. Circulation 61:296–301

41. Serruys PW, Lablance JM, Reiber JHC, Bertrand ME, Hugenholtz PG (1983) Contribution of dynamic vascular wall thickening to luminal narrowing during arterial vasomotion. Z Kardiol 72 (Suppl 3): 116–123

42. Heusch G, Deussen A, Schipke J, Thämer V (1984) Alpha-1 and alpha-2 adrenoceptor mediated vasoconstriction of large and small canine coronary arteries in vivo. J Cardiovasc Pharmacol 6:961–968

43. Schroeder JS, Bolen JL, Quint RA, Clark DA, Hayden WG, Higgins CB, Wexler L (1977) Provocation of coronary spasm with ergonovine maleate. Am J Cardiol 40:487–491

44. Heupler FA, Proudfit WL, Razavi M, Shirey EK, Greenstreet R, Sheldon WC (1978) Ergonovine maleate provocative test for coronary arterial spasm. Am J Cardiol 41:631–640

45. Holtz J, Held W, Sommer O, Kühne G, Bassenge E (1982) Ergonovine-induced constrictions of epicardial coronary arteries in conscious dogs: alpha-adrenoceptors are not involved. Basic Res Cardiol 77:278–291

46. Henry PD, Yokohama M (1980) Supersensitivity of atherosclerotic rabbit aorta to ergonovine. J Clin Invest 66:306–313
47. Heistad DD, Armstrong ML, Marcus ML, Piegors DJ, Mark AL (1984) Augmented responses to vasoconstrictor stimuli in hypercholesterolemic and atherosclerotic monkeys. Circ Res 54:711–718
48. Ginsburg R, Bristow MR, Kantrowitz N, Baim S, Harrison DC (1981) Histamine provocation of clinical coronary artery spasm: implications concerning pathogenesis of variant angina pectoris. Am Heart J 102:819–822
49. Furchgott RF, Zawadzki JV (1980) The obligatory role of endothelial cells in the relaxation of arterial smooth muscle by acetylcholine. Nature 288:373–376
50. Furchgott RF (1983) Role of endothelium in responses of vascular smooth muscle. Circ Res 53:557–573
51. Young MA, Vatner SF (1986) Enhanced adrenergic constriction of iliac artery with removal of endothelium in conscious dogs. Am J Physiol 250:H892–H897
52. Schipke JD, Heusch G, Deussen A, Thämer V (1985) Acetylcholine induces constriction of epicardial coronary arteries in anesthetized dogs after removal of endothelium. Drug Res 35:926–929
53. Holtz J, Giesler M, Bassenge E (1983) Two dilatory mechanisms of anti-anginal drugs on epicardial coronary arteries in vivo: indirect, flow-dependent, endothelium-mediated dilation and direct smooth muscle relaxation. Z Kardiol 72 (Suppl 3):98–106
54. Holtz J, Förstermann U, Phol U, Giesler M, Bassenge E (1984) Flow-dependent, endothelium-mediated dilation of epicardial coronary arteries in conscious dogs: effects of cyclooxygenase inhibition. J Cardiovasc Pharmacol 6:1161–1169
55. Hintze TH, Vatner SF (1984) Reactive dilation of large coronary arteries in conscious dogs. Circ Res 54:50–57
56. Chierchia S, Davies G, Berkenboom G, Crea F, Crean P, Maseri A (1984) Alpha-adrenergic receptors and coronary spasm: an elusive link. Circulation 68:8–14
57. Winniford MD, Filipchuk N, Hillis LD (1983) Alpha-adrenergic blockade for variant angina: a long-term, double-blind, randomized trial. Circulation 67:1185–1188
58. De Caterina R, Carpeggiani C, L'Abbate AL (1984) A double-blind, placebo-controlled study of ketanserin in patients with Prinzmetal's angina. Circulation 69:889–894
59. Gewirtz H, Brautigan DL, Olsson RA, Brown P, Most AS (1983) Role of adenosine in the maintenance of coronary vasodilation distal to a severe coronary artery stenosis. Circ Res 53:42–51
60. Johannsen UJ, Mark AL, Marcus ML (1982) Responsiveness to cardiac sympathetic nerve stimulation during maximal coronary dilation produced by adenosine. Circ Res 50:510–517
61. Buffington CW, Feigl EO (1981) Adrenergic coronary vasoconstriction in the presence of coronary stenosis in the dog. Circ Res 48:416–423
62. Gorman MW, Sparks HV Jr (1982) Progressive coronary vasoconstriction during relative ischemia in canine myocardium. Circ Res 51:411–420
63. Canty JM, Klocke FJ (1985) Reduced regional myocardial perfusion in the presence of pharmacologic vasodilator reserve. Circulation 71:370–377
64. Aversano T, Becker LC (1985) Persistence of coronary vasodilator reserve despite functionally significant flow reduction. Am J Physiol 248:H403–H411
65. Pantely GA, Bristow JD, Swenson LJ, Ladley HD, Johnson WB, Anselone CG (1985) Incomplete coronary vasodilation during myocardial ischemia in swine. Am J Physiol 249:H638–H647
66. Heusch G, Deussen A (1983) The effects of cardiac sympathetic nerve stimulation on perfusion of stenotic coronary arteries in the dog. Circ Res 53:8–15
67. Heusch G, Deussen A (1984) Nifedipine prevents sympathetic vasoconstriction distal to severe coronary stenoses. J Cardiovasc Pharmacol 6:378–383
68. Heusch G (1985) Sympathische Herznerven und Myokardischämie. Thieme Verlag Stuttgart – New York
69. Tölle TR, Schipke JD, Schulz R, Thämer V, Haase J (1986) The nociceptive stimulation induced myocardial ischemia is prevented by fentanyl. Neuroscience Letter, Suppl 26:522
70. Heusch G, Deussen A, Thämer V (1985) Cardiac sympathetic nerve activity and progressive vasoconstriction distal to coronary stenoses: feed-back aggravation of myocardial ischemia. J Auton Nerv Syst 13:311–326
71. Heusch G, Schipke JD, Thämer V (1985) Clonidine prevents the sympathetic initiation and aggravation of poststenotic myocardial ischemia. J Cardiovasc Pharmacol 7:1176–1182

72. Seitelberger R, Guth BD, Heusch G, Katayama K, Lee JD, Ross J Jr (1988) Intracoronary α_2-adrenergic receptor blockade attenuates ischemia in conscious dogs during exercise. Circ Res 62: 436–442
73. Heusch G, Guth BD, Seitelberger R, Ross J Jr (1987) Attenuation of exercise-induced ischemia in dogs with recruitment of coronary vasodilator reserve by nifedipine. Circulation 75:482–490
74. Müller HS, Rao PS, Rao PB, Gory DJ, Mudd JG, Ayres SM (1982) Enhanced transcardiac ι-norepinephrine response during cold pressor test in obstructive coronary artery disease. Am J Cardiol 50:1223–1128
75. Mudge GH, Grossmann W, Mills RM Jr, Lesch M, Braunwald E (1976) Reflex increase in coronary vascular resistance in patients with ischemic heart disease. New Engl J Med 295:1333–1337
76. Mudge GH, Goldberg S, Gunter S, Mann T, Grossmann W (1979) Comparison of metabolic and vasoconstrictor stimuli on coronary vascular resistance in man. Circulation 59:544–550
77. Malacoff RF, Mudge GH, Holman BL, Idoine J, Bifolck L, Cohn PF (1983) Effects of the cold pressor test on regional myocardial blood flow in patients with coronary artery disease. Am Heart J 106:78–84
78. Berkenboom GM, Abramowicz M, Vandermoten P, Degre SG (1986) Role of alpha-adrenergic coronary tone in exercise-induced angina pectoris. Am J Cardiol 57:195–198
79. Chierchia S, Pratt T, De Coster P, Maseri A (1985) Alpha-adrenergic control of collateral flow: another determinant of coronary flow reserve. Circulation 72 (Suppl 3):190
80. Motulsky HJ, Snavely MD, Hughes RJ, Insel PA (1983) Interaction of verapamil and other calcium channel blockers with alpha-1 and alpha-2 adrenergic receptors. Circ Res 52:226–231
81. Maseri A (1986) Coronary blood flow and myocardial perfusion in humans: mechanism of acute transient myocardial ischemia. J Cardiovasc Pharmacol 8 (Suppl 3):S17–S20
82. Rowe GG (1970) Inequalities of myocardial perfusion in coronary artery disease („coronary steal"). Circulation 42:193–194
83. Heusch G, Yoshimoto N (1983) Effects of heart rate and perfusion pressure on segmental coronary resistance and collateral perfusion. Pflügers Arch 397:284–289
84. Gallagher KP, Osakada G, Matsuzaki M, Kemper WS, Ross J Jr (1982) Myocardial blood flow and function with critical stenosis in exercising dogs. Am J Physiol 243:H698–H707
85. Gallagher KP, Matsuzaki M, Osakada G, Kemper WS, Ross J Jr (1983) Effects of exercise on the relationship between myocardial blood flow and systolic wall thickening in dogs with acute coronary stenosis. Circ Res 52:716–729
86. Gallagher KP, Matsuzaki M, Koziol JA, Kemper WS, Ross J Jr (1984) Regional myocardial perfusion and wall thickening during ischemia in conscious dogs. Am J Physiol 247:H727–H738
87. Matsuzaki M, Gallagher KP, Patritti J, Tajimi T, Kemper WS, White FC, Ross J Jr (1984) Effects of a calcium-entry blocker (diltiazem) on regional myocardial flow and function during exercise in conscious dogs. Circulation 69:801–814
88. Matsuzaki M, Patritti J, Tajimi T, Miller M, Kemper WS, Ross J Jr (1984) Effects of beta-blockade on regional myocardial flow and function during exercise. Am J Physiol 247:H52–H60
89. Guth BD, Heusch G, Seitelberger R, Ross J Jr (1987) Mechanism of beneficial effect of beta-blockade on exercise-induced myocardial ischemia in conscious dogs. Circ Res 60:738–746
90. Guth BD, Heusch G, Seitelberger R, Ross J Jr (1987) Elimination of exercise-induced regional myocardial dysfunction by a bradycardiac agent in dogs with chronic coronary stenosis. Circulation 75:661–669
91. Osakada G, Kumada T, Gallagher KP, Kemper WS, Ross J Jr (1981) Reduction of exercise-induced ischemic regional myocardial dysfunction by verapamil in conscious dogs. Am Heart J 101:707–712
92. Matsuzaki M, Guth B, Tajimi T, Kemper WS, Ross J Jr (1985) Effect of the combination of diltiazem and atenolol on exercise-induced regional myocardial ischemia in conscious dogs. Circulation 72:233–243
93. Guth BD, Tajimi T, Seitelberger R, Lee JD, Matsuzaki M, Ross J Jr (1986) Experimental exercise-induced ischemia: drug therapy can eliminate regional dysfunction and oxygen supply-demand imbalance. J Am Coll Cardiol 7:1036–1046
94. Jacobus WE, Pores IH, Lucas SK, Kallmann CH, Weisfeldt ML, Flaherty JT (1982) The role of intracellular pH in the control of normal and ischemic myocardial contractility: a 31P nuclear magnetic resonance and mass spectrometry study. In: Intracellular pH: its measurement, regulation and utilization in cellular functions. Alan R Liss. New York, pp. 537–565

95. Schipke JD, Burkhoff D, Schäfer J (1986) Änderung des ventrikulären mechanischen Wirkungsgrades bei reduzierter Koronardurchblutung. Z Kardiol 75. Suppl. 4:43
96. Guth BD, Martin JF, Heusch G, Ross J Jr (1987) Regional myocardial blood flow, function and metabolism using 31P NMR spectroscopy during ischemia and reperfusion in dogs. J Am Coll Cardiol 10, 673–681

Authors' address:

Prof. Dr. Gerd Heusch
Abteilung für Pathophysiologie
Zentrum für Innere Medizin
Medizinische Klinik und Poliklinik
Universitätsklinikum Essen
Hufelandstraße 55
4300 Essen 1

Discussion

GÜLKER

It has been shown in humans that poststenotic coronary blood flow is increased under calcium antagonists, but not under nitrates and – as far as I know – not under β-blockers. How is that explained?

HEUSCH

In fact, nitrates appear not to increase absolute subendocardial blood flow. This may be because nitrates are not functional antagonists of α-adrenoceptors in coronary resistance vessels, whereas calcium antagonists are. For the anti-ischemic effect of β-blockers not the coronary arterial inflow which is clinically measured, but the transmural distribution of blood flow is important. β-blockade may increase subendocardial blood flow and decrease subepicardial blood flow, resulting in no change in coronary arterial inflow but an attenuation of subendocardial ischemia.

SPECCHIA

Your hypotheses are very attractive. I have two questions: How do you explain the different reactions to nifedipine in patients with chronic stable angina, i.e. some patients showing good improvement whereas others show none at all. Do you think that in man a steady state of severe ischemia is possible at all?

HEUSCH

I emphasized that the two essential underlying mechanisms of exercise-induced myocardial ischemia are tachycardia and α-adrenoceptor mediated coronary constriction. Patients with marked tachycardia will then, of course, not benefit from nifedipine but rather from β-blockers or negative chronotropic calcium antagonists. Conversely, patients with a predominant coronary constriction will benefit more from nifedipine.
The term steady state in the context of ischemia is certainly problematic. In principle, ischemia is a progressive process leading to infarction. However, it is unclear how and when the balance between myocardial blood flow and function is turned into an imbalance, which then compromises the vitality and integrity of myocardial cells.

The status of calcium antagonists in the drug treatment of coronary heart disease

H. Gülker

University Hospital, Department of Cardiology-Angiology, Münster

Introduction

Up to now it has not been possible to treat the underlying cause of coronary artery disease, namely arteriosclerosis, so it has been necessary to resort to the indirect approach of minimizing and preventing "risk factors" (10, 18, 19). Symptomatic and palliative therapies, including the antianginal use of antianginal drugs, percutaneous or intra-operative trans-luminal coronary angioplasty and surgical revascularization by aortocoronary bypass, or implantation of the mammary artery are the first choice approaches to the treatment of overt disease.

Drug treatment

The drugs used for treating coronary heart disease are beta-blockers, calcium antagonists, molsidomine and nitrates, either alone or in combination.

Aims of treatment are:

1. to improve the oxygen balance of the heart by increasing myocardial oxygen supply and/ or reducing myocardial oxygen demand; this improves the clinical signs and symptoms by reducing the frequency and severity of angina pectoris and increasing exercise tolerance.
2. to provide cardioprotection by increasing the heart's ability to tolerate ischaemia;
3. to prevent complications, namely:
   - life-threatening arrhythmias,
   - myocardial infarction,
   - cardiac death.
4. to provide vasoprotection, that is to halt progression of arteriosclerosis and encourage regression of arteriosclerotic damage.

Factors such as frequency of tablet-taking, incidence and severity of adverse reactions, and the associated issue of patient compliance, are also important practical considerations.

First aim of treatment: to improve myocardial oxygen balance and thus improve clinical signs and symptoms of ischemia

Angina pectoris is caused by coronary insufficiency, an imbalance between myocardial oxygen supply and demand. *Supply of oxygen* to the myocardium is determined by the coronary perfusion pressure, extravascular and intravascular coronary resistance and by blood viscosity, haemoglobin concentration and arterial oxygen saturation. The diameter of a coronary artery, even one with organic stenosis, can usually vary to some extent, depending on the degree of contraction or relaxation of responsive segments of the vessel wall. The *uptake of oxygen* by the heart depends essentially on heart rate, wall tension, contractility and peripheral arterial resistance. The most important determinant of oxygen uptake in the non-failing myocardium of normal size is the heart rate at rest and during exercise. On the other hand, the most important factor in the enlarged heart with elevated intracardiac pressures and volumes is wall tension.

Calcium antagonists and nitrates increase the supply of oxygen to the myocardium (Table 1). These drugs cause direct, dose-dependent dilation of coronary arteries, arterioles and interarterial connections. In contrast, beta-blockers only increase coronary blood flow indirectly, by prolonging the duration of the coronary blood flow relevant diastole. The advantages of calcium antagonists over nitrates are, firstly, that they have a more marked, dose-related vasodilatation, and, secondly, that they increase blood flow in the poststenotic vascular bed. Nitrates fail to increase poststenotic coronary flow (29).

Beta-blockers reduce heart rate and contractility at rest and during exercise (Table 2); as a result they are likely to have an oxygen-sparing effect, particularly in patients who have a myocardium of normal size which is not failing, but have a hpyerkinetic circulatory picture at rest and/or during exercise, and in patients with hypertension and myocardial hypertrophy. As nitrates are strongest in reducing wall tension, they can predominantly be used to control acute rises of diastolic intracardiac pressure and volume during anginal attacks, and to treat patients with a dilated myocardium which has been failing chronically.

Table 1. Effect of coronary drugs on the oxygen supply to the heart

	desired effect	beta-blockers	nitrates	verapamil gallopamil diltiazem	dihydrobenz-pyridines
Oxygen supply:	↑	−	↑	↑	↑
Coronary perfusion pressure	↑	↓	−	↓	↓
Intravascular coronary resistance	↓	(↑)	↓	↓	↓
Extravascular coronary resistance	↓	(↑)	↓	−	−
Relevant period of diastole	↑	↑	↓	↑	↓
Poststenotic coronary flow	↑	−	−	↑	↑
Haemoglobin,					
O$_2$ saturation,					
Viscosity	−	−	−	−	−

↑ increase   ↓ decrease   − no effect

Table 2. Effect of coronary drugs on oxygen uptake by the heart

	desired effect	beta-blockers	nitrates	verapamil gallopamil diltiazem	dihydrobenz-pyridines
Oxygen uptake:	↓	↓	↓	↓	↓
Heart rate	↓	↓	↑	−↑	−↑
Contractility	↓	↓	−	↓	−
Peripheral arterial resistance	↓	−↑	↓	↓	↓
Wall tension	↓	↑	↓	−	−

↑ increase   ↓ decrease   − no effect

Calcium antagonists reduce cardiac oxygen requirement by lowering peripheral arterial resistance. Verapamil, gallopamil and diltiazem reduce heart rate and contractility, particularly during exercise, that means they save even more oxygen if the heart is not failing. Dihydropyridines do not have these effects; particularly when combined with nitrates, this group of calcium antagonists appears to offer an advantage for treating patients with an enlarged, failing myocardium, since the resulting reduction of arterial resistance contributes to reducing wall tension without any cardiodepressant effect being produced.

In practice there are not always clear-cut distinctions between the main indications for the various coronary drugs. Calcium antagonists are mainly used to treat the following groups of patients:

1. Patients with exclusively or predominantly vasospastic symptoms (21, 32 and other references) that is to say patients with typical angina at rest whose exercise tolerance is not impaired. Dihydropyridines have the most powerful vasodilator effect and are therefore the drugs of choice for these patients.

2. Patients with unstable angina pectoris (9, 26 and other references) that is to say patients with newly developed severe angina pectoris and patients whose attacks of pain are becoming more frequent and severe and who are becoming less responsive to nitrates. The underlying cause is usually high-grade vascular stenosis. Cardioactive calcium antagonists, namely verapamil, gallopamil and diltiazem, appear to be particularly suitable for patients with normal resting pressures, since apart from relaxing responsive segments of vessels, these drugs reduce oxygen uptake by the heart by reducing heart rate and contractility. However, drugs of the nifedipine type are preferred for patients with myocardial failure. Nitrates are an alternative; maximum anti-anginal effects are achieved by combining both types of drugs.

3. Patients with stable coronary stenosis and exercise-induced angina (2, 7 and other references). Here, the cardio-active calcium antagonists are the first drugs to consider for patients without myocardial failure. Beta-blockers are the alternative. The advantage of calcium antagonists is that they do not reduce maximal exercise capacity to the same degree as beta-blockers. However, the dihydropyridines, as an alternative to nitrates, or in combination with nitrates, are preferred for patients with elevated intracardiac pressures or volumes.

Second aim of treatment: to improve the heart's ability to tolerate ischaemia in patients with transient acute coronary insufficiency; this is known as "cardioprotection"

Cardioprotection means an improvement in the ability of the myocardium to tolerate intermittent ischaemia without irreversible cell damage. There are many reports documented in the literature that both beta-blockers and calcium antagonists have cardioprotective effects (see refs. 6, 23, 24 and others). Given prophylactically, these drugs are capable of preventing or significantly reducing ischaemia-induced cell damage due to myocardial hypoxia or anoxia, and reperfusion-induced cell lesions. Cardioprotection is particularly important with respect to the frequent occurrence of "silent ischaemia". Treatment to prevent these episodes of ischaemia may well reduce secondary damage to the structure of the myocardium.

Third aim of treatment: to prevent complications

a) Arrhythmias

It can be demonstrated in animals that ventricular arrhythmias, including ventricular fibrillation, in the first minutes of acute myocardial ischaemia, can be almost completely prevented by prophylactic administration of beta-blockers which have no intrinsic sympathomimetic activity, or by cardio-active calcium antagonists, namely verapamil, gallopamil and diltiazem (Table 3). These drugs have proved superior to local anaesthetics and class-III anti-arrhythmic agents in these circumstances. Nifedipine and its derivatives have no electrophysiological effects on the heart in situ and thus they have no direct anti-arrhythmic or antifibrillatory acitivity (11, 12).

There is no doubt that the results of these animal experiments can be extrapolated to humans. The improved survival of postinfarction patients under some beta-blockers and under verapamil (see Table 4) may be due to some degree to direct antifibrillatory effects of these drugs, and the fact that beta-blockers (22) and verapamil (13) have been shown to prevent exercise-induced and ischaemia-related ventricular arrhythmias in patients with coronary heart disease can be seen as further corroborative evidence of this assumption.

b) Myocardial infarction

Long-term treatment with some beta-blockers, including metoprolol, timolol and propranolol, has been shown to reduce the incidence of reinfarction in postinfarction patients. There is also evidence that verapamil probably reduces the reinfarction rate. The incidence of reinfarction between the 21st and 180th day of treatment was 7% in the control patients as opposed to 3.3% in patients under verapamil (8). The corresponding figures after 6–12 months were 8.3% and 7% respectively (30). However, by this time the differences were not statistically significant.

c) Cardiac mortality

The beta-blocker prevention studies and the verapamil postinfarction study showed that in addition to prophylaxis of reinfarction, there was also a reduction in cardiac mortality. In the prevention study with verapamil, cardiac mortality was reduced by 42% between the 21st and 180th day after starting the treatment. However, after 6–12 months the differences were

Table 3. Antiarrhythmic and antifibrillatory effects of coronary drugs in animals with experimentally-induced, reversible myocardial ischaemia

	beta-blockers	nitrates	verapamil gallopamil diltiazem	dihydrobenz-pyridines
Acute myocardial ischaemia following coronary occlusion				
anti-arrhythmic effect	+	−	+ +	−
fibrillation prophylaxis	+ +	−	+ +	−
Acute myocardial ischaemia reperfusion				
anti-arrhythmic effect	+ *	−	+ *	+ *
fibrillation prophylaxis	−	−	−	−

+ definite effect   + + pronounced effect   − no effect
* indirect action as a result of cardioprotective effects

Table 4. Secondary prevention studies in postinfarction patients with evidence that beta-blockers and verapamil increase the likelihood of survival

Author/year	Drug	Study conditions	Start of treatment	Observation period	Dosage	Control deaths	Active drug deaths
Noris 1968	Propranolol	DB	< 72 h	3 weeks	80 mg/d	24/228	31/226
Wilhelmson 1974	Alprenolol	DB	1st–3rd week	2 years	400 mg/d	14/116	7/114
Multicentre 1975	Practolol	DB	1–4 weeks	1–3 years	400 mg/d	117/1514	94/1524
MIAMI 1980	Metoprolol	DB	at admission	< 15 days	15 mg i.v. 200 mg/d	137/2901	120/2877
Hjalmarson 1981	Metoprolol	DB	about 11.3 h	3 months	15 mg i.v. + 2200 mg/d	62/697	40/698
BHAT 1982	Propranolol	DB	5–21 days	12–30 months	180–240 mg/d	118/1921	138/1916
Hansteen 1982	Propranolol	PR	4–6 days	1 year	160 mg/d	37/282	25/278
Boyle 1983	Metoprolol	DB	< 6 h	1 year	15 mg i.v. + 300 mg/d	52/384	49/416
Herlitz 1986	Metoprolol	DB	< 48 h$\bar{x}$ = 8 h	2 years	5 mg t.i.d., i.v. + 200 mg/d	120/698	92/697
ISIS 1986	Atenolol	PR	< 12 h$\bar{x}$ = 5 h	7 days	5–10 mg i.v. 200 mg/d	365/7990	313/8037
ISIS 1986	Atenolol	PR	< 12 h$\bar{x}$ = 5 h	1 year	5–10 mg i.v. 200 mg/d	1120/7990	1071/8037
Multicentre 1981	Timolol	DB	17–28 days	1–3 years	200 mg/d	152/939	98/945
MILLIS	Propranolol	R	8.5 h	E = 36 months	0.1 mg/kg i.v. + 20–600 mg/d	not significant	
Dan. Study Group 1984	Verapamil	DB	at admission	after 6 months in all	0.1 mg/kg i.v. + 360 mg/d	100/719	92/717
Dan. Study Group 1984	Verapamil	DB	at admission	after 12 months in all	0.1 mg/kg i.v. + 360 mg/d	118/719	110/717
Fischer-Hansen 1986	Verapamil	DB	at admission	21st–180th day	0.1 mg/kg i.v. + 360 mg p.o.	38/719	12/717

not statistically significant; at these times the reduction of overall mortality was only about 8%. Altogether, the results are evidence that the cardioactive calcium antagonists have a protective effect in postinfarction patients, but the findings need to be confirmed by further clinical trials.

The results of the prevention studies in postinfarction patients are an important argument in favour of the use of beta-blockers, and in future perhaps also of cardio-active calcium antagonists for the basic treatment of coronary diseases, since it seems likely that, apart from their effect on symptoms, these drugs prevent the most important complications. There is no evidence of comparable protective effects with dihydropyridines or nitrates (33), so these drugs can only be considered as symptomatic treatments.

Fourth aim of treatment: vasoprotection that is to halt progression of arteriosclerosis and to encourage regression of arteriosclerotic damage

There is evidence from animal experiments that coronary arteriosclerosis caused by hypertension, can largely be prevented by long-term treatment with calcium antagonists. The vasoprotective effects of calcium antagonists are evidently specific and can be achieved with verapamil-type drugs and with nifedipine derivatives. We do not yet know whether the experimental results can be extrapolated to humans and therapeutic dosage. Several investigators have reported regression of arteriosclerotic lesions under long-term treatment with verapamil (20). However, in view of the small number of patients assessed hitherto, the extraordinary variability in the spontaneous progression of arteriosclerosis (27) and the as yet short observation periods, the possibility that the results might have been misinterpreted can not be ruled out.

Adverse reactions

The frequency and severity of adverse reactions are important considerations when evaluating a long-term drug treatment for chronic illnesses. Generally, as long as the contraindications are observed, none of the marketed beta-blockers for coronary treatment, calcium antagonists or nitrates have serious adverse effects on any organs, but they do differ as regards the incidence of subjective side effects. Beta-blockade modifies a variety of organ functions, and patients frequently report side effects. Particularly important from the point of view of circulatory physiology is the reduction in the exercise capacity. With nitrates, the incidence of subjective side effects, mainly persistent headaches, is also significant. The incidence of individual side effects of calcium antagonists is low: at less than 15% (35), which is in the anticipated placebo range (Table 5).

Table 5. Adverse reactions to coronary treatment with calcium antagonists, taking gallopamil (data in % : n = 18627 patients)

Gastro-intestinal reactions	7.20
Cardiovascular reactions	2.17
Cardiac reactions	1.6
Other adverse reactions	2.59
No adverse reactions	86.44

Summary

To sum up, the status of calcium antagonists in the treatment of coronary heart disease may be defined as follows:

1. Calcium antagonists are the drugs of choice for patients with, predominantly, angina at rest or with unstable forms of angina.
2. For certain patients with predominantly or exclusively exercise-induced angina, calcium antagonists should be considered as an alternative to beta-blockers and nitrates. Cardioactive calcium antagonists are preferred for patients without myocardial failure. Dihydropyridines are the front-line drugs for patients with a dilated heart and increased resting pressures.
3. Calcium antagonists supplement and extend the spectrum of action of beta-blockers and nitrates. This makes them suitable for combined treatment.
4. In terms of cardioprotection, prophylaxis of ischaemia-induced ventricular arrhythmias, prophylaxis of reinfarction and deaths of cardiac origin, the cardioactive calcium antagonists appear to offer advantages over the dihydropyridines. However, their effect is not superior to that of the beta-blockers.
5. The low incidence of adverse reactions, and correspondingly good patient compliance, are important practical arguments in favour of calcium antagonists. Subjective side effects are less frequent and less severe than those reported under beta-blockers and nitrates.
6. Experimental evidence that calcium antagonists protect the vessels from arteriosclerotic damage may in future give new impetus to the use of these compounds as coronary drugs.

References

1. A Multicentre International Study (1975) Improvement in prognosis of myocardial infarction by long term beta-adrenoceptor blockade using Practolol. Br Med J 297:735.
2. Bala Subramanian V, Raftery EB (1982) An objective comparison of verapamil and placebo in chronic stable angina. Clin Exp Pharmacol Physiol (Suppl 6):51
3. Beta Blocker Heart Attack Trial Research Group (1981) A randomized trial of propranolol in patients with acute myocardial infarction: I. Mortality results. JAMA 247:1707
4. Boyle DM, Barber JM, Mc Ilmoyle El, Salathia KS, Evans AE, Cran G, Elwood JH, Shanks RG (1983) Effect of very early intervention with metoprolol on myocardial infarct size. Br Heart J 49:229
5. Fleckenstein A (1971) Specific inhibitors and promoters of calcium action in the excitation-contraction coupling of the heart muscle and their role in the prevention or production of myocardial lesions. In: Harris P, Opie L (eds) Calcium and the heart. Proceedings of the meeting of the European Section of the International Study Group for Research in Cardiac Metabolism. Academic Press, London New York, pp. 135–188
6. Fleckenstein A, Frey M, Fleckenstein-Grün G (1985) Myocardial vascular damage by intracellular calcium-overload. Preventive actions of calcium antagonists. In: Godfraind T, Vanhoutte PM, Govoni S, Paoletti R (eds) Calcium Entry Blockers and Tissue Protection. Raven Press, New York, pp 91–105
7. Fischer-Hansen J, Gryther C, Thomsen St, Sigurd B (1982) Verapamil and ß-adrenoceptor blockade in the treatment of stable angina pectoris. Clin Exp Pharmacol Physiol (Suppl 6):31
8. Fischer-Hansen JF (1988) Sekundärprävention des Myokardinfarktes. In: Bender F, Fleckenstein A (eds) Therapie und Prävention mit Kalziumantagonisten: Hypertonie – Koronare Herzkrankheit – Arteriosklerose. Steinkopff, Darmstadt.
9. Gerstenblith G, Ongang P, Achuff SC, Bulkley BH, Becker LE, Mellits ED, Baugham KL, Weiss JL, Flaherty JT, Kallmann CH, Llewellyn M, Weisfeld Ml (1982) Nifedipine in instable angina. A double blind, randomized trial. New England J Med 306:885

10. Gleichmann U, Mannebach H, Gleichmann S (1984) Prävention der Koronaren Herzkrankheit – praktische Gesichtspunkte. Z Kardiol 73 (Suppl 2):143
11. Gülker H, Thale J (1986) Ischämische Herzrhythmusstörungen: Einflüsse des autonomen Nervensystems auf elektrophysiologische Befunde und Pharmakotherapie. Z Kardiol 75 (Suppl 5):15
12. Gülker H (1989) Antiarrhythmische Pharmakotherapie bei Myokardischämie und Myokardnekrose. Steinkopff, Darmstadt, in press
13. Gülker H, Heuer H, Behrenbeck Th, Bender F (1987) Prophylaxe belastungsinduzierter ventrikulärerArrhythmien durch Verapamil. Z Kardiol 76:404
14. Hansteen V, Moinicher E, Lorentsen E (1982) One year's treatment with propranolol after myocardial infarction: Preliminary report of Norwegian multicenter trial. Br Med J 284:155
15. Herlitz J, Elmfeldt D, Holmberg S, Malek I, Nyberg G, Pennert K, Ryden L, Swedberg K, Vedin A, Waagstein F, Waldenström A, Waldenström J, Wedel M, Wilhelmssen L, Wilhelmssen C, Hjalmarson A (1984) Göteborg Metoprolol Trial: Mortality and causes of death. Am J Cardiol 53:8D-15D
16. Hjalmarson A, Elmfeld D, Herlitz J, Homberg S, Malek I, Nyberg J, Ryden L, Swedberg K, Vedin A, Waagstein F, Waldenström J, Wedel H, Wilhelmsen L, Wilhelmsson C (1981) Effect on mortality of metoprolol in acute myocardial infarction. A double blind randomized trial. Lancet 11:823
17. ISIS (International Study of Infarct Survival) (1986) Randomized trial of intravenous Atenolol among 16027 causes of suspected acute myocardial infarction: ISIS I. Lancet II:57
18. Kannel WB, Dawber TR, Kagan A, Revotskie N, Stokes J (1961) Factors of risk in the development of coronary heart disease – six year follow-up experience. Ann Intern Med 55:33
19. Keys A (1953) Prediction and possible prevention of coronary disease. Am J Publ Hlth 43:1399
20. Kober G, Nickelsen T, Jakobs B, Kaltenbach M (1986) Der Einfluß einer Langzeittherapie mit Calcium-Antagonisten auf die Entwicklung der stenosierenden Koronarsklerose. In: Rosenthal J (ed) Calcium-Antagonisten und Hypertonie – aktueller Stand. Excerpta Medica. Amsterdam, pp. 98–107
21. Maseri A, Severi S, De Nes M, L'Abbate A, Chierchia S, Marzilli M, Balestra AM, Parodi O, Biagini A, Distante A (1978) "Variant" angina: one aspect of a continuous spectrum of vasospastic myocardial ischemia, Pathogenetic mechanisms, estimated incidence, clinical and coronarographic findings in 138 patients. Am J Cardiol 42:1019
22. Meinertz TH (1987) Wirkung von Gallopamil auf stumme Myokardischämien. In this book, p. 150
23. Makotoff DM, Quinones MA, Miller RR (1980) Exercise induced ventricular tachycardia: clinical features, relation to chronic ventricular ectopy and prognosis. Chest 77:10
24 Nayler WG (1978) Prolonged protective effect of propranolol on hypoxic heart muscle. Am J Cardiol 42:217
25. Nayler WG, Ferrari F, Slade A (1980) Cardioprotective actions of calcium antagonists in myocardial anoxia and ischemia. In: Fleckenstein A, Roskamm H (eds) Calcium Antagonismus. Springer, Berlin Heidelberg New York, pp 119–137
26. Norris RM, Caughey DE, Scott PJ (1968) Trial of propranolol in acute myocardial infarction. Br Med J II:398–400
27. Parodi O, Maseri A, Simonetti I (1979) Management of instable angina at rest by verapamil: a double blind cross over study in CCU. Br Heart J 41:167
28. Rafflenbeul W, Nellesen U, Galvao P, Kreft M, Peters S, Lichtlen P (1984) Progression and Regression der Koronarsklerose im angiographischen Bild. Z Kardiol 73, Suppl 2:33
29. Rude RE, Buja M, Willerson JT (1986) Propranolol in acute myocardial infarction: The MILIS experience. Am J Cardiol 57:38F–42F
30. Simon R (1984) Calcium-Antagonisten: Wirkung auf periphere und koronare Hämodynamik. Z Kardiol 73, Suppl 2:79
31. The Danish Study Group on Verapamil in Myocardial Infarction (1984) Verapamil in acute myocardial infarction. Eur Heart J 5:516–528
32. The MIAMI Trial Research group (1985) Metoprolol in acute myocardial infarction. A randomized placebo controlled trial. Eur Heart J 6:199–226
33. Waters DD, Theroux P, Szlachic J, Dauwe F (1981) Provocative testing with ergonovine to assess the efficacy of treatment with nifedipine, diltiazem and verapamil in variant angina. Am J Cardiol 48:123

34. Wilcox RG, Hampton JR, Banks DC, Birkhead J, Brooksby I, Burns-Cox C, Haves AJ, Joy M, Malcolm AD, Mather HG, Rowley JM (1986) Trial of early nifedipine treatment in patients with suspected myocardial infarction (the TRENT study). Br Med J 293:1204–1208
35. Wilhelmsson C, Vedin JA, Wilhelmsen L, Tubblin G, Werkö L (1974) Reduction of sudden death after myocardial infarction by treatment with Alprenolol, Lancet II:1157
36. Wolf EH (1986) KHK: Operation oder Medikamente: neuere Calcium-Antagonisten senken das Risiko der Langzeittherapie. Fortschr Med 45:104

Author's address:

Prof. Dr. med. Hartmut Gülker
Medizinische Universitätsklinik
Albert-Schweitzer-Str. 33
D–4400 Münster
West Germany

Discussion

STAUCH

Perhaps the statement about unstable angina should be modified by saying that in the light of the results of the calcium antagonists studies in comparison with metoprolol, nifedipine was so poor in respect of mortality and incidence of reinfarction that the study had to be stopped. Admittedly, these results were only obtained recently, but they are still important because they indicate that distinctions between the calcium antagonists should be drawn even more clearly than before, and we should stop using the broad classifications "verapamil type" and "nifedipine type". I do not know whether studies of this sort have been carried out with verapamil or gallopamil.

Haemodynamic effects of gallopamil in patients with coronary heart disease and/or pulmonary hypertension

P. Richter, M. Stauch

Department of Cardiovascular and Respiratory Medicine, University of Ulm

Introduction

Calcium antagonists are of proven use for the treatment of coronary heart disease. As is evident from published reports on nifedipine and verapamil (2, 3, 5), like other vasodilators they are also used for the treatment of pulmonary hypertension. Gallopamil, a calcium antagonist of the verapamil type, is a potent vasodilator and caution is required when administering this drug intravenously because its effect on the systemic circulation may result in a fall of blood pressure, and because it has a marked effect on bioelectrical conduction.

The response of pulmonary resistance and pulmonary pressures to gallopamil may vary from patient to patient. The powerful dilator effect on the systemic circulation, which is exploited when, for example, verapamil is used to treat a hypertensive crisis, might also be useful for treating pulmonary hypertension.

On the other hand, the impairment of myocardial contractility anticipated on theoretical grounds with calcium antagonists of the verapamil type might result in a rise of pulmonary pressure as a consequence of a deterioration of left ventricular function. However, this might, in turn, be offset or masked by a reduction of left ventricular afterload. Moreover, the relative prominence of the effects which are to be discussed in detail also depends on the specific degree of hypoxaemia and global cardiac function in each patient (1, 3). In order to take a closer look at the effect of gallopamil on the pulmonary circulation we studied two groups of patients. One group had coronary disease (CHD) without pulmonary disease and without pulmonary pressures and various cardiac diseases.

Method

The first group comprised 13 patients with coronary heart disease. After diagnostic coronary angiography, at least 30 minutes after ventriculography these patients were given 3 mg gallopamil administered slowly into the right atrium (Table 1). The previous medication was

Tabl. 1 Composition of group I

13 patients with CHD
6 with transmural infarctions EF > 45%   4 with one-vessel disease   9 with several significant stenoses   Investigation at rest; 3 mg gallopamil administered into the right atrium; measurement after 0, 5, 10, 15 min

stopped the day before examination. Cardiac output (CO) and the pressures in the pulmonary circulation were measured with the aid of a Swan-Ganz 7F thermodilution catheter. None of the patients had pulmonary hypertension; while they had at least significant one-vessel disease, none presented with severely impaired global function. Six patients had had transmural infarctions. None had aneurysms.

For the second group we selected patients with raised pulmonary pressures. For this group we increased the dose of gallopamil to 5 mg, again administered slowly (no faster than 1 mg/min) into the right atrium. Table 2 shows the composition of group II. The previous medication of all the patients was stopped for at least 24 hours with the patients fasted. All the patients were familiar with the test procedure because they had previously done exercise tests on a bicycle ergometer. They were tested in the supine position on the bicycle ergometer with the work load being increased in 25 W increments every 4 minutes. Cardiac output and pressures in the pulmonary circulation were measured, again by thermodilution. The estimated mean aortic pressure (pressures measured with a sphygmomanometer, $1/3 \times$pulse pressure $+$ BP_{dia}) was used to calculate total peripheral resistance $(TPR = Ao_m\text{-}Pad_m/CO \times 80)$. After exercising at the maximum level of loading, the patient was allowed enough time to recover, usually 15 minutes depending on his general condition and heart rate, before gallopamil was administered. After the injection and a further 10-minute pause, another staged exercise test was carried out. One patient could not repeat the exercise test; in this patient, who had a patent ductus arteriosus, there was pressure equalization and cross-over shunt and the reduction in systemic resistance elicited by gallopamil increased the right-left shunt fraction. The patient recovered within an hour. No other patient experienced any adverse effects or impairment of exercise tolerance.

Table 2. Composition of group II

7 patients with raised pulmonary resistance:
1 patient ductus arteriosus
3 with secondary pulmonary hypertension associated with CHD and impaired left ventricular function
1 had had recurrent pulmonary embolism
1 sarcoidosis stage III
1 severe chronic obstr./restr. pulmonary disease with pulmonary heart disease

Results

In the group of patients with coronary heart disease the EF was, in the worst case, 47%; on average it was 55%. The left ventricular end diastolic pressures were about 10 mm Hg. They did not rise, even during the 15 minutes after the injection. The pulmonary pressures also remained the same, while the systemic pressure fell by 10% in the first 5 minutes, rising slightly again later (Figure 1).

There was an appreciable change in cardiac output. It rose from 5.9 l/min to a maximum of 7 l/min after 5 minutes and then fell back virtually to the baseline value again at 6 l/min after 15 minutes. There was no initial fall in any of the patients (Figure 2). The calculated total peripheral resistance values showed a corresponding response: they fell significantly from 1350 dynseccm^{-5} to 1165 dynseccm^{-5} and remained significantly depressed throughout the 15-minute measurement period. The heart rate did not change.

96

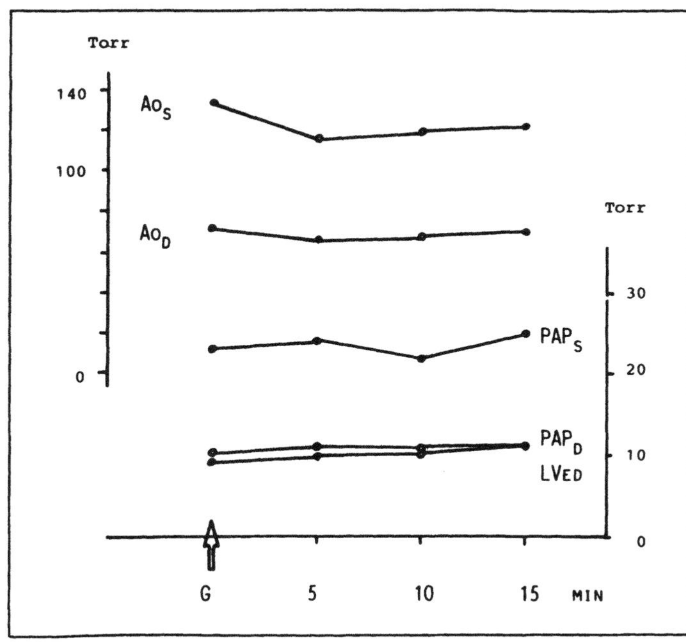

Figure 1. Systolic (Ao_s) and diastolic (Ao_d) aortic and pulmonary (PAP_s, PAP_d) pressures and left ventricular enddiastolic pressures (LVed) after injecting 3 mg gallopamil into the right atrium

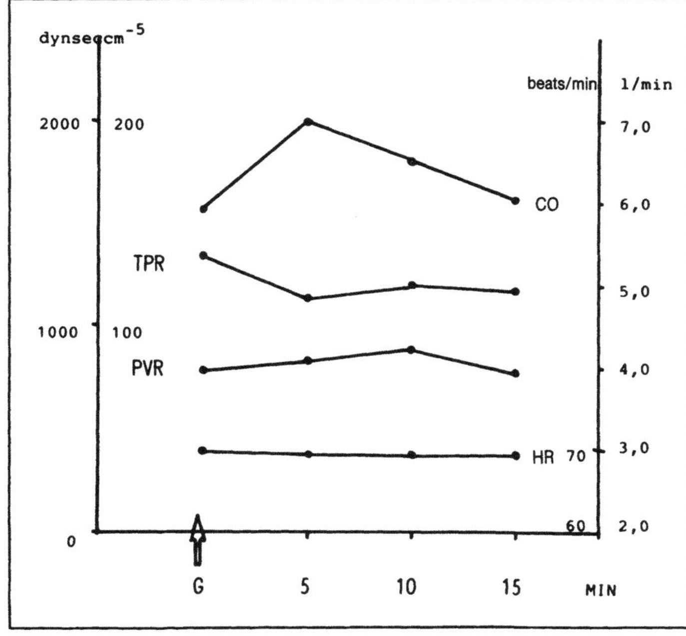

Figure 2. Cardiac output (CO), heart rate (HR), total peripheral resistance (TPR) and pulmonary vascular resistance (PVR) after 3 mg gallopamil

97

There was no significant change in pulmonary vascular resistance ($PVR = PAP_m\text{-}PC_m/CO \times 80$) during the measurement period: it rose slightly from an initial 78 dynseccm^{-5} to 89 dynseccm^{-5} after 10 minutes and had fallen to the baseline again after 15 minutes (Table 3). Figures 3 and 4 and Table 4 show the results without and with medication in the group of patients with pulmonary hypertension:

The resting systemic blood pressures were at most 45% and on average 23% lower. The pulmonary pressures were not significantly lower after gallopamil, but they did show a more

Table 3. Means and standard deviations for each parameter

	before	5 min	10 min	15 min	
LVDIA	9 ± 3	10 ± 4	10 ± 3	11 ± 4	mmHg
AO_{sys}	134 ± 15	118 ± 15	120 ± 14	121 ± 13	mmHg
AO_{dia}	72 ± 15	66 ± 9	67 ± 8	69 ± 9	mmHg
PAP_s	23 ± 4	24 ± 4	22 ± 4	25 ± 5	mmHg
PAP_d	10 ± 3	11 ± 2	11 ± 2	11 ± 3	mmHg
CO	5.9 ± 1.6	7 ± 3	6.6 ± 2.4	6.1 ± 1.2	l/min
HR	69 ± 6	68 ± 6	67 ± 4	67 ± 6	/min
TPR	1357 ± 395	1165 ± 255	1220 ± 267	1175 ± 318	dynseccm^{-5}
PVR	78 ± 52	83 ± 72	89 ± 74	77 ± 71	dynseccm^{-5}

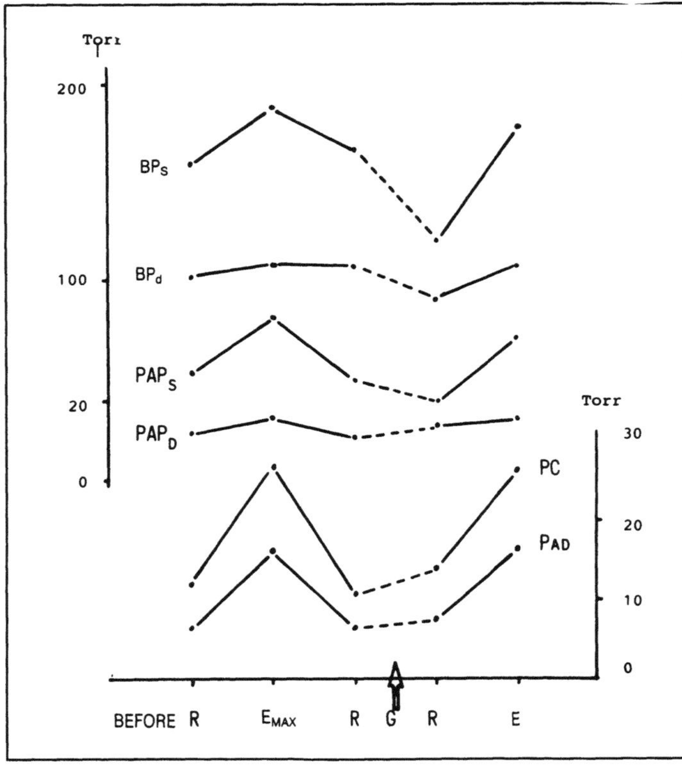

Figure 3. Systemic (BP) and pulmonary (PAP) pressures (syst. and diast.), pulmonary capillary pressure (PC) and right atrial pressure (PAD) at rest and at the patient-specific maximum work load (E_{max}) without medication and after administration of 5 mg gallopamil i.v. (G)

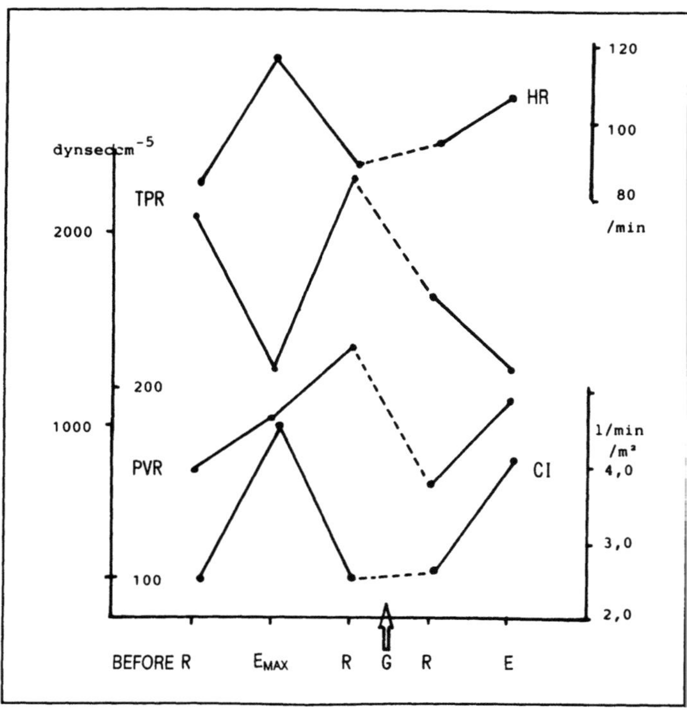

Figure 4. Heart rate (HR), cardiac index (CI), total peripheral resistance and pulmonary vascular resistance after administration of 5 mg gallopamil (as Fig. 3)

Table 4. Means and standard deviations for each parameter

	R	E$_{MAX}$	before G	R 2	E 2	
BP$_s$	161 ± 20	189 ± 38	169 ± 19	123 ± 33	181 ± 37	mmHg
BP$_d$	104 ± 11	109 ± 20	108 ± 15	93 ± 10	108 ± 33	mmHg
PAP$_s$	55 ± 40	82 ± 29	48 ± 34	40 ± 12	72 ± 19	mmHg
PAP$_d$	24 ± 24	32 ± 9	20 ± 18	28 ± 9	32 ± 11	mmHg
PC	12 ± 5	27 ± 17	11 ± 1	14 ± 7	27 ± 18	mmHg
PAD	6.5 ± 4	16.4 ± 9	6.4 ± 5	7.6 ± 7	16.7 ± 12	mmHg
TPR	2100 ± 724	1299 ± 757	2300 ± 1160	1688 ± 727	1345 ± 665	dynseccm⁻⁵
PVR	156 ± 54	184 ± 36	223 ± 96	150 ± 69	194 ± 47	
CI	2.5 ± 0.6	4.6 ± 1.9	2.5 ± 0.8	2.6 ± 0.4	4.1 ± 1.5	l/min/m²
HR	84 ± 15	116 ± 17	88 ± 16	94 ± 20	108 ± 27	/min

marked, short-lived fall during the injection. The pulmonary capillary pressure (PC) and the right atrial pressure (PAD) were the same before and after gallopamil. The resting heart rate rose slightly after gallopamil, but cardiac output barely increased.

Although conducted in an identical manner, the second exercise test produced lower values for heart rate and cardiac output, although the differences were not significant.

There was a significant difference in the TPR values at rest (2100 vs. 1688 dynseccm⁻⁵). Gallopamil produced no significant changes in PVR either at rest (156 vs. 150 dynseccm⁻⁵) or during exercise (184 vs. 194 dynseccm⁻⁵).

Discussion

The haemodynamic findings in the first group correspond to those reported by Sesto et al. (7) in comparable patients. After gallopamil, there was a significant reduction in peripheral resistance throughout the 15-minute measurement period. Thus, an increase in stroke volume associated with a lower afterload might have been responsible for the increase in cardiac output, and the increase in pumping function is a consequence of the reduction in afterload. There were no significant changes in pulmonary vascular resistances and there was no evidence that gallopamil had any pulmonary vascular effects. There was no deterioration of left or right ventricular myocardial properties of the sort reported by Packer (4) for verapamil, since the filling pressures remained the same (the right ventricular filling pressure was determined from the atrial pressure). Our study on patients without severely compromised right ventricular function shows that, in contrast to the systemic vasodilator response, at rest there was no pulmonary vasodilator response immediately after injection of 3 mg gallopamil and there was no evidence of a negative inotropic effect either on the right or on the left ventricle (1, 5, 8).

Administering 5 mg gallopamil to patients with pulmonary hypertension and various degrees of impaired left ventricular function elicited systemic circulatory changes at rest and during exercise similar to those observed in patients without pulmonary hypertension, namely a reduction in afterload. On the other hand, there was no evidence of a clear-cut reduction of right ventricular filling pressures under gallopamil, so pulmonary vascular resistance, which does not change under gallopamil, probably accounts for the bulk of the afterload. The rise of pulmonary capillary pressure and mean right atrial pressure into the pathological range during the control exercise test could be interpreted as an increase in filling pressures associated with deteriorating ventricular function. In fact, the rise in pulmonary capillary pressure was more marked in patients with CHD, whereas right atrial pressure rose equally in all the patients. Repeating the measurements after gallopamil did not reveal any significant changes vs. the control, so there was no evidence that gallopamil impaired left or right ventricular function. The clear-cut rise in pulmonary vascular resistance, which was also apparent from the reduction in the arterial oxygen partial pressure (65 mm Hg vs. 57 mm Hg), in the recovery phase after the control exercise test may be attributed to hypoxic vasoconstriction. Where cardiac output has previously been raised by exercising, it is arguable that, independently of drug-induced relaxation of vessel myocytes, previously unused vascular beds open up, with a consequential decrease in pulmonary resistance. Comparison with the control examination at rest did not reveal any change in oxygen saturation under gallopamil (65 mm Hg vs. 63 mm Hg).

While gallopamil was being injected there was a short lived, fairly marked reduction of pulmonary and systemic pressures. Since this was accompanied by a transient rise in right atrial pressures, it must be assumed that there was transient change in right ventricular function which disappeared shortly afterwards.

Conclusions

The reduction of left ventricular afterload as a result of peripheral vasodilation was significant and led to an initial rise in cardiac output. The peripheral vasodilator response was sustained, whereas cardiac output had fallen back to the baseline 15 minutes after injection.

100

In contrast, there was only a short-lived reduction of pulmonary pressures after injection of gallopamil. There was no evidence of a significant reduction of pulmonary resistance or of a more sustained reduction of right ventricular afterload.

There was no evidence from the haemodynamic data of any significant impairment of left or right ventricular function.

As is recommended for all drugs which may be used as specific medications (6), it would appear rational to prescribe gallopamil for patients with pulmonary hypertension only after testing and checking its effectiveness individually in each patient and at intervals.

References

1. Burrows B, Kettel LJ, Niden AH, Rabinowitz M, Diener CF (1972) Patterns of cardiovascular dysfunction in chronic obstructive lung disease. New Engl J Med Apr: 912–917
2. Henrichs KJ, Erbel R, Meyer J (1985) Wirkung von parenteraler Nifedipingabe bei pulmonaler Hypertonie. In: Meyer, Erbel (eds) Intravenöse und intrakoronare Anwendung von Adalat. Springer, Berlin Heidelberg New York Tokyo, pp. 73–79
3. Landmark K, Refsum AM, Simonsen S, Storstein O (1978) Verapamil and pulmonary hypertension. Acta Med Scand 204: 299–302
4. Packer M, Medina N, Yushak M, Wiener I (1984) Detrimental effects of verapamil in patients with primary pulmonary hypertension. Br Heart J 52: 106–111
5. Packer M, Medina N, Yushak M (1984) Adverse hemodynamic and clinical effects of calcium channel blockade in pulmonary hypertension secondary to obliterative pulmonary vascular disease. JACC 4: 890–901
6. Packer M (1985) Vasodilator therapy for primary pulmonary hypertension. Ann Int Med 103: 258–270
7. Sesto M, Invancic R, Custovic F (1983) Die Wirkung von Gallopamil auf die Hämodynamik bei Patienten mit KHK. In: Kaltenbach M, Hopf R (eds.) Gallopamil. Pharmakologisches und klinisches Wirkungsprofil eines Kalziumantagonisten. Springer, Berlin Heidelberg New York Tokyo, pp. 97–100.
8. Simon R (1984) Kalziumantagonisten: Wirkung auf periphere und koronare Hämodynamik. Z Kardiol 73, Suppl 2:79–88

Author's address:

Dr. med. P. Richter
Sektion Kardiologie,
Angiologie und Pulmologie
Zentrum für Innere Medizin
Klinikum der Universität Ulm
D–7900 Ulm
West Germany

The effect of gallopamil p.o. on global and regional ventricular function in patients with coronary heart disease

G. Großmann, M. Stauch, A. Schmidt, J. Waitzinger[1]

Department of Cardiovascular and Respiratory Medicine and
[1] Department of Nuclear Medicine, Clinical Centre, University of Ulm, FRG

Introduction

On the basis of its pharmacodynamic profile, gallopamil, a methoxy derivative of verapamil, is a specific calcium antagonist (8). Its anti-anginal efficacy has been demonstrated in a number of trials involving patients with coronary heart disease (CHD) in which the assessment criterion was the exercise ECG (6, 12, 16, 21, 23, 35, 37). However, a study using emission tomography has also shown that myocardial microperfusion improves under gallopamil (10).

Radionuclide ventriculography (RNV) is another established, non-invasive technique for obtaining objective evidence of myocardial ischaemia (1, 2, 3, 5, 25). Since, by this technique, it is possible to carry out sequential investigations over hours or days with good reproducibility (11, 13, 32), it would appear to be very suitable for testing the effects of drugs. Here, the measurement parameter is left ventricular function, which can be analysed both globally and regionally (1). The link between this and a disorder of myocardial perfusion is that under ischaemic conditions there are usually regional disorders of wall motion which, given enough circumferential spread, also result in a measurable reduction of global function, evident as a fall in the left ventricular ejection fraction (18).

The study reported here set out to obtain objective evidence, by means of RNV, of the short-term effects of the calcium antagonist gallopamil p.o. on global and regional ventricular function in patients with CHD. This raised the implied question as to how far a measurable response might be attributed to the anti-ischaemic effect of the drug.

Patients and method

The effect of gallopamil was studied in 33 patients (31 men and 2 women) with CHD confirmed by coronary angiography. The average age of the patients was 54 and they were on average 172 cm tall and 77 kg in weight. They were allocated to one of two groups, according to whether or not they showed signs of exercise-induced ischaemia.

The first group, the ischaemia group, comprised 16 patients who showed a significantly positive exercise ECG, a typical history of angina pectoris and a fall in the left ventricular ejection fraction (EF) during exercise of at least 5% in the first RNV carried out under medication-free conditions. Nine of these patients had a history of anterior wall infarction (AWI) and 6 had a history of posterior wall infarction (PWI); one patient had not had an infarction. The second group, the no-ischaemia group, comprised 17 patients. Seven of these patients had no postinfarction angina and had a negative exercise ECG. Five patients had a history of anginal symptoms, but their exercise ECG was normal at the workload achieved during RNV. In 5 other patients the exercise ECG was positive, with exercise-induced horizontal ST-segment depressions of more than 0.1 mV; three of these patients also had a history of angina pectoris. However, under control conditions without any medication the left ventricular EF did not fall by 5% or more in the RNV during exercise in any of the 17 patients in group 2 so, based on three parameters there was no significant exercise-induced ischaemic response under control conditions. Six of the 17 patients had previously had an AWI and 8 had had a PWI; there was no history of infarction in 3 patients. Based on the symptoms and ECGs, at the time of the study there was no evidence of myocardial ischaemia at rest in any of the 33 patients.

In accordance with the trial protocol, an exercise ECG was first recorded with the patients supine on a bicycle ergometer; in a few cases this was done a few days before RNV, but in most cases it was done on the same day, before RNV. RNV was also performed with the patients supine, first with them at rest, and then during exercise on the bicycle ergometer. Usually, the highest work load achieved in the exercise ECG was selected. The erythrocytes were labelled with 20 mCi ^{99m}technetium in vivo with the patients recumbent, about 10 min before the recording at rest. The gamma camera (ON-400) was positioned over the heart in a left anterior oblique (LAO) projection of 30–45° to provide orthograde visualization of the interventricular septum to differentiate between the left and right ventricle. After the initial RNV measurement at rest and during exercise, all the patients took 75 mg gallopamil p.o. Two hours later the investigation was repeated at rest and during exercise at the identical work load. Depending on the counting rate before the second recording at rest, a second, suitable dose of ^{99m}technetium was injected. Other anti-anginal drugs and digitalis preparations had been stopped long enough before all the investigations to ensure an adequate wash-out period.

Regional analysis

In addition to calculating global left ventricular parameters, including the EF, we also carried out a computerized analysis of regional left ventricular motility at rest and during exercise. To do this, the left ventricle was divided into segments numbered from 0 to 8; seven of these segments were analysed. Segments 1 and 8 cannot be analysed in more detail because of masking effects, particularly by the left atrium (Fig. 1); (9). The amplitude of the segmental time-activity curve, after Fourier transformation, was taken as a measure of motility in a defined segment. These "Fourier amplitudes" were stated in standard deviations from the mean values for a group of healthy volunteers. Of the 7 segments stated, we defined for each patient two segments which at the control RNV before gallopamil, showed the greatest exercise-induced fall or the smallest exercise-induced rise in Fourier amplitude. In other words segments were selected, which showed the most marked deterioration or the least improvement in regional motility during exercise. These were designated as the segments with the poorest exertional dynamics (SpE). Conversely, the two segments of each patient which under the conditions stated above showed the greatest exercise-induced improvement or the smallest exercise-induced deterioration in Fourier amplitudes, were designated as having the best exertional dynamics (SbE) (see Fig. 1).

The statistical analysis was carried out with the Wilcoxon test for related samples, and with the Wilcoxon-Mann-Whitney test for unrelated samples. The data were tested for significant differences between more than two samples by means of Friedman's test for related samples, and by one-way non-balanced analysis of variance for unrelated samples.

104

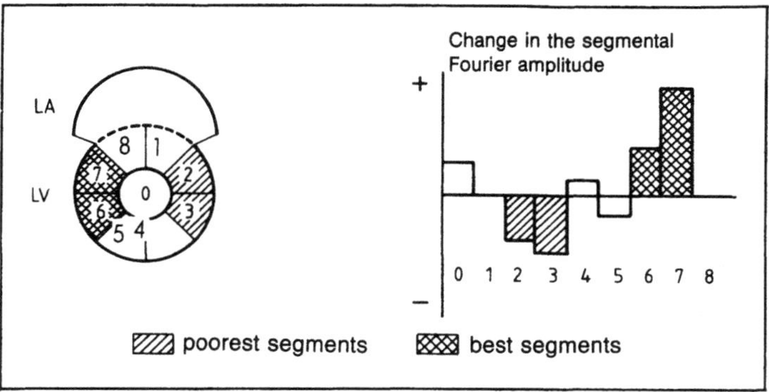

Fig. 1. Diagram to illustrate how the two segments with the best exertional dynamics (SbE) and the two with the poorest exertional dynamics (SpE) are identified. Segments 1 and 8 are not assessed. The exercise-induced change in the segmental Fourier amplitude was used as a measure of the exertional dynamics.
LA = left atrium, LV = left ventricle.

Results

Blood pressure, heart rate

At baseline there were no significant differences between the two groups of patients with regard to blood pressure and heart rate at rest and during exercise. Under medication the resting systolic blood pressure (BP) was significantly lower in the patients without exercise-induced ischaemia than in the ischaemia group ($p < 0.05$). Correspondingly, the systolic blood pressure at rest and during exercise was only reduced significantly ($p < 0.01$) by the medication in the patients who did not suffer from exercise-induced ischaemia. In the ischaemia group the systolic BP readings were only slightly lower under gallopamil. Generally speaking, there was only a trend towards a reduction in the diastolic BP readings under gallopamil. The heart rate at rest was higher after gallopamil; this was only significant ($p < 0.01$) in the patients who did not suffer from exercise-induced ischaemia. On the other hand, the heart rate during exercise tended to be lower in both groups. The results are shown in Table 1.

Cardiac output, stroke volume, enddiastolic volume

In the no-ischaemia group, gallopamil caused a significant ($p < 0.05$) increase in cardiac output at rest, but a slight decrease during exercise. It had a similar effect in the patients with exercise-induced ischaemia, although the difference was not significant even at rest (see Table 1). There were no significant drug-induced changes of stroke volume; however, under gallopamil there was a slight fall in the value during exercise in the group without exercise-induced ischaemia, whereas there was a slight rise after gallopamil in the group with exercise-induced ischaemia. Fig. 2 shows the effect on the end diastolic volume; there were no significant differences.

Table 1. Effect of gallopamil on the heart rate (HR), systolic blood pressure (BP sys), cardiac output (CO) and stroke volume of the left ventricle (SV) at rest and during exercise in the patients without and in those with exercise-induced ischaemia

	Without ischaemia n=17			With ischaemia n=16		
	Control	Gallopamil	p<	Control	Gallopamil	p<
HR rest [beats/min]	64 ± 10	68 ± 10	0.01	69 ± 10	74 ± 14	n.s.
HR exercise	120 ± 16	119 ± 17	n.s.	130 ± 18	124 ± 18	n.s.
BP rest [mmHg] sys	140 ± 14	128 ± 15	0.01	150 ± 26	142 ± 13	n.s.
BP exercise	195 ± 26	188 ± 25	0.01	189 ± 32	188 ± 28	n.s.
CO rest [l/min]	4.98 ± 1.1	5.31 ± 1.0	0.05	6.23 ± 1.3	6.55 ± 1.7	n.s.
CO exercise	10.7 ± 3.1	10.2 ± 2.2	n.s.	10.8 ± 2.9	10.6 ± 3.1	n.s.
SV rest [ml]	78 ± 16	79 ± 15	n.s.	91 ± 18	89 ± 19	n.s.
SV exercise	88 ± 18	86 ± 16	n.s.	83 ± 15	85 ± 17	n.s.

Left ventricular ejection fraction (EF)

In the patients without exercise-induced ischaemia, under gallopamil the EF increased slightly both at rest and during exercise (Fig. 3). The exercise-induced rise in the EF was

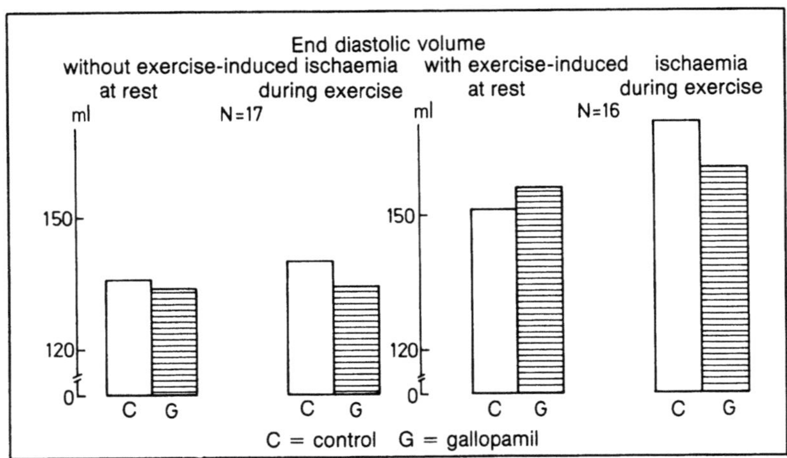

Fig. 2. Effect of gallopamil on the enddiastolic left ventricular volumes at rest and during exercise in patients without (on the left) and those with (on the right) exercise-induced ischaemia.

unchanged under medication (Fig. 4). In the patients who had exercise-induced ischaemia, the EF at rest was significantly lower under gallopamil (p < 0.05); on the other hand, gallopamil increased the ejection fraction during exercise significantly (p < 0.05) (Fig. 5). Although gallopamil did not completely reverse the marked exercise-induced fall of EF in this group, it did bring about a highly significant reduction (p < 0.001) (see Fig. 4). The results are summarized in Table 2.

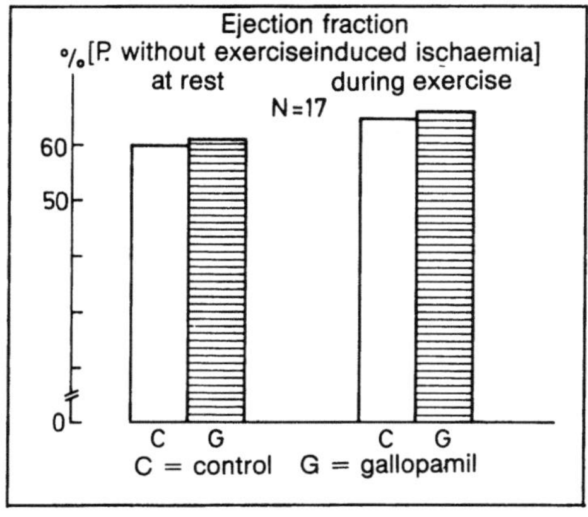

Fig. 3. Effect of gallopamil on the left ventricular ejection fraction at rest and during exercise in patients without exercise-induced ischaemia

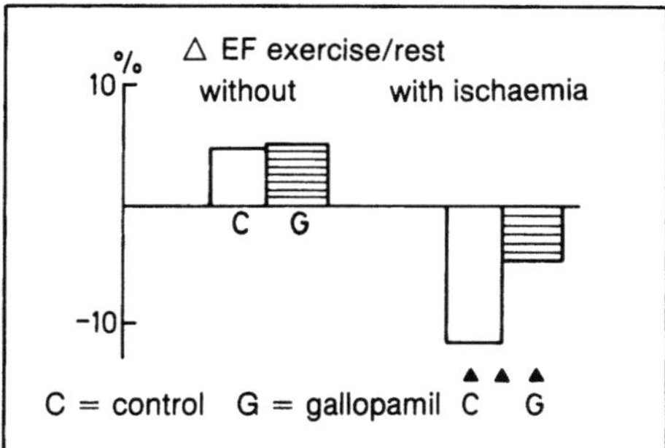

Fig. 4. Exercise-induced change in the left ventricular ejection fraction (EF) in the control test and after gallopamil in patients without and in those with exercise-induced ischaemia.
▲ ▲ ▲ = p < 0.001

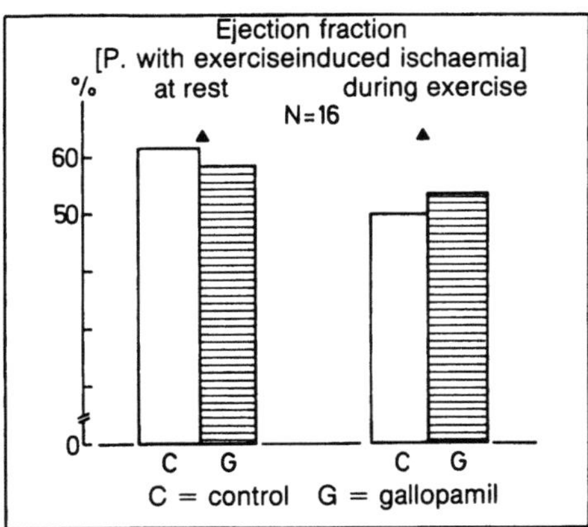

Fig. 5. Effect of gallopamil on the left ventricular ejection fraction at rest and during exercise in patients with exercise-induced ischaemia.
▲ = p < 0.05

Table 2. Effect of gallopamil on the left ventricular ejection fraction (EF) and on segmental contractility, expressed as segmental Fourier amplitude (FA), at rest and during exercise. The table shows the regional data, analysed into segments with the best (SbE) and the poorest (SpE) exertional dynamics in the control test. The table also shows the effect of the drug on the exercise-induced change in the ejection fraction (ΔEF) and in the Fourier amplitudes in the SbE and SpE (ΔFA)

	Patients without ischaemia			Patients with ischaemia		
	Control	Gallopamil	$p<$	Control	Gallopamil	$p<$
EF rest [%]	58.9 ± 10.9	60.0 ± 8.6	n.s.	61.9 ± 11.2	58.9 ± 9.9	0.05
EF exercise	63.9 ± 9.8	65.3 ± 10.1	n.s.	50.4 ± 11.5	54.2 ± 10.2	0.05
ΔEF	$+5.5 \pm 5.5$	$+5.3 \pm 4.9$	n.s.	-11.5 ± 6.1	-4.5 ± 5.6	0.001
FA SbE [SD] rest	-1.2 ± 1.3	-1.0 ± 1.3	n.s.	-1.2 ± 1.2	-1.3 ± 1.2	n.s.
FA SpE	-1.2 ± 1.2	-1.2 ± 1.0	n.s.	-0.7 ± 1.1	-1.0 ± 1.1	0.05
FA SbE [SD] exercise	-0.4 ± 1.3	-0.4 ± 1.1	n.s.	-1.8 ± 1.4	-1.4 ± 1.4	0.01
FA SpE	-1.2 ± 1.1	-0.9 ± 1.3	n.s.	-2.6 ± 1.0	-2.0 ± 1.0	0.001
ΔFA SbE [SD]	$+0.9 \pm 0.6$	$+0.6 \pm 1.2$	n.s.	-0.6 ± 0.5	-0.1 ± 0.8	n.s.
ΔFA SpE	0.0 ± 0.7	40.3 ± 0.9	n.s.	-1.9 ± 0.7	-1.0 ± 0.9	0.01

Regional motility

Gallopamil did not produce any significant changes of regional motility in the patients who did not have exercise-induced ischaemia (Fig. 6). In the ischaemia group gallopamil resulted

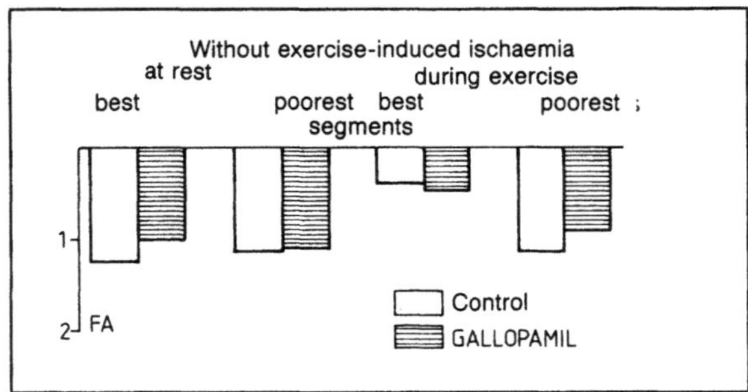

Fig. 6. Effect of gallopamil on contractility in the segments with the best and poorest exertional dynamics. The Fourier amplitude (FA) of the time-activity curve for the particular segment was calculated as a measure of the segmental contractility and expressed as standard deviations from the mean values for a population of healthy volunteers. The figure shows the results obtained from the patients without exercise-induced ischaemia

in a deterioration of regional motility in the segments with the poorest exertional dynamics (SpE) and in the segments with the best exertional dynamics (SbE) under resting conditions. This deterioration was significant in the SpE ($p < 0.05$). On the other hand, during exercise gallopamil brought about a significant or highly significant improvement in regional motility in the SbE ($p < 0.01$) and SpE ($p < 0.001$) (Fig. 7). Gallopamil did not significantly modify the rest-to-exercise change in regional motility in the patients without exercise-induced ischaemia (Fig. 8). On the other hand, in the group of patients with exercise-induced ischaemia the exercise-induced deterioration of regional motility was reduced both in the SbE and SpE. This change was highly significant ($p < 0.001$) for the SpE (see Fig. 8). The data are shown in Table 2.

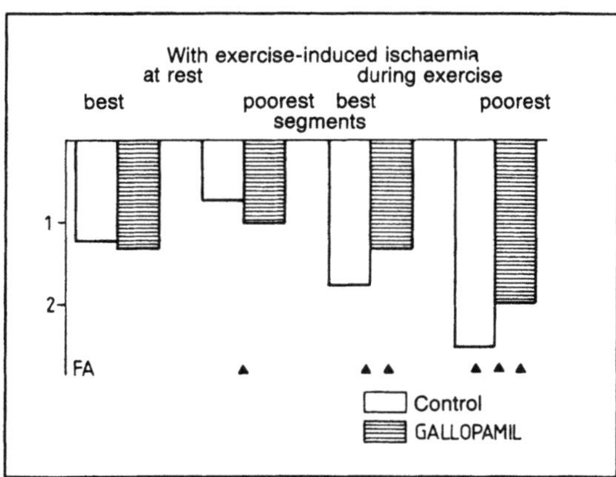

Fig. 7. Effect of gallopamil on segmental contractility in patients with exercise-induced ischaemia. See Fig. 6 for explanation. ▲▲ = $p < 0.01$

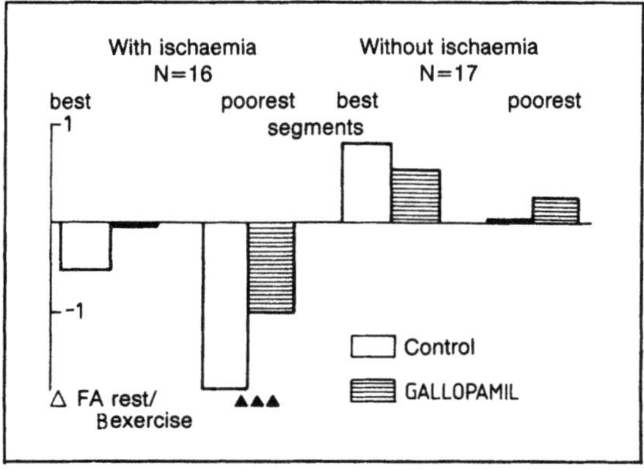

Fig. 8. Exercise-induced changes in regional contractility in the segments with the best and poorest exertional dynamics, before and after gallopamil. The figure shows the data for both groups of patients.

Analysis of the four selected segments for all the patients (n = 33) together revealed a significant correlation between the effect of gallopamil on regional motility during exercise and the segmental response in the baseline control test (p < 0.01). Segments which showed an exercise-induced fall of more than 0.5 standard deviations in Fourier amplitude before gallopamil improved during exercise under the calcium antagonist, whereas segments which showed an exercise-induced rise of more than 0.5 standard deviations in Fourier amplitude in the control test did not benefit from the medication (Fig. 9). The picture was the reverse

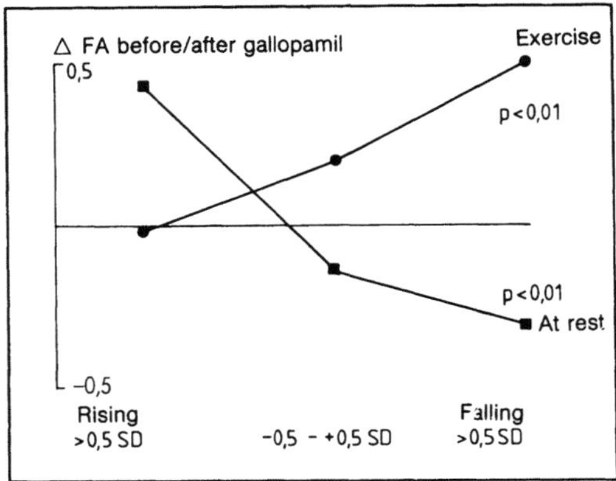

Fig. 9. Effect of gallopamil on segmental contractility at rest and during exercise (ordinate) as a function of the exercise-induced change in the segmental Fourier amplitude before medication (abscissa). The segments of all 33 patients were used for the analysis.

under resting conditions: the segments which showed an exercise-induced fall in Fourier amplitude in the control test deteriorated after medication, whereas the other segments improved. Again, the responses were significantly different (p < 0.01) (see Fig. 9).

Discussion

Although RNV is a very sensitive procedure for detecting coronary insufficiency due to CHD, it is not very specific (3). In order to minimize the chances of obtaining false positive measurements, patients recruited for the ischaemia group had to show a fall of EF during exercise of at least 5% in the control test, and their medical history and ECG during exercise had to show evidence of exercise-induced myocardial ischaemia. In this way we obtained an intrinsically consistent, well-defined group of patients of this type. It is possible that at least 3 volunteers with slight exertional coronary insufficiency were allocated to the no-ischaemia group.

Data on the effect of verapamil on global left ventricular function in patients with CHD were obtained some time ago. Two RNV studies conducted during oral treatment with verapamil at doses of 360 and 480 mg/day respectively revealed an improvement in left ventricular EF during exercise and a reduction in the exercise-induced fall of EF, while the EF at rest remained the same (15, 36). Another research group observed a reduction of exercise-induced regional hypokinesia after oral verapamil, but only when it was combined with propranolol; in these patients there was no significant reduction of the global EF during

110

exercise, even without medication (14). In contrast, Bonow et al. (4) observed a reduction in the left ventricular EF at rest under verapamil, whereas there was no change in the exertional EF. The drug only improved diastolic filling and the authors postulated that this might be one of the principal reasons for the symptomatic improvement in CHD patients under verapamil.

In our RNV study on gallopamil, the patients who did not have exercise-induced ischaemia showed a slight, non-significant rise in the EF at rest and during exercise. Comparison with the data from the patients who did have exercise-induced ischaemia revealed that at rest, as long as there were no signs of myocardial ischaemia, there was a slight, just significant reduction of EF. It is not clear why this should be so, but it is noticeable that in this group the resting blood pressure did not fall significantly as in the other volunteers, so here there was perhaps no compensation for a direct negative inotropic effect of the drug (8), because there was no corresponding reduction of afterload. The EF during exercise, which showed a marked fall before gallopamil, rose significantly under gallopamil. The effect of the drug was even more clear-cut if we take into account the exercise-induced fall of the EF. There was a highly significant reduction in the mean fall of the EF from -11.5% to -4.5%. Assuming that the exercise-induced fall of the EF is a measure of myocardial ischaemia (3), there is evidence that gallopamil has an anti-ischaemic effect which is evident as a measurable improvement in left ventricular function. As with other drugs, left ventricular function did not return to normal, and likewise under gallopamil, on average, the fall of the EF was at the borderline of statistical significance.

Thus, our results correlate well with the results of two of the studies with verapamil quoted above and with those of two studies on gallopamil in which the effect of i.v. administration on left ventricular EF was investigated by ventriculography (29, 30). The effect of the drug was evident principally as a reduction in the exercise-related fall of the EF. The data obtained without provoked ischaemia did not reveal any appreciable changes after medication. Evidently the drug had little direct cardiac depressant effect or, if it did, the effect was offset by indirect peripheral effects such as the reduction of afterload. On the basis of the available data it is impossible to state how far this can be extrapolated to patients with markedly compromised ventricular function, who are a special problem group among CHD patients. Only two of our patients, one with and one without exercise-induced ischaemia, had a resting EF of less than 40%. Neither deteriorated under gallopamil. However, in light of the results obtained by Sesto et al. (30) by ventriculography, and general considerations as to the profile of action of calcium antagonists (7, 19), caution is advised.

The effect of calcium antagonists, notably those of the verapamil type, on global left ventricular function must be seen as a complex function made up of a number of factors: in addition to a coronary dilatation and a direct negative inotropic effect, these drugs affect afterload and there may be associated, compensating beta-adrenoceptor-mediated effects, which may in turn modify the characteristics of myocardial contraction (31). It was therefore logical to build up a more complete profile of the effect of gallopamil on the function of areas of the left ventricle affected to varying extents, or not at all, by the disease, by analysing regional left ventricular motility. Furthermore, changes of regional function are more sensitive indicators of the occurrence of myocardial ischaemia than changes in global function (18). Data from animal experiments and clinical studies show that this improved sensitivity of regional analysis with respect to ischaemia-induced dysfunction can be extrapolated to RNV measurements (9, 27), since it enables regional disorders of wall motion to be detected and quantified with sufficient accuracy (20, 26). Thus, this appears to be a reliable way of detecting the anti-ischaemic effect of various drugs, irrespective of the underlying mechanisms of action (22).

The regional analysis can be quantified by determining the Fourier amplitudes of the regional sectors over the left ventricle individually (2). This enables a "dynamic analysis" to be carried out which was used as part of the evaluation of pentoxifylline, but without eliminating the less reliable sectors 1 and 8 (34). It is reported that this dynamic analysis also used in this study provides a more specific selection of the ischaemic sectors and of the sectors with little or no ischaemia, and this enables the effect of drugs to be analysed more accurately even where there were interactions (33). This is particularly necessary for drugs such as gallopamil which are not like, for example, the preload reducers, which fairly certainly alter ventricular function by exerting a marked peripheral action. This may increase the EF just by changing the geometry, that is by reducing the end diastolic volume, if the stroke volume remains the same.

Gallopamil did not significantly alter regional function in the patients who did not suffer from exercise-induced ischaemia. It was the segments with the poorest exertional dynamics (SpE) which improved slightly during exercise after medication, whereas the segments with the best exertional dynamics (SbE) did not; this was probably because in some of the patients the effects of exercise-induced ischaemia were only regional and these patients were assessed as non-ischaemic on the basis of a global analysis. In the ischaemia group there were highly significant to significant improvements in the SpE and SbE. In this group the SbE also showed a clear-cut ischaemia-induced deterioration of function during exercise resulting from myocardial ischaemia in these segments, and there was an improvement under gallopamil. However, the response to the drug was significantly better in the SpE and there was a discernible correlation between the degree of the regional, ischaemia-induced dysfunction and the improvement in motility under gallopamil. However, under resting conditions there was a deterioration of regional contractility and this deterioration was actually significant in the SpE.

Comparable results were also obtained from the combined assessment of all four segments for the 33 patients. The greater the exercise-induced reduction of segmental contractility in the control test, i.e. the more marked the ischaemia-induced deterioration of function, the more obvious was the effect of gallopamil in improving function. Under resting conditions the response was the reverse. Segments with good exertional dynamics improved after gallopamil, possibly as a result of reduction of afterload, whereas regional contractility was reduced in segments with poor exertional dynamics, most of which were found in patients of the exercise-induced ischaemia group. We can only speculate as to the reasons for this, and we have already touched on this topic in the discussion about the global EF. It may be because the drug had an accentuated negative inotropic effect on the segments with poor exertional dynamics, which was not offset by a reduction of afterload (in the patients with exercise-induced ischaemia) or because it caused an unfavorable redistribution of regional perfusion in these segments. It has been shown in animals that nifedipine causes a regional redistribution of perfusion in ischaemic areas of the myocardium without compromising regional function; this effect was not observed with verapamil (38). It is also conceivable that it was the first exercise test which caused clear-cut ischaemia in these particular segments. The results might then be explained by a delay in the recovery of myocardial function in areas which had previously been markedly ischaemic (28), although there were 2 hours between the measurements.

We may conclude that the improvement in global left ventricular function during exercise under gallopamil is due principally to an improvement in the function of ischaemic areas of the myocardium, whereas there was little or no improvement in the other areas. The positive correlation between the degree of ischaemia-induced dysfunction and the improvement under gallopamil demonstrated not only by comparing the groups of patients, but also independently of this, by studying areas of the myocardium with different exertional dynamics is unequivocal evidence of the anti-ischaemic effect of this drug. Regional analysis provided clearer evidence of the drug-induced changes, that is to say the level of statistical significance was higher, because the areas in which there were no signs of ischaemia, did not dilute the effects on the ischaemia segments. A deterioration in left ventricular EF under gallopamil, which was only observed at rest in the group with exercise-induced ischaemia, was due to a deterioration of regional contractility in the segments which previously had shown the most pronounced exercise-induced ischaemia. It is not clear to what extent this can actually be regarded as an effect of the drug.

From the data available at present it is easier to rule out rather than confirm a particular mechanism as being responsible for the anti-ischaemic effect of gallopamil. Gallopamil probably does not emulate the nitrates in reducing preload, since the end diastolic volume, which can be measured accurately enough by radionuclide ventriculography (24), did not change significantly under gallopamil in either of the groups. In the ischaemia group, which benefited most from the medication, there was very little effect on the heart rate and blood pressure or on the stroke volume of the left ventricle.

A plausible conclusion to be drawn from the studies is that the anti-ischaemic effect, which improves cardiac function during exercise, is due to the specific calcium-antagonising effect on the myocardial cells; this might also explain why the reverse effect is seen under resting conditions. However, the reduction of afterload and the coronary dilatation (which was not measured directly here) (17, 29) probably contribute to the overall effect (23).

Summary

Radionuclide ventriculography (RNV) is a non-invasive technique which enables the global and regional function of the left ventricle to be determined repeatedly, at rest and during exercise. The technique is suitable for measuring the effect of anti-anginal drugs on left ventricular function. This technique was used to investigate the effect of gallopamil (GA), a calcium antagonist of the verapamil type, on the global ejection fraction (EF) and the regional Fourier amplitudes in 33 patients with CHD confirmed by angiography. Sixteen patients had exercise-induced ischaemia (EI), 17 patients did not.

In terms of global function, there were no significant changes in the EF or the Fourier amplitudes in the patients without EI. In the patients with EI, there was a slight reduction of EF at rest from 61.9 ± 11.2 to $58.7 \pm 9.9\%$, $p < 0.05$. During exercise the EF rose from 50.4 ± 11.5 to 54.2 ± 10.2 ($p < 0.05$). The difference between the resting and exercise values is considered to be a measure of ischaemia. Gallopamil reduced this difference from -11.5 ± 6.1 to $-4.5 \pm 5.6\%$; this reduction was highly significant ($p < 0.001$). In each patient, the two sectors with no, or with the least marked signs of ischaemia, and the two sectors with the most marked signs of ischaemia, based on the difference between the contractility at rest and during exercise without GA were selected for the regional analysis. A reduction of function was present at rest under GA in the sectors with the poorest exertional function in patients with EI. On the other hand, these sectors showed the most marked improvement during exercise. No significant changes in regional contractility could be observed in patients without EI.

Thus, during exercise, GA improved function in zones with exercise-induced ischaemia and the potential negative inotropic effect of the calcium antagonist was only evident at rest. It is not possible to state for certain whether the improvement in function was due primarily to the myocardial or vascular component of action of GA. The slight negative inotropic effect at rest is evidence that the myocardial component makes an important contribution to the beneficial overall effect. However, in patients who did not suffer from exercise-induced ischaemia there was neither a negative nor a positive inotropic effect.

References

1. Adam WE, Stauch M (1985) Radionuclide Methods. In: Abshagen U (ed) Clinical Pharmacology of Antianginal Drugs. Springer, Berlin Heidelberg New York Tokyo, pp. 213–237
2. Adam WE, Tarkowska F, Bitter F, Stauch M, Geffers H (1979) Equilibrium (gated) radionuclide ventriculography. Cardiovasc Radiol 2: 161–173
3. Austin EH, Cobb FR, Coleman RE, Jones RH (1982) Prospective Evaluation of Radionuclide Angiocardiography for the Diagnosis of Coronary Artery Disease. Am J Cardiol 50:1212–1216
4. Bonow RO, Leon MB, Rosing DR, Kent KM, Lipson LC, Bacharach SL, Green MV, Epstein SE (1981) Effects of Verapamil and Propranolol on Left Ventricular Systolic Function and Diastolic Filling in Patients with Coronary Artery Disease: Radionuclide Angiographic Studies at Rest and During Exercise. Circulation 65:1337–1350
5. Borer JS, Kent KM, Bacharach SL, Green MV, Rosing DR, Seides SF, Epstein SE, Johnston GS (1979) Sensitivity. Specificity and Predictive Accuracy of Radionuclide Cineangiography During Exercise in Patients with Coronary Artery Disease. Circulation 60:572–580
6. Bouzo H (1983) Gallopamil und Propranolol bei stabiler belastungsinduzierter Angina pectoris. Therapiewoche 33:6465–6468
7. Colucci WS, Fifer MA, Lorell BH, Wynne J (1985) Calcium Channel Blockers in Congestive Heart Failure: Theoretic Considerations and Clinical Experience. Am J Med 78, Suppl 2B:9–17
8. Fleckenstein A, Fleckenstein B, Späh F, Byon YK (1983) Gallopamil (D600) – ein Kalziumantagonist von hoher Wirkungsstärke und Spezifität. Effekt auf Myocard und Schrittmacher. In: Kaltenbach M, Hopf R (eds) Gallopamil. Springer, Berlin Heidelberg New York Tokyo, pp. 1–34
9. Gibbons RJ, Morris KG, Lee K, Coleman RE, Cobb FR (1984) Assessment of Regional Left Ventricular Function Using Gated Radionuclide Angiography. Am J Cardiol 54:294–300
10. Gutmann M, Eichstätt H (1985) Tomoszintigraphische Untersuchungen zur myokardialen Mikroperfusion unter dem Kalziumantagonisten Gallopamil. Herz/Kreislauf 7:363–368
11. Hecht HS, Josephson MA, Hopkins JM, Singh BN (1982) Reproducibility of equilibrium radionuclide ventriculography in patients with coronary artery disease: Response of left ventricular ejection fraction and regional wall motion to supine bicycle exercise. Am Heart J 104:567–574
12. Hopf R, Drews H, Kaltenbach M (1984) Die antianginöse Wirkung von Gallopamil im Vergleich mit einem anderen Calciumantagonisten und Placebo. Z Kardiol 73:578–585
13. Jeremy R, Tokuyasu Y, Coong CYP, Bautovich G, Hutton BF, Shen W-F, Kelly DT, Harris PJ (1985) The reproducibility of nongeometric analysis of cardiac output and left ventricular volume by radionuclide angiography. Am Heart J 110:1020–1026
14. Johnston DL, Gebhardt VA, Donald A, Kostuk WJ (1983) Comparative effects of propranolol and verapamil alone and in combination on left ventricular function and volumes in patients with chronic exertional angina: a double-blind, placebo-controlled, randomized, crossover study with radionuclide ventriculography. Circulation 68:1280–1289
15. Hecht HS, Hopkins JM, Singh BN (1981) Oral Verapamil vs Propranolol in Coronary Artery Disease: Evaluation of Left Ventricular Function by Exercise Radionuclides Ventriculography. Am J Cardiol 47:463
16. Khurmi NS, O'Hara MJ, Bowles MJ, Subramanian VB, Raftery EB (1984) Randomized Double-Blind Comparison of Gallopamil and Propranolol in Stable Angina Pectoris. Am J Cardiol 53:684–688

17. Kovach AGB, Ligeti L, Bakos M, Rubanyi G, Koller A (1983) In-vitro- und In-vivo-Untersuchungen über die Wirkung von Gallopamil and Koronargefäßen. In: Kaltenbach M, Hopf R (eds.) Gallopamil. Springer, Berlin Heidelberg New York, pp. 61–68
18. Krayenbühl HP, Hess OM, Hirzel HO, Carrol JD (1984) Hämodynamik unter Ischämie. Systolische Phase. Z Kardiol 73, Suppl 2:119–126
19. Low RI, Takeda P, Mason DT, DeMaria AN (1982) The Effects of Channel Blocking Agents on Cardiovascular Function. Am J Cardiol 49:547–553
20. Maddox DE, Wynne J, Uren R, Parker JA, Idoine J, Siegel LC, Neill JM, Cohn PF, Holman BL (1979) Regional Ejection Fraction: A Quantitative Radionuclide Index of Regional Left Ventricular Performance. Circulation 59:1001–1009
21. Mitrovic V, Niemelä L, Neuss H, Schlepper M (1982) Zur antianginösen Wirkung des Kalziumantagonisten Gallopamil. Herz/Kreislauf 11:611–616
22. Pfisterer M, Glaus L, Burkart F (1983) Comparative Effects of Nitroglycerin, Nifedipine and Metoprolol on Regional Left Ventricular Function in Patients with One-vessel Coronary Disease. Circulation 67:192–301
23. Rettig G, Sen S (1983) Akut- und Langzeiteffekte von Gallopamil bei Patienten mit stabiler Angina pectoris. In: Kaltenbach M, Hopf R (eds.): Gallopamil. Springer, Berlin Heidelberg New York Tokyo, pp. 141–147
24. Richter P, Sigel H, Nechwatal W, Adam WE, Stauch M (1986) Vergleich der enddiastolischen Volumina des linken Ventrikels, bestimmt mittels der Radionuklidventrikulographie, der Kontrastmittelventrikulographie und einer geometrieunabhängigen Methode. Z Kardiol 75:107–112
25. Salel AF, Berman DS, DeNardo GL, Mason DT (1976) Radionuclide Assessment of Nitroglycerin Influence on Abnormal Left Ventricular Segmental Contraction in Patients with Coronary Heart Disease. Circulation 53:975–982
26. Sauer E, Sebening H, Hör G, Lutilsky L, Dressler J, Bofilias I, Weber N, Pabst HW, Blömer H (1978) Nichtinvasive Erfassung der Dynamik des linken Ventrikels. Dtsch Med Wochenschr 103:1199–1206
27. Schneider RM, Roberts KB, Morris KG, Stanfield JA, Cobb FR (1984) Relation Between Radionuclide Angiographic Regional Ejection Fraction and Left Ventricular Regional Ischemia in Awake Dogs. Am J Cardiol 53:294–301
28. Schneider RM, Weintraub WS, Klein LW, Seelaus PA, Agarwal JB, Helfant RH (1986) Rate of Left Ventricular Functional Recovery by Radionuclide Angiography after Exercise in Coronary Artery Disease. Am J Cardiol 57:927–932
29. Sebening H, Sauer E (1983) Beeinflussung der Koronararterien und Hämodynamik durch Gallopamil. In: Kaltenbach M, Hopf R (eds) Gallopamil. Springer, Berlin Heidelberg New York Tokyo, pp. 117–118
30. Sesto M, Ivanic R, Custovic F (1983) Die Wirkung von Gallopamil auf die Hämodynamik bei Patienten mit KHK. In: Kaltenbach M, Hopf R (eds) Gallopamil. Springer, Berlin Heidelberg New York Tokyo, pp. 97–100
31. Simon R (1984) Kalziumantagonisten. Wirkung auf periphere und koronare Hämodynamik. Z Kardiol 73, Suppl. 2:79–88
32. Slutsky R, Karliner J, Battler A (1979) Reproducibility of ejection fraction and ventricular volume by gated radionuclide angiography after myocardial infarction. Radiology 132:155
33. Stauch M, Haerer W, Rogg-Dussler G, Sigel H, Adam WE (1985) Effects of molsidomine on regional contraction and global function of the left ventricle. Am Heart J 109: 653–658
34. Stauch M, Richter P, Roth J, Herrmann T, Schmutz C, Henze E, Adam WE (1986) Cardiac effects of pentoxylline in patients with coronary heart disease at rest and during exercise. Herz/Kreislauf 10:489–495
35. Subramanian VB (1985) Vergleichende Untersuchung von Gallopamil und 6 weiteren Kalziumantagonisten mit Placebo und Propranolol bei Patienten mit chronisch stabiler Angina pectoris. Herz/Kreislauf 1:9–20
36. Tan ATH, Sadick N, Kelly DT, Harris PJ, Freedman SB, Bautovich G (1982) Verapamil in Stable Effort Angina: Effects on Left Ventricular Function Evaluated With Exercise Radionuclide Ventriculography. Am J Cardiol 49:425–430
37. Theisen F, Jahrmärker H (1983) Wirkung von Gallopamil (D600) auf das Belastungs-EKG bei koronarer Herzerkrankung. In: Kaltenbach M, Hopf R (eds) Gallopamil. Springer, Berlin Heidelberg New York Tokyo, pp. 120–126

38. Weintraub WS, Hattori S, Agrarwal JB, Bodenheimer MM, Banka VS, Helfant RH (1983) Contrasting effects of nifedipine and verapamil on myocardium and vascular smooth muscle at two levels of coronary occlusion in the dog. Am Heart J 106:1347–1352

Author's address:

Dr. med. G. Großmann
Sektion Kardiologie, Angiologie und Pulmonologie
Zentrum für Innere Medizin
Steinhövelstr. 9
D–7900 Ulm
FRG

Discussion

BENDER

You found that myocardial function deteriorated at rest and improved during exercise in the same group of patients. How do you explain that?

STAUCH

That is the question which causes us concern. Is this a genuine effect or an incidental finding? Assuming that it is genuine, it could be that the negative inotropic effect of gallopamil, which was mentioned a number of times here, is only evident at rest, whereas during exercise it is masked by the improvement in oxygen supply (I hardly dare use the word supply here; at any rate by an improvement in the ischaemic picture) so that any negative inotropic effect is completely masked or does not show up at all. On the other hand, under resting conditions, a negative inotropic effect becomes apparent in this damaged area, that is to say in those areas in which there is little increase in contractility in response to exercise. However, this is probably of no clinical relevance. What interested us was that an effect of this sort can be detected at all, even if only under resting conditions and in certain segments.

MEINERTZ

You have shown an LAO projection and the original ventriculographs. If your patients have anterior ischaemia, do you still use the 30°C LAO projection for determining regional wall motion?

STAUCH

We always have to use the LAO projection, otherwise we have the right ventricle, or more precisely the blood pool in the right ventricle, projecting into the foreground. This is of course the disadvantage of the method. We have a sum of regional functions which are more representative of the anterior wall region, firstly because they are closer to the camera and secondly because the amplitude of anterior wall motion is usually greater. The radioactive particles in the posterior wall are further away, so the method is not all that suitable purely for detecting coronary disease in the posterior wall region; it is actually a function-based technique which can be used to assess the global and possibly regional function. There is certainly no regional resolution as is achieved in an angiogram, because there is always superimposition of the anterior and posterior wall. At best it is genuinely regional in the lateral wall area, although the anterior and posterior wall of the lateral area have to be viewed together.

Treatment of chronic stable angina pectoris with gallopamil

D. Scrutinio, S. Iliceto*, R. Lagioia, D. Accettura, N. Preziusi, F. Mastropasqua, A. Chiddo*, P. Rizzon*

"Clinica del Lavoro" Foundation, Hospital and Research Institute, Medical Rehabilitation Centre, Department of Cardiology, Cassano Murge, Bari, Italy
* Department of Cardiology, University of Bari, Italy

Introduction

In the last few years the number of calcium antagonists available for treatment has increased rapidly since these drugs were shown to be effective in the treatment of stable and unstable angina pectoris. Gallopamil is a new calcium antagonist which appears to be three to four times more potent in animals than verapamil (3, 4). About 90% of the dose of gallopamil is absorbed and its bioavailability is about 25% (21). Studies in patients give a mean half-life of 2.8 to 4.8 hours (21), with the concentrations of the unchanged substance peaking one to 2 hours after administration (20). After intravenous administration, this drug dilates the arteries and veins (5, 14), reduces peripheral arterial resistance and the work of the heart (−13%), and myocardial oxygen uptake (−10%), (12). It also dilates the epicardial coronary vessels and prevents vasospasm (10, 11): Gallopamil reduces sino-atrial node excitability and slows conduction in the AV node (4, 6).
The study reported here assessed the efficacy of gallopamil in the treatment of chronic, stable, exercise-induced angina.

Patients and methods

Eighteen male inpatients between 45 and 70 years of age (mean age 59) were recruited for the study after they had given their informed consent. All the patients had a history of chronic, stable, exercise-induced angina and complied with the criteria for inclusion. The criteria for inclusion and exclusion are shown in Table 1. Ten patients had had a myocardial infarction. Coronary angiography performed on 13 patients revealed one-vessel disease (stenosis ≥75%) in 3 patients, two-vessel disease in 7 patients and three-vessel disease in 3 patients.
Starting 10 days before the study the previous anti-anginal medications were gradually discontinued, but the patients were still permitted to take nitroglycerin sublingually p.r.n.
The examinations before the study were the medical history, physical examination, ECG at rest, 24-hour ECG monitoring and two baseline exercise tests on a bicycle ergometer, performed on two days, to assess the reproducibility of the exercise data. Patients who showed a variability exceeding one minute in the period of exercising in the two baseline exercise tests and 3000 for the maximum rate-pressure product, or a difference in the two measurements for each parameter of more than 20% were not accepted for the study (18, 19).

Table 1. Criteria for inclusion and exclusion

Criteria for inclusion
– chronic exercise-induced angina pectoris
– pain alleviated by resting and/or sublingual nitrates
– occurrence of classic anginal pain and a horizontal or descending ST-segment depression of at least 1 mm during exercise
– coronary heart disease confirmed on the basis of previous myocardial infarction or by coronary angiography
Criteria for exclusion
– patient reluctant to give consent to take part
– patient unable to perform exercise test on bicycle
– acute myocardial infarction within the last 3 months
– severe ventricular arrhythmias or spontaneous silent myocardial ischaemia (silent ischaemic episodes) evident in the 24-hour ECG
– bundle-branch block or repolarization disorders which interfere with the interpretation of the exercise ECG
– heart failure
– resting blood pressure over 160/100 mmHg
– valvular heart disease
– treatment with digitalis or anti-arrhythmic drugs indicated
– intermittent claudication
– bronchospastic or obstructive lung disease

Study protocol

SHORT-TERM STUDY. The short-term study was carried out double-blind with 12 patients on four consecutive days. On each day, before administration of the trial medication, each patient performed an exercise test. After administration of the trial medication, which was either one placebo tablet, 80 mg propranolol, 50 mg gallopamil or 100 mg gallopamil, the exercise test was repeated after 2 hours (phase 1) or after 7 hours (phase 2). The trial treatments were allocated in a randomized sequence.

LONG-TERM STUDY. Six patients took part in the long-term study, which was divided into three consecutive treatment phases each of 7 days. The treatment consisted either of placebo, 50 mg gallopamil t.i.d. or 75 mg gallopamil t.i.d. given in random sequence. The exercise test was performed on the 7th day of each treatment phase, about 2 hours after the last dose of the medication. Two-dimensional echocardiography and 24-hour ECG monitoring were performed on the 6th day.

The trial physicians did not know which medication had been allocated to which patient until the end of the study.

Protocol for the exercise tests

The exercise tests were carried out with the patients seated on a bicycle ergometer (Elema-Shonander model 380B) with a computerized Avionics system. The patients pedalled at a constant rate of 50 rpm. After a two-minute warm-up period, the test began at a work load of 30 watts. The work load was increased in 10-watt increments each minute until anginal symptoms occurred, or the ST segment was depressed by > 4 mm, or the patient was exhausted. The exercise test did not have to be stopped prematurely in any of the patients because of arrhythmia. During the exercise test and for 10 minutes thereafter, the ECG,

heart rate and ST-segment depression were monitored continuously and the blood pressure
was taken every minute in mm Hg with a sphygmomanometer. The following parameters
were analysed: period of exercising, −1 mm time (= time taken for the ST segment to fall
1 mm below the resting value), ST-segment depression (measured in the CM5 bipolar lead)
at the highest average level of loading and at the maximum work load, heart rate (HR) and
the rate-pressure product (RPP) at rest, at the highest average work load, at the time of
−1 mm ST-segment depression and at the maximum work load.

Analysis of the data

The statistical significance of the results was determined by two-way variance analysis with
treatments and measurement times as factors. Differences between the groups were
evaluated by the Newman-Keuls test (24). A p value ≤0.05 was considered significant. The
values are expressed as means ± standard deviation (SD).
Patients whose exercise period was at least 20% longer than under placebo were regarded as
responders.

Results

Baseline exercise tests

All the baseline exercise tests had to be stopped because of anginal symptoms. There were
no significant differences in the period of exercising or RPP at maximum work load in the 18
patients selected for the study.

Short-term study

Exercise tests before treatment

All the exercise tests carried out before the start of treatment had to be stopped because of
anginal symptoms.
There was no evidence of any significant increase in stamina from the 1st to the 4th day; the
average periods of exercising before treatment were 381 ± 100 s (1st day), 395 ± 137 s
(2nd day), 415 ± 125 s (3rd day) and 418 ± 141 s (4th day). These times are not
significantly different from those obtained in the baseline exercise tests.

Placebo

All the patients experienced exercise-induced anginal symptoms; the period of exercising
ranged from 270 to 600 s in phase 1 and from 240 to 600 s in phase 2, with a mean ± SD of
387 ± 123 s and 400 ± 120 s, respectively. Comparison with the exercise tests before the
start of treatment and the two baseline exercise tests did not reveal any significant change in
the period of exercising under placebo. The −1 mm time varied between 150 and 410 s in
phase 1 and between 150 and 390 s in phase 2, with a mean ± SD of 285 ± 106 s and
269 ± 85 s respectively.
The placebo data are shown in Table 2; there were no significant differences between the
results from phase 1 and those from phase 2.

Table 2. Data obtained from exercise tests after placebo

Placebo	2 hours	7 hours
Period of exercising	387 ± 123	400 ± 120
−1 mm time	285 ± 106	269 ± 85
HR at rest	69 ± 9	74 ± 11
HR at highest average level of loading	114 ± 19	114 ± 20
HR at maximum work load	127 ± 17	122 ± 20
RPP at rest	7.4 ± 1.4	8 ± 1.3
RPP at highest average level of loading	18.1 ± 4	18.5 ± 5
RPP at time of −1 mm ST depression	16.1 ± 2.3	16 ± 2.7
RPP at maximum work load	20.3 ± 4	20.9 ± 6
ST depression at highest average level of loading	1.6 ± 0.7	1.8 ± 1
ST depression at maximum work load	2.2 ± 0.8	2.4 ± 0.7

Propranolol

Compared with placebo, propranolol increased the mean period of exercising to 474 ± 98 s (+22%; ns) and 470 ± 110 s (+17%; ns) 2 and 7 hours, respectively, after medication. Six patients responded to the treatment in phase 1 and 5 responded in phase 2, with increases in the period of exercising ranging from 22% to 78% in phase 1 and from 25% to 100% in phase 2. In 2 patients there was a 60 s reduction. Six patients in phase 1 and 5 patients in phase 2 had no anginal symptoms.
The mean −1 mm time increased to 388 ± 84 s (+36%; p< 0.05) and to 357 ± 98 s (+32%; ns) 2 and 7 hours, respectively, after administration of the trial drug.
The data for propranolol are shown in Table 3; there were no differences between the results from phase 1 and those from phase 2.

50 mg gallopamil

Compared with placebo, 50 mg gallopamil increased the mean period of exercising to 525 ± 150 s (+36%; p < 0.05) and to 467 ± 128 s (+17%; ns) 2 and 7 hours, respectively, after medication (2h versus 7h; ns). Eight patients responded to the treatment in phase 1 and 6 responded in phase 2, with increases in the period of exercising ranging from 21% to 100% in phase 1 and from 21% to 28% in phase 2. In 2 patients there was a 60 s reduction in phase 2. Four patients in phase 1 and 4 in phase 2 were symptom-free. The mean −1 mm time increased to 422 ± 120 s (+48%; p < 0.05) and 304 ± 69 s (+13%; ns) 2 and 7 hours, respectively, after administration of the trial drug. The data for the 50 mg dose of gallopamil are shown in Table 3.

100 mg gallopamil

Compared with placebo, 100 mg gallopamil increased the mean period of exercising to 550 ± 164 s (+42%; p < 0.05) and to 490 ± 151 s (+22%; ns) 2 hours and 7 hours, respectively, after medication (2h versus 7h; ns). Nine patients responded to the treatment in phase 1 and 7 responded in phase 2, with increases in the period of exercising ranging from 22% to 122% in phase 1 and from 20% to 100% in phase 2. In 2 patients there was a 60 s reduction in phase 2. Six patients in phase 1 and 6 in phase 2 were symptom-free. The

Table 3. Data obtained from exercise tests after propranolol or gallopamil

Propranolol	2 hours		7 hours	
Period of exercising	474 ± 98	(+22%)	470 ± 120	(+17%)
– 1 mm time	* 388 ± 84	(+36%)	357 ± 98	(+32%)
HR at rest	* 59 ± 9	(−14%)	* 60 ± 7	(−19%)
HR at highest average level of loading	97 ± 17	(−15%)	94 ± 16	(−17%)
HR at maximum work load	108 ± 19	(−11%)	104 ± 17	(−15%)
RPP at rest	* 6.3 ± 17	(−15%)	6.3 ± 1	(−20%)
RPP at highest average level of loading	14.9 ± 3.7	(−20%)	13.9 ± 3.5	(−24%)
RPP at time of –1 mm ST depression	15.9 ± 3.4	(− 1%)	14.8 ± 2.5	(− 7%)
RPP at maximum work load	18.5 ± 4.5	(− 9%)	17.4 ± 4.4	(−17%)
ST depression at highest average level of loading	* 0.6 ± 1	(−62%)	0.8 ± 1	(−55%)
ST depression at maximum work load	1.6 ± 1	(−27%)	1.7 ± 1	(−29%)

Gallopamil 50 mg	2 hours		7 hours	
Period of exercising	* 525 ± 150	(+36%)	467 = 128	(+17%)
– 1 mm time	* 422 ± 120	(+48%) p<0.05	304 = 69	(+13%)
HR at rest	68 ± 11	(− 1%)	71 = 11	(− 4%)
HR at highest average level of loading	106 ± 17	(− 7%)	111 = 23	(− 2%)
HR at maximum work load	128 ± 23	(− 6%)	130 = 22	(+ 6%)
RPP at rest	7.3 ± 1.6	(− 1%)	7.7 ± 1.8	(− 4%)
RPP at highest average level of loading	15.8 ± 5	(−12%)	17.3 ± 6.2	(− 6%)
RPP at time of –1 mm ST depression	18.9 ± 5.7	(+17%)	16.3 ± 4	(+ 2%)
RPP at maximum work load	22.6 ± 7.1	(+11%)	22.6 = 6.5	(+ 8%)
ST depression at highest average level of loading	* 0.6 ± 0.7	(−62%) p<0.05	1.3 = 0.6	(−28%)
ST depression at maximum work load	1.9 ± 1	(−14%)	2.6 = 0.9	(+8%)

Gallopamil 100 mg	2 hours		7 hours	
Period of exercising	550 ± 16	(+42%)	490 ± 151	(+22%)
– 1 mm time	*** 490 ± 159	(+71%) p<0.01	362 ± 111	(+34%)
HR at rest	69 ± 12	(+10%)	69 ± 11	(− 6%)
HR at highest average level of loading	102 ± 16	(−10%)	104 ± 18	(− 9%)
HR at maximum work load	125 ± 21	(+ 6%)	124 ± 25	(+ 2%)
RPP at rest	7.2 ± 1.6	(− 1%)	7.4 = 1.5	(− 7%)
RPP at highest average level of loading	15.3 ± 4.4	(−15%)	16.1 ± 5.2	(−13%)
RPP at time of –1 mm ST depression	** 21.2 ± 7.1	(+32%)	16.8 ± 4	(+ 5%)
RPP at maximum work load	23.1 ± 7.4	(+13%)	22.6 ± 8	(+ 8%)
ST depression at highest average level of loading	* 0.6 ± 0.8	(−62%) p<0.05	1.1 ± 0.9	(−39%)
ST depression at maximum work load	1.4 ± 1	(−36%)	2.2 ± 1.1	(− 8%)

* p<0.05   ** p<0.02   *** p<0.01

RPP = rate-pressure product; (%) = percentage changes versus placebo mean -1 mm time increased to 490 $\pm$ 150 s ($+71\%$; p $<$ 0.01) and to 362 $\pm$ 111 s ($+34\%$; ns) 2 hours and 7 hours, respectively, after administration of the trial drug. The data for the 100 mg dose of gallopamil are shown in Table 3.

Comparison of the trial medications with each other showed no significant differences in any of the time intervals. However, in 10 patients, 2 hours after medication the increase in the period of exercising was much longer after gallopamil than after propranolol (in 7 patients this difference was evident after the 50 mg and after the 100 mg dose of gallopamil; in 3 patients it was only evident after the 100 mg dose); 2 patients were able to exercise longer after propranolol. Seven hours after administration the period of exercising of 4 patients was longer under gallopamil than under propranolol (in 3 patients this difference was evident after the 50 mg and after the 100 mg dose of gallopamil and in one patient it was only evident after the 100 mg dose), whereas under propranolol 2 patients were able to exercise for longer than under the 50 mg dose of gallopamil and 5 patients were able to exercise for longer than under the 100 mg dose of gallopamil.

Effect on the heart rate at rest and AV conduction

There were no adverse reactions under placebo or the 50 mg dose of gallopamil. Under propranolol, 4 patients showed pronounced sinus bradycardia, with a heart rate of 47–49 beats/min. After the 100 mg dose of gallopamil there was isorhythmic AV dissociation with heart rates of 63, 59 and 50 beats/min, in 3 patients.

Long-term study (interim results)

Compared with placebo, administration of 50 mg gallopamil t.i.d. increased the mean period of exercising from 430 $\pm$ 158 to 540 $\pm$ 186 s ($+26\%$) and the mean -1 mm time from 315 $\pm$ 140 to 430 $\pm$ 149 s ($+27\%$). Five patients responded to the treatment and 3 of these responders became symptom-free; the increase in the period of exercising varied between 25% and 40%.

75 mg gallopamil t.i.d. increased the period of exercising to 540 $\pm$ 203 s ($+26\%$) and the mean -1 mm time to 456 $\pm$ 198 s ($+45\%$).

Four patients responded to the treatment and 3 of these responders became symptom-free; the increase in the period of exercising ranged from 25% to 66%.

24-hour ECG monitoring revealed intermittent isorhythmic AV dissociation in one patient treated with 225 mg gallopamil daily.

The ejection fraction, measured by two-dimensional echocardiography, was 56 $\pm$ 5% (range: 50%–63%) under placebo, 54 $\pm$ 4% (range: 49%–60%) under 150 mg gallopamil daily and 58 $\pm$ 3% (range: 50%–63%) under 225 mg gallopamil daily.

Discussion

Over the past 20 years, beta-blockers have been widely used for treating angina pectoris. In certain patients these drugs only afforded partial and inadequate control of the anginal symptoms, and they were ineffective in vasospastic angina (7, 15). Potentially, calcium antagonists offer more complete control of the anginal symptoms, with none of the adverse effects of beta-blockers. Consequently, more and more calcium antagonists are becoming available. Our study was to assess the anti-anginal effect of gallopamil, a new calcium antagonist, in patients with chronic, stable, exercise-induced angina.

Short-term study

Propranolol

Propranolol increased the mean period of exercising by 22% and 17% 2 hours and 7 hours, respectively, after administration. Six patients responded to the treatment in phase 1 and 5 patients responded in phase 2. Although the increase in the period of exercising was of the same order of magnitude as reported in previous studies (1, 2, 7, 16), in our study the increases were not statistically significant. The most beneficial effect of propranolol was found in exercise tolerance, with an increase in the -1 mm time of 36% in phase 1 and 32% in phase 2 and a smaller ST-segment depression at the highest average work load (62% and 55%). Although the differences in the increase in -1 mm time and reduction of the ST depression after 2 hours and 7 hours were only moderately pronounced and not clinically significant, the difference versus placebo was statistically significant after 2 hours.
Under propranolol, the mean heart rate and mean rate-pressure product were appreciably lower (15% and 20% reduction, respectively) during the exercise tests. This is evidence of a primary effect of beta-blockers, which is due to a reduction of myocardial oxygen uptake during exercise. On the other hand, the fact that the rate-pressure product was unchanged at the time of the -1 mm ST depression confirms that beta-blockers have no effect on myocardial oxygen supply.

Gallopamil

Several studies have been carried out recently to assess the anti-anginal effect of this new calcium antagonist. They showed that gallopamil (100 mg to 150 mg daily) reduced nitroglycerin consumption and the number of anginal attacks each week. It also significantly improved exercise tolerance and reduced the exercise-induced ST depression by 40% to 50% (8, 13, 22, 23).
A recent, long-term, placebo-controlled study by Khurmi et al. in which 150 mg gallopamil daily was compared with 240 mg propranolol revealed an increase in the mean period of exercising of 87% under the calcium antagonist and of 74% under the beta-blocker, and increases in the mean -1 mm time of 73% and 94%, respectively (9).
In our short-term study, the measurements taken 2 hours after administering 50 mg and 100 mg gallopamil revealed significant increases in the mean period of exercising of 36% and 41%, respectively, and in the mean -1 mm time of 48% and 71%, respectively, whereas the beta-blocker was slightly less effective than the 50 mg dose of gallopamil. At the highest average level of loading, the reduction in the ST depression (62%) was significant and comparable under gallopamil and under propranolol. In comparison with the lower dose of gallopamil and with propranolol, there was a further, but not significant, improvement in exercise tolerance under the 100 mg dose of gallopamil after 2 hours, demonstrated by an increase in the period of exercising and in the -1 mm time.
The increase in the period of exercising we observed under gallopamil and propranolol was less than that observed by Khurmi (9). However, it must be borne in mind that the type of

study chosen, long-term or short-term, may affect the exercise-test parameters. Also, the patients in the Khurmi study exercised on a treadmill; our patients were on a bicycle ergometer. The differences may also have been due to the use of a different patient population and/or the smaller number of patients in our study. As with 50 mg gallopamil, the improvement under the 100 mg dose of gallopamil was more pronounced after 2 hours than after 7 hours, although the values were only significant for the -1 mm time and the ST-segment depression at the highest average level of loading. Seven hours after administration, the beneficial effect of 100 mg gallopamil was much the same as that of propranolol, but was still more marked than that of 50 mg gallopamil. The reduction in the rate-pressure product at the highest average level of loading is evidence of a reduction in myocardial oxygen demand after gallopamil and after propranolol (gallopamil < propranolol). On the other hand, the increase in the rate-pressure product at the highest work load and more particularly at the time of the -1 mm ST depression 2 hours after administration of gallopamil is evidence that this drug may also exert its anti-anginal effect by improving myocardial oxygen supply. Data from patients with coronary stenosis showed a 26% increase in vessel diameter under gallopamil, although the lumen was originally narrowed, on average by 83%. Conversely, the maximum rate-pressure product was reduced by propranolol in spite of the increased exercise time and the rate-pressure product was substantially unchanged at -1 mm ST depression.

Long-term study

The interim results of our long-term study, which is still in progress, go some way towards confirming the short-term efficacy of gallopamil for the treatment of exercise-induced angina. Although as yet too few patients on the long-term treatment have been assessed to provide a long-term versus short-term comparison or to enable any final conclusions to be drawn, there is already evidence of a promising trend. Although the duration of exercising only increased by on average 25%, in 3 patients it increased by between 25% and 66% and they no longer experienced anginal symptoms. The beneficial effect of gallopamil was more obvious from the 36% increase in the -1 mm time after 150 mg gallopamil daily and the 45% increase after 225 mg daily. We conclude from our study that gallopamil is an effective treatment for stable, exercise-induced angina and that a better response can be achieved with the higher dose of gallopamil. The beneficial effect of this drug appears to be due to a reduction of oxygen demand during exercise and an improvement in the supply of oxygen to the myocardium.

References

1. Alderman EL, Davies RO, Crowley JJ et al. (1975) Dose response effectiveness of Propranolol for the treatment of angina pectoris, Circulation 51:964–975
2. Anderson JL, Wagner JM, Datz FL, Christian PE, Bray BE, Taylor AT (1984) Comparative effects of Diltiazem, Propranolol and Placebo on exercise performance using radionuclide ventriculography in patients with symptomatic coronary artery disease: results of a double-blind, randomized, crossover study. Am Heart J 107:698–706.
3. Fleckenstein A, Tritthart H, Fleckenstein B, Herbst A, Grün G (1969) Eine neue Gruppe kompetitiver Ca^{++}-Antagonisten (Iproveratril, D 600, Prenylamin) mit starken Hemmeffekten auf die elektromechanische Koppelung im Warmblutmyokard. Pflügers Arch Ges Physiol 307:R25

4. Fleckenstein A, Fleckenstein B, Späth F, Byon YK (1984) Gallopamil (D 600) – a calcium antagonist of high potency and specificity. Effects on the myocardium and pacemakers. In: Kaltenbach M, Hopf R (eds) Gallopamil. Pharmacological and clinical profile of a calcium antagonist. Springer, Berlin Heidelberg New York Tokyo, pp. 1–32

5. Fleckenstein-Grün G, Fleckenstein A (1984) Blockade of the Ca^{++}-dependent bioelectrical automaticity and electromechanical coupling of smooth muscle cells by gallopamil (D 600). In: Kaltenbach M, Hopf R (eds) Gallopamil. Pharmacological and clinical profile of a calcium antagonist. Springer, Berlin Heidelberg New York Tokyo, pp. 33–48

6. Fleckenstein A (1980) Steuerung der myokardialen Kontraktilität, ATP-Spaltung, Atmungsintensität und Schrittmacherfunktion durch Calcium-Ionen-Wirkungsmechanismus der Calcium-Antagonisten. In: Fleckenstein A, Roskamm H (eds) Calcium-Antagonisten. Springer, Berlin Heidelberg New York, pp. 1–28

7. Frishman WH, Klein NA, Strom JA, Willens H, Lejemtel TH, Jentzer J, Siegel L, Klein P, Kirschen N, Silverman R, Pollack S, Doyle R, Kirsten E, Sonnenblick EH (1982) Superiority of Verapamil to Propranolol in stable angina pectoris: a double-blind, randomized crossover trial. Circulation 65 (Suppl):51–59

8. Hopf R, Drews H, and Kaltenbach M (1984) Anti-anginal effect of gallopamil as compared with nifedipine. In: Kaltenbach M, Hopf R (eds) Gallopamil. Pharmacological and clinical profile of a calcium antagonist. Springer, Berlin Heidelberg New York Tokyo, pp. 123–131

9. Khurmi NS, O'Hara MJ, Bowles MJ, Bala Subramanian V, and Raftery EB (1984) Randomized double-blind comparison of Gallopamil and Propranolol in stable angina pectoris. Am J Cardiol 53:684–688

10. Kohlhardt M, Bauer B, Krause H, Fleckenstein A (1972) Differentiation of the transmembrane Na^+ and Ca^{++} channel in mammalian cardiac fibres by the use of specific inhibitors. Pflügers Arch Ges Physiol 335:309

11. Kovách AGB, Ligeti L, Bakos M, Rubanyi G, Koller A (1984) Studies in vitro and in vivo on the effects of gallopamil on coronary vessels. In: Kaltenbach M, Hopf R (eds) Gallopamil. Pharmacological and clinical profile of a calcium antagonist. Springer, Berlin Heidelberg New York Tokyo, pp. 58–65

12. Lehmann HU, Taegener-Torge C, Witt E, Beck OA, Hochrein M (1979) Antiarrhythmischer Wirkungsvergleich zwischen Gallopamil (D 600) und Verapamil. Angiocard 2:103–111

13. Mitrović K, Nimelä L, Neuss N, and Schlepper M (1984): Antianginal effect of the calcium antagonist gallopamil. In: Kaltenbach M, Hopf R (eds) Gallopamil. Pharmacological and clinical profile of a calcium antagonist. Springer, Berlin Heidelberg New York Tokyo, pp. 107–113

14. Raschack M, Gries J, Bühler V, Maurer R (1984) Studies of the cardiovascular effects of gallopamil. In: Kaltenbach M, Hopf R (eds) Gallopamil. Pharmacological and clinical profile of a calcium antagonist. Springer, Berlin Heidelberg New York Tokyo, pp. 72–80

15. Robertson RM, Wood AJJ, Vaughan WK, and Robertson D (1982) Exacerbation of vasotonic angina pectoris by Propranolol. Circulation 65:281–285

16. Sadick NN, Tan ATH, Fletcher PJ, Morris J, Kelly DT (1982) A double-blind randomized trial of Propranolol and Verapamil in the treatment of effort angina. Circulation 66:574–579

17. Sesto M, Ivancić R, Custović F (1984) The effect of gallopamil on the haemodynamics of patients with coronary heart disease. In: Kaltenbach M, Hopf R (eds) Gallopamil. Pharmacological and clinical profile of a calcium antagonist. Springer, Berlin Heidelberg New York Tokyo, pp. 94–99

18. Smoker PE, MacAlpin RN, Alvaro A, Kattus AA (1972) Reproducibility of a multi-stage near maximal treadmill test for exercise tolerance in angina pectoris. Circulation 48:346

19. Starling MR, Moody M, Crawford MH, Levi B, O'Rourke RA (1984) Repeat treadmill exercise testing: variability of results in patients with angina pectoris. Am Heart J 107:298–303

20. Stieren B, Bühler V, Hege HG, Hollmann M, Neuss H, Schlepper M, and Weymann J (1984) Pharmacokinetics and metabolism of gallopamil. In: Kaltenbach M and Hopf R (eds) Gallopamil. Pharmacological and clinical profile of a calcium antagonist. Springer, Berlin Heidelberg New York Tokyo, pp. 88–93

21. Sučić MJ, Bühler V, Kehrhahn OH and Stieren B (1980) Zur Pharmakokinetik und Pharmakodynamik von Gallopamil. Report VP/FMK/FMH 8005 dated 28. 10. 80. Medical Research and Development Department, Pharmaceuticals Division, BASF Aktiengesellschaft

22. Sučić MJ, Schiemann J (1984) Results of an open multicentre study with 455 patients with coronary heart disease, treated with gallopamil for 1 year. In: Kaltenbach M, Hopf R (eds) Gallopamil, Pharmacological and clinical profile of a calcium antagonist. Springer, Berlin Heidelberg New York Tokyo, pp. 132–135
23. Theisen F, Jahrmärker H (1984) Effect of gallopamil (D 600) on the ECG during exercise in coronary heart disease. In: Kaltenbach M, Hopf R (eds) Gallopamil. Pharmacological and clinical profile of a calcium antagonist. Springer, Berlin Heidelberg New York Tokyo, pp. 117–122
24. Zar J (1974) Biostatistical Analysis. Englewood Cliffs, New York, Prentice Hall

Author's address:

Dr. med. Sabino Iliceto
Divisone di Cardiologia
Policlinico Universitario
I–70124 Bari
Italy

Discussion

From the audience:

Am I right in understanding that after 100 mg of gallopamil the heart rate was higher than after placebo?

ILICETO

At the highest level of loading the heart rate did show a slight, but not significant, rise after both 50 mg and 100 mg.
From the audience:
How long did the effect of gallopamil last?

ILICETO

We carried out two tests, one after 2 hours and one after 7 hours. After 7 hours the response after various drugs was a very flat curve and I believe that most of the short-term effects were actually over by that time. Perhaps tests conducted at shorter intervals would answer this question. However, after 7 hours there were no differences, at any rate no clinically discernible differences.

BALA SUBRAMANIAN

What was the protocol used for the exercise tests in your study? Was this increase in the period of exercising related to the work load at each level of loading; in other words, was it a percentage increase? Did you use a bicycle ergometer or a treadmill?

ILICETO

We used a bicycle ergometer. The work load was increased by 10 watts per minute.

Time course of the response to gallopamil in the steady state in the exercise ECG of patients with coronary heart disease

D. Fleischmann

Medical Department, Lahr District Hospital

Introduction

Short-term and long-term studies carried out in recent years by a number of authors (2, 3, 4, 5, 6, 8, 9) have demonstrated that the ischaemic ECG changes observed during an exercise test in patients with coronary heart disease show a significant improvement 1–3 hours after administration of 50 mg gallopamil. In these studies, the clinical effect of 50 mg gallopamil proved to be comparable to that of 20 mg nifedipine and 80 mg propranolol. Several authors have also verified the anti-ischaemic effect of gallopamil in the steady state during long-term trials; according to Mitrovíc et al. (4), with regular administration of 50 mg gallopamil t.i.d., the steady state is reached after about 7 days. Unlike the above authors, we were interested in the time course of the response to gallopamil under steady-state conditions with the patients taking 50 mg gallopamil t.i.d., that is to say during an 8-hour interval between doses. The study is still in progress, but the provisional results from 10 patients are reported below.

Method

Ten patients, 8 men and 2 women, on average 55 ± 7.7 years of age, took part in the study. The patients had coronary heart disease diagnosed on the basis of a history of typical angina pectoris (n = 10), the ECG findings during an exercise test (n = 10) and the results of coronary angiography (n = 7), which revealed one-vessel disease in 3 patients, two-vessel disease in 2 patients and three-vessel disease in 2 patients.

Beta-blockers and long-term medications were stopped 3 days before the study, which was carried out single-blind, with placebo control. The patient were first given one placebo t.i.d. for 3 days. On the 3rd day of the placebo phase, between 10.00 and 11.00 a.m. 2–3 hours after breakfast, an ECG was recorded whilst the patients were exercising in the supine position on a bicycle ergometer. At the end of the placebo phase the patients took 50 mg gallopamil t.i.d., with an 8-hour interval between doses (8.00 a.m./4.00 p.m.midnight) for 7 days.

On the 7th day an exercise ECG was recorded at 7.30 a.m., that is 30 min before the next dose of gallopamil, and 2, 4 and 6 hours after gallopamil. The exercise test was started at 25 watts and the work load was increased by 25 watts every 2 minutes. The ECG was recorded with a 6-channel recorder and the blood pressure was measured at one-minute intervals up to the 6th minute after the exercise test. Blood was sampled before the exercise test and during the gallopamil phase for determining the plasma level of gallopamil.

The clinical parameters, frequency of anginal attacks and nitrate consumption and the objective parameters ST-segment depression during exercise, heart rate and blood pressure, at maximum work load was determined. For this, the arithmetic mean of the ST-segment depression in leads V4–V6 at the maximum work load which the patient could achieve under placebo was compared with the mean ST-segment depression at the corresponding work load under gallopamil. The ST-segment depression was determined 80 ms after the J point.

Results

The frequency of anginal attacks fell from 4.8 ± 3.4/week (n = 9) during the placebo phase to 1.1 ± 1.5/week (n = 10) during the gallopamil phase. Nitrate consumption fell from 6.4 ± 4.0 doses/week to 0.7 ± 1.1 doses/week. While they were on gallopamil, there was a clear-cut improvement in the patients' physical capabilities and exercise tolerance as they coped with the routine of hospital life, which included climbing stairs and going for a walk, and the majority of them were symptom-free.

In the exercise tests, the threshold work load for angina improved. This correlated with a reduction in the ST-segment depression at the maximum comparable work load (Fig. 1). The reduction in the ischaemic ST-segment depression was greatest 2 hours after administration of 50 mg gallopamil.

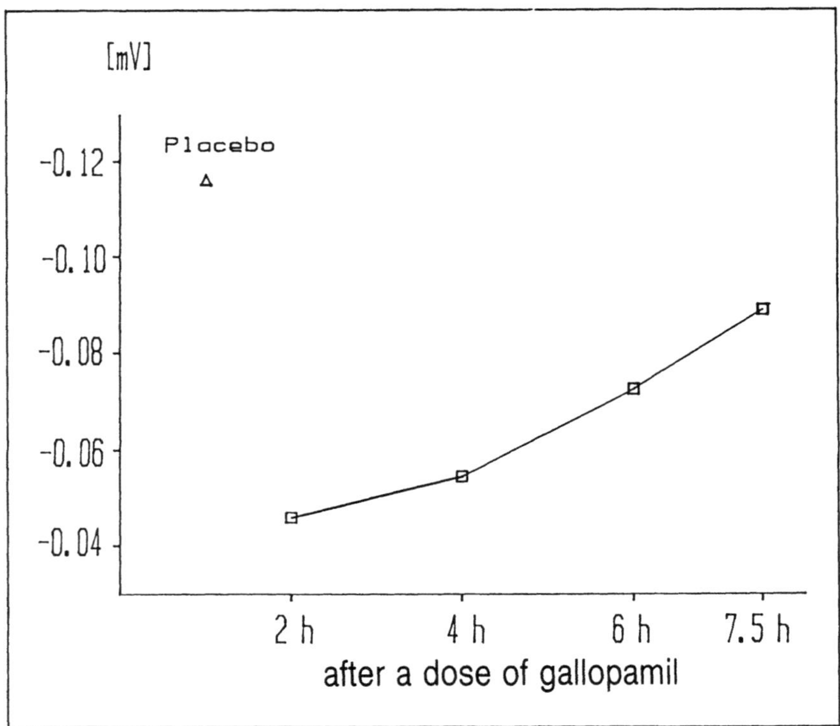

Figure 1. Relationship between the ST-segment depression at the maximum comparable work load under placebo and 2, 4, 6 and 7.5 hours after 50 mg gallopamil, during an interval between doses in the steady state. The mean comparable ST-segment depression was calculated; means from 10 patients with coronary heart disease

The mean ST-segment depression at the maximum comparable work load was 0.116 mV (n = 10) under placebo and it fell to 0.046 mV (n = 10) 2 hours after gallopamil. Four and 6 hours after gallopamil the ST-segment depression, at 0.053 mV and 0.073 mV respectively, was still distinctly below the placebo value. Just before the next dose of gallopamil, that is 7.5 hours after the previous dose, the ST-segment depression was 0.089 mV, which was still less than the ST-depression in the placebo phase, although by that time the signs of ischaemia were increasing again. The plasma gallopamil levels, which were measured in 7 patients, peaked 2 hours after the dose of gallopamil had been taken, at an average of 63.4 ng/ml. The plasma levels then fell rapidly, to an average of 24.3 ng/ml 4 hours after administration of gallopamil, to 13.5 ng/ml after 6 hours and to 10.6 ng/ml after 7.5 hours (Fig. 2).

During the treatment phase the heart rate at the maximum comparable work load fell slightly from an average of 114.9/min to 108.3/min 2 hours after gallopamil (Fig. 3). 7.5 hours after gallopamil the heart rate had risen to 110/min. The systolic and diastolic pressure at the maximum comparable work load also tended to be lower under gallopamil (Fig. 3) although the changes were modest.

During the trial, in no case did the gallopamil medication have to be stopped because of adverse reactions. There was a definite increase of the PQ interval in one patient. However, it was not deemed necessary to reduce the dose or stop the medication.

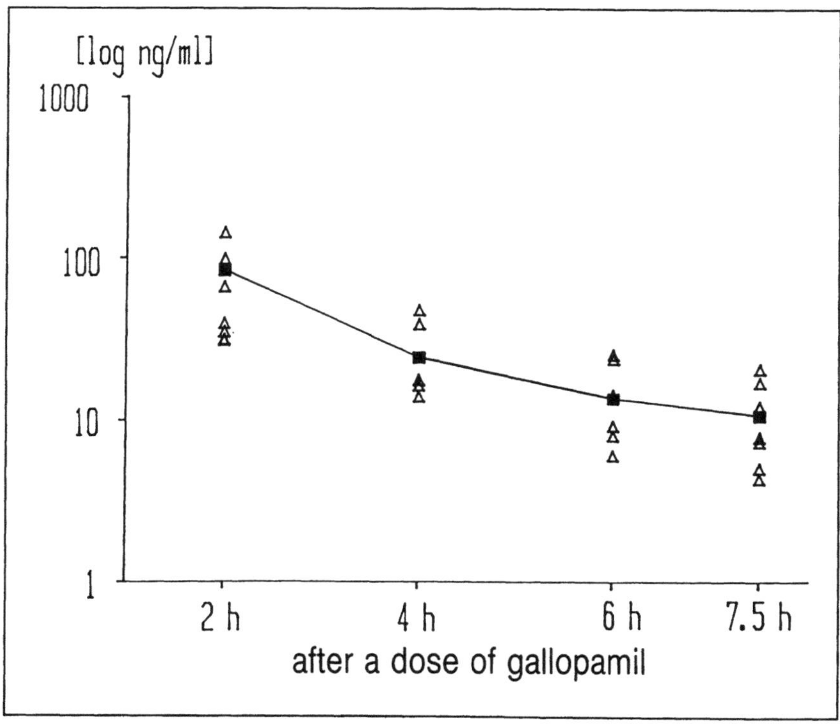

Figure 2. Relationship between the plasma level of gallopamil (ng/ml) and time after administration of 50 mg gallopamil, during an interval between medication

Discussion

In this trial 10 patients with coronary heart disease took the calcium antagonist gallopamil regularly at a dosage of 50 mg t.i.d. It was found that, in the steady state, gallopamil exhibited an anti-ischaemic effect in exercise tests for up to 6 hours after administration. Since the study is still in progress, the results have not yet been verified by statistical tests. The reduction of the ST-segment depression observed during the exercise tests was most clear-cut 2 hours after medication. This significant response 2 hours after gallopamil has already been reported by several authors (2, 3, 5, 6, 8, 9). Our results also show that there was still a clear-cut anti-ischaemic effect on the exercise-induced depression of the ST-segment and the threshold for angina, 4 and 6 hours after gallopamil. However, the improvement of the ST-segment depression steadily diminished during the interval between doses and was only just discernible shortly before the next dose (see Fig. 1). Scrutinio et al. (6) have also reported that the anti-ischaemic effect is much less marked 7 hours after a single dose of 50 mg or 100 mg gallopamil than 2 hours after administration. The rapid fall in the plasma level of gallopamil after the 2-hour peak might explain the decline in the anti-ischaemic effect of gallopamil observed in the exercise tests during the interval between doses (see Fig. 2). The plasma-level profile of gallopamil described here is somewhat similar to that reported by Stieren et al. (7) after a single oral dose of 50 mg ^{14}C-gallopamil

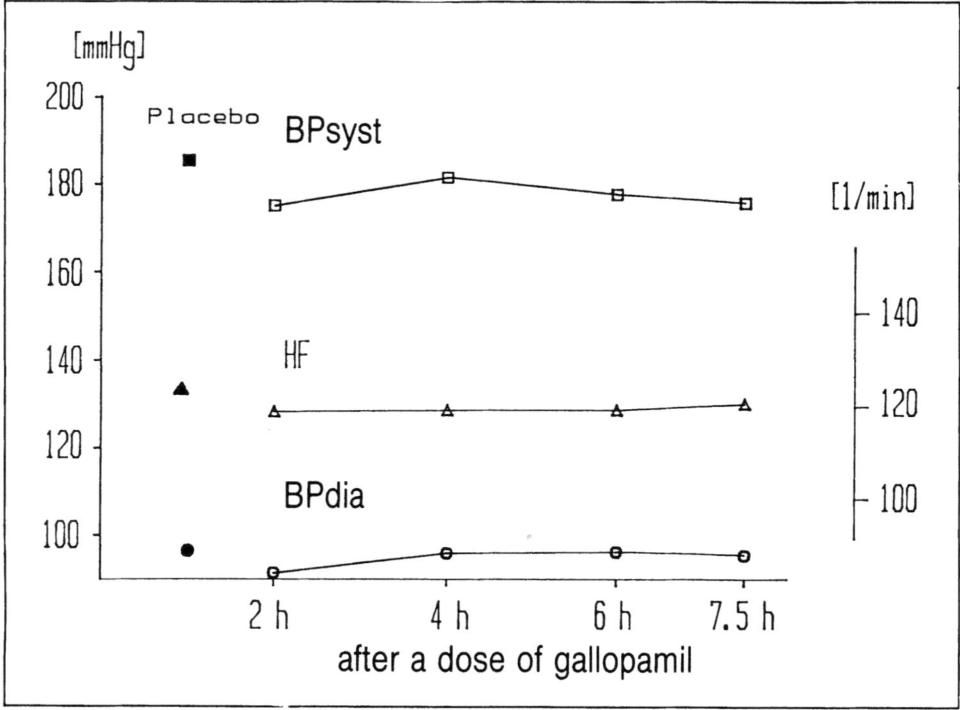

Figure 3. Relationship between heart rate (HR), systolic pressure (BP syst.) and diastolic pressure (BP dia.) after administration of 50 mg gallopamil, during an interval between medication

hydrochloride. With regular administration of 50 mg gallopamil, in the steady state, after 2–3 hours these authors found a mean level of 68.3 ng/ml in 6 volunteers; this is consistent with the mean 2-hour level of 63.4 ng/ml in 7 patients in our study.

Although the anti-ischaemic effect of gallopamil observed in the exercise tests declined during the interval between doses, the anti-anginal effect of 50 mg gallopamil t.i.d. evidently enabled the patients to cope with the routine of hospital life. There was a marked reduction of anginal attacks and nitrate consumption. Most of the patients were symptom-free during their stay in hospital and were able to tolerate exercise, such as climbing stairs, better. In no case did the dose have to be reduced or the medication stopped because of adverse reactions.

These results do not provide any additional information about the mechanism of action of gallopamil in exercise-induced coronary insufficiency.

The trend towards a reduction of the heart rate and systolic and diastolic blood pressure at the maximum comparable work load is evidence of a haemodynamic effect. In addition to the direct, calcium-antagonising effect of gallopamil on the myocardial cells, the reduction of oxygen uptake resulting from the reduction of heart rate and blood pressure may add to the improvement in coronary insufficiency during exercise.

Summary

In a single-blind, placebo-controlled study the time course of the anti-ischaemic effect of gallopamil was investigated during an interval between doses in 10 patients with coronary heart disease who were receiving regular medication with 50 mg t.i.d. In the steady state, with the patients supine, an exercise ECG was recorded 2, 4, 6 and 7.5 hours after administering 50 mg gallopamil. Blood was sampled at the same times to determine the plasma level of gallopamil. The highest plasma levels of gallopamil and the most marked anti-ischaemic effect in the exercise tests were found 2 hours after the patients had taken gallopamil. Thereafter, the plasma levels of gallopamil fell rapidly. However, the anti-ischaemic effect of gallopamil was still clearly discernible 4 and 6 hours after the tablet had been taken. In line with the sustained anti-ischaemic effect of gallopamil under stress conditions in the interval between doses, during the 7-day gallopamil phase the majority of patients remained symptom-free whilst coping with the routine of hospital life.

References

1. Gutmann M, Eichstädt H (1985) Tomoszintigraphische Untersuchungen zur myokardialen Mikroperfusion unter dem Calciumantagonisten Gallopamil. Herz/Kreisl 17:363–368
2. Hopf R, Drews H, Kaltenbach M (1984) Die antianginöse Wirkung von Gallopamil im Vergleich mit einem anderen Calciumantagonisten und Placebo. Z. Kardiol 73:578–585
3. Khummi NS, O'Hara MJ, Bowles MJ, Bala Subramanian V, Raftery EB (1984) Randomized Double-Blind Comparison of Gallopamil and Propranolol in Stable Angina Pectoris. Am J Cardiol 53:684–688
4. Mitrovíc V, Niemelä I, Neuss H, Schlepper M (1983) Zur antianginösen Wirkung des Kalziumantagonisten Gallopamil. In: Kaltenbach M, Hopf R (eds) Gallopamil. Springer, Berlin Heidelberg New York Tokyo, pp. 109–116
5. Rettig G, Sen S, Schieffer H, Bette I (1983) Akut- und Langzeitwirkungen von Gallopamil (D 600) bei stabiler Angina pectoris – Eine randomisierte Doppelblindstudie. Z Kardiol 72:746–754
6. Scrutinio D, Lagioia R, Accettura D, Preziusi N, Mastropasqua F, Rizzon P (1985) Dose-Response Effectiveness Of Gallopamil For The Treatment Of Chronic Stable Effort Angina Pectoris: Camparison With Propranolol. Curr Therap Res 37:830–842

7. Stieren B, Bühler V, Hege HG, Hollmann M, Neuss H, Schlepper M, Weymann J (1983) Pharmakokinetik und Metabolismus von Gallopamil. In: Kaltenbach M, Hopf R (eds) Gallopamil. Springer, Berlin Heidelberg New York Tokyo, pp. 90–96

8. Bala Subramanian V (1985) Vergleichende Untersuchung von Gallopamil und 6 weiteren Ca^{++}-Antagonisten mit Placebo und Propranolol bei Patienten mit chronisch stabiler Angina pectoris. Herz/Kreisl 17:9–20

9. Theisen F, Jahrmärker H (1983) Wirkung von Gallopamil (D 600) auf das Belastungs-EKG bei koronarer Herzkrankheit. In: Kaltenbach M, Hopf R (eds) Gallopamil. Springer, Berlin Heidelberg New York Tokyo, pp. 120–126

Author's address:

Prof. Dr. med. D. Fleischmann
Innere Abteilung des Kreiskrankenhauses
Klostenstraße 19
D–7630 Lahr
West Germany

Discussion

MEESMANN

I would like to make a general comment about the plasma levels of gallopamil which you have shown in relation to the declining responses in the exercise ECG. This applies not only to gallopamil, but to other calcium antagonists as well. In pharmacokinetic terms we certainly have to assume that we have a multicompartment system in which the plasma level is of little relevance and certainly does not equate with the intensity and duration of the cardiac responses. We have been able to study this with the calcium antagonist anipamil, although unfortunately not yet with gallopamil because the concentrations of gallopamil in myocardial tissue are comparatively low and cannot yet be determined with sufficient accuracy. After an i.v. dose of anipamil, as the plasma level falls the level of anipamil in myocardial tissue rises and actually goes even higher when, eventually, the plasma level of anipamil is barely measurable. The level in the myocardium correlates with the duration of the cardiac responses such as the effect on the ischaemia-induced rise in extracellular potassium and the anti-arrhythmic effect. The explanation for this is that the calcium antagonists bind to varying extents to myocardial proteins in the calcium channels. This protein binding, and how long it lasts, evidently determines the duration of action of the calcium antagonists. This being so, there is no point in attempting to relate the effects of calcium antagonists to their plasma levels at the time.

Your results showed that two hours after oral administration of gallopamil there was a large between-patient variation in the plasma levels, which ranged from about 30 to 140 ng/ml; the comparatively low mean value declined as time went on, and there was a conspicuous reduction in the variation.

This profile could well be explained by initial, between-patient differences in the times of the peak plasma concentrations of gallopamil as a result of different absorption times. The ensuing exponential decline in the individual concentration vs. time curves would then displace the different absorption times correspondingly to the right. The plasma levels of gallopamil probably peak well before the 2-hour value. I mention this because apparently a great deal of clinical effort is being expended on attempts to correlate the plasma levels of gallopamil or of other calcium antagonists with the level of the response. However, there is no point in doing this if the key factor is the concentration in myocardial tissue.

FLEISCHMANN

Your general points are probably correct. With the marked between-patient variations in the 2-hour value, between 31 and 124 ng/ml, which we found there is probably an appreciable first-pass effect to consider. Also, as we are aware in respect of other medications, patients vary in terms of being responders or "metabolic responders". One the other hand, there was indeed a rapid fall in the blood levels and there was a positive correlation between this fall and the exercise ECG.

132

Effects of gallopamil in patients with severe coronary heart disease: Investigations by radionuclide ventriculography

B. Brisse, M. Weber, F. Bender

Medical Department C, Münster University Hospital

Introduction

Calcium antagonists reduce clinical symptoms in many patients with coronary heart disease by altering haemodynamics and myocardial metabolism (6, 7, 11). The overall balance of the effects on the coronary system, pump function and oxygen uptake is crucial in these patients if left ventricular function is compromised. So, as a general principle, heart failure in a patient with coronary heart disease has to be regarded as a contra-indication. However, in hospital, these patients with severely compromised ventricular function often pose a problem. On the one hand a further reduction of left ventricular performance as a result of a drug-related negative inotropic effect is unacceptable, while on the other hand the effects of calcium antagonists on the coronary system and, to some degree, also on heart rate and afterload are desirable. In the study reported below we therefore set out to ascertain the overall asset-to-liability ratio of gallopamil in this group of patients.

Patients and procedure

Fifteen patients, 14 men and one woman, between 41 and 68 years of age, average age 56.67 ($s = 8.2$), took part in the study. All patients had coronary heart disease confirmed by angiography. Five patients suffered from a one-vessel disease, one patient from a two-vessel and 9 patients from a three-vessel disease.

After a 20-minute resting period, the patients were given a bolus injection of 10–15 mCi of a Tc^{99m}-albumin solution intravenously. Left ventricular function was then measured by radionuclide stethoscopy (1, 2, 4) and the resting ECG was recorded at the same time. The patients were then subjected to volume load by positioning them supine on a bicycle ergometer with their feet stationary in the pedals. ECG's were again recorded and left ventricular function measured with the patients in this position. An exercise test was then carried out; all the patients exercised at the 25-watt work load, but because of the severity of the coronary heart disease only 8 patients achieved 50 watts. There was a comparatively high drop-out rate at higher work loads, so that the measurements obtained at these work loads were not included in the assessment or statistical analysis. All the patients carried out this exercise test at 25 watts for 2 minutes and the ECG was recorded continuously. During the 2nd minute left ventricular function was again measured by radionuclide stethoscopy. Eight patients of this group were able to exercise similarly in the 3rd and 4th minutes at 50 watts. The ECG was also recorded continuously for 15-minutes during the recovery phase and left ventricular function was measured simultaneously by radionuclide ventriculography after 5 minutes, 10 minutes and 15 minutes. After this investigation each patient received 2×50 mg gallopamil orally. Two hours later the above mentioned procedure was repeated completely, except for the injection.

Before the study all patients had given their consent to take part. The results were analysed statistically by Wilcoxon's test for paired samples.

Results

All the patients had a normal heart rate and a sinus rhythm. The mean rate at rest was 75 ($s = 11$) and it did not alter appreciably during volume load ($\bar{x} = 75/min$, $s = 9$). At a work load of 25 watts heart rate rose to 110/min ($s = 12$) on an average and at 50 watts to 120/min ($s = 12$). During the recovery phase heart rate was 80 ($s = 10$) after 5 minutes, 78 ($s = 9$) after 10 minutes and 78 ($s = 8$) after 15 minutes. Under gallopamil, after 2 hours the resting heart rate was not appreciably different from the baseline rate ($\bar{x} = 73$, $s = 10$). Also, there was no difference during volume load ($\bar{x} = 74$, $s = 11$). However, at a work load of 25 watts the rise in the *heart rate* was reduced; the rate only rose to 104/min ($s = 10$). The difference was statistically significant with $p = 0.011$. At a work load of 50 watts the *heart rate* rose to 113/min ($s = 8$). Here again, the difference was statistically significant with $p = 0.01$. In the recovery phase the values corresponded to the baseline data.

Before gallopamil the *systolic blood pressure* at rest was 134 mm Hg ($s = 17$), under volume loading it was 139 mm Hg ($s = 18$), at 25 watts it increased to 155 mm Hg ($s = 20$) and at 50 watts it rose to 165 mm Hg ($s = 18$). After a 5-minute rest phase it was 142 mm Hg ($s = 21$), it was 134 mm Hg ($s = 18$) after 10 minutes and 132 mm Hg ($s = 18$) after 15 minutes. After gallopamil, even the resting systolic pressure differed from the pre-gallopamil value (Table 1); under gallopamil it was 118 mm Hg ($s = 9$, $p = 0.001$). Under volume loading it did not alter appreciably, being 119 mm Hg ($s = 10$, $p = 0.001$). At a work load of 25 watts the systolic pressure rose less than before gallopamil, to just 142 mm Hg ($s = 22$, $p = 0.018$). At 50 watts it was similar to the pre-gallopamil value, at 163 mm Hg ($s = 20$, $p = 0.34$). Five minutes after the exercise test, at rest the systolic pressure was distinctly lower than the pre-gallopamil value, at 124 mm Hg ($s = 9$, $p = 0.003$); after 10 minutes it was 116 mm Hg ($s = 9$, $p = 0.004$) and after 15 minutes it was 115 mm Hg ($s = 10$, $p = 0.001$).

The mean *diastolic* blood pressure before gallopamil was 83 mm Hg ($s = 6$) at rest, under volume load it was 83 mm Hg ($s = 6$), after exercise at 25 watts it was 92 mm Hg ($s = 7$) and after 50 watts it was 97 mm Hg ($s = 9$). In the recovery phase the diastolic pressure was

Table 1. Changes under *gallopamil in patients with severe CHD:* comparison of the values obtained before and under treatment (100 mg orally)

	At rest	Volume loading	25–50 watts
Heart rate	=	=	▽
Systolic pressure	▽	▽	▽
Diastolic pressure	▽	▽	▽
Double product	=	=	▽
Stroke volume	=	=	=
Ejection fraction	=	=	=

134

82 mm Hg (s = 7) after 5 minutes, 80 mm Hg (s = 6) after 10 minutes and 80 mm Hg (s = 6) after 15 minutes. After gallopamil the diastolic pressure at rest was reduced to 72 mm Hg (s = 6, p = 0.001) and under volume load it was reduced to 73 mm Hg (s = 6, p = 0.001). During the exercise test the diastolic pressure also rose less: after 25 watts it was 86 mm Hg (s = 7, p = 0.003) and after 50 watts it was 92 mm Hg (s = 5, p = 0.041). In the recovery phase the diastolic pressure was 71 mm Hg (s = 4, p = 0.001) after 5 minutes, 70 mm Hg (s = 7, p = 0.001) after 10 minutes and 70 mm Hg (s = 5, p = 0.001) after 15 minutes.

This reduction in the heart rate rise during exercise and the reduction in systolic pressure resulted in a change in the *double product*, as shown in Table 2. There was a clear-cut, statistically significant reduction of the rise in the rate-pressure product at work loads of 25 and 50 watts.

Because of severe left ventricular dysfunction before gallopamil the *ejection fraction* at rest was comparatively low, at 40% (s = 11). Under volume loading it was 37% (s = 11). At 25 watts it fell to 31% (s = 12) and at 50 watts it was 37% (s = 13). After 5 minutes recovery the ejection fraction was 46% (s = 18), it was 46% (s = 16) after 10 minutes and 48% (s = 17) after 15 minutes. After gallopamil the value at rest was identical, 40% (s = 10) and the change under volume loading was similar to that observed before medication (35%, s = 10). During the exercise test the values were similar to those observed before gallopamil, 32% (s = 10) after 25 watts and 33% (s = 9) after 50 watts. Five minutes after the exercise test the ejection fraction was 44% (s = 14). It was 40% (s = 13) 10 minutes after exercise and 37% (s = 14) 15 minutes after exercise. Thus, the values at rest and those obtained under volume loading, during the exercise tests and in the early recovery phase before and after medication were not significantly different.

Before gallopamil the *stroke volume* at rest was 50 ml (s = 18). It was 48 ml (s = 20) under volume load, 39 ml (s = 19) at 25 watts work load and 49 ml (s = 22) at 50 watts. Five minutes after the exercise test the stroke volume was 64 ml (s = 39), 10 minutes after exercise it was 64 ml (s = 33) and 15 minutes after exercise it was 66 ml (s = 33). After

Table 2. *Change of the double product* in patients with severe coronary heart disease under volume loading and during exercise tests on a bicycle ergometer. Comparison of the values obtained before and under treatment with 100 mg gallopamil orally

	At rest	At rest/ under volume load.	At rest/ 1st–2nd min 25 watts	At rest/ 3rd–4th min 50 watts*	At rest/ 5 min	At rest/ 10 min	At rest/ 15 min
						after exercise	
Before gallopamil							
x̄	0	143	6024	9608	1120	103	29
s		906	2539	3266	1382	986	1277
After gallopamil (100 mg orally)							
x̄	0	315	4876	8114	932	120	−118
s		547	2271	1572	1041	890	623
Comparison of the values (Wilcoxon's test)							
p =		ns	0.004	0.002	ns	ns	ns

n = 15, except for * n = 8

Table 3. Comparison of systolic and diastolic changes in patients with severe coronary heart disease under volume loading and during exercise tests. Comparison of the values obtained before and under treatment with 100 mg gallopamil orally

	At rest	Volume loading	25–50 watts
Heart rate	=	=	▽
Period of systole	=	=	=
Period of diastole	=	=	△
% emptying of LV during first half of systole	=	=	=
% filling of LV during first half of diastole	=	△▽	△▽
Rapid filling time as % of diastole	=	▽	▽

gallopamil the stroke volume at rest was 47 ml (s = 16), during volume load it was 44 ml (s = 16), at 25 watts work load it was 38 ml (s = 13) and at 50 watts it was 42 ml (s = 15). In the recovery phase the stroke volume was 50 ml (s = 21) after 5 minutes, 50 ml (s = 18) after 10 minutes and 49 ml (s = 20) after 15 minutes. There were no significant differences either at rest, under volume load during the exercise tests or the early recovery phase.

The *period of systole* before gallopamil was 358 ms (s = 30) at rest, 345 ms (s = 33) under volume loading, 287 ms (s = 37) after 25 watts, 260 ms (s = 34) after 50 watts, 332 ms (s = 30) 5 minutes after the exercise test, 332 ms (s = 23) 10 minutes after exercise and 334 ms (s = 43) 15 minutes after exercise. There were no significant changes after gallopamil (Table 3). The values were 346 ms (s = 41) at rest, 344 ms (s = 33) under volume load, 290 ms (s = 48) at 25 watts, 272 ms (s = 40) at 50 watts, 325 ms (s = 35) 5 minutes after the exercise test, 340 ms (s = 26) after 10 minutes and 332 ms (s = 37) after 15 minutes. Comparison of the values before and after gallopamil did not reveal any statistically significant differences. During the exercise tests there was a reduction of the *period of diastole* corresponding to the rise in heart rate. Before gallopamil the values were 517 ms (s = 117) at rest, 450 ms (s = 102) under volume load, 274 ms (s = 45) after 25 watts, 240 ms (s = 29) at 50 watts, 444 ms (s = 100) 5 minutes after the exercise tests, 490 ms (s = 138) 10 minutes after exercise and 458 ms (s = 98) 15 minutes after exercise. After gallopamil the period of diastole was 540 ms (s = 132) at rest, 472 ms (s = 141) under volume loading, 312 ms (s = 44) after 25 watts, 276 ms (s = 39) after 50 watts, 477 ms (s = 96) 5 minutes after the exercise test, 452 ms (s = 102) 10 minutes after exercise and 470 ms (s = 110) 15 minutes after exercise. Comparison of the values obtained before and after gallopamil revealed a significant difference at 25 watts work load (p = 0.007) and at 50 watts (p = 0.019). Under both conditions gallopamil increased the duration of diastole.

Before gallopamil the *percentage ejection of the left ventricular volume during the first half of systole* was 46% (s = 13) at rest, 50% (s = 10) under volume load, 49% (s = 7) at 25 watts work load, 56% (s = 8) at 50 watts, 46% (s = 13) 5 minutes after the exercise test, 52% (s = 14) after 10 minutes and 48% (s = 12) 15 minutes after exercise. The values after gallopamil were not significantly different from the corresponding pre-gallopamil values. They were 38% (s = 12) at rest, 45% (s = 11) under volume load, 51% (s = 10) at 25 watts, 48% (s = 11) at 50 watts, 70% (s = 10) 5 minutes after the exercise test, 41% (s = 11) 10 minutes after exercise and 44% (s = 17) 15 minutes after exercise.

Before gallopamil the *percentage filling of the left ventricle during the first half of diastole* was 64% (s = 16) at rest, 67% (s = 12) under volume load, 62% (s = 9) at 25 watts work load, 57%

(s = 15) at 50 watts, 62% (s = 11) 5 minutes after the exercise test, 62% (s = 19) after 10 minutes and 55% (s = 16) after 15 minutes. After gallopamil the percentage filling was 71% (s = 14) at rest, 74% (s = 14) under volume load, 64% (s = 13) after 25 watts work load, 72% (s = 13) after 50 watts, 68% (s = 13) 5 minutes after the exercise test, 70% (s = 12) 10 minutes after exercise and 66% (s = 10) 15 minutes after exercise. The statistical comparisons of the values obtained before and under treatment revealed an increase under volume load after treatment at a significance level of p = 0.05 and an increase at 50 watts work load, again at a significance level of 0.05. All the values obtained after exercise were also significantly higher under medication, with p = 0.08 after 5 minutes, 0.03 after 10 minutes and p = 0.06 after 15 minutes.

The *rapid filling time as a percentage of the period of diastole* was significantly different after gallopamil both under volume load and during the exercise test. The detailed results are shown in Table 4.

Discussion

Our patients suffered from severe coronary heart disease. Consequently, even at rest left ventricular ejection fraction was markedly depressed and declined both under volume load and during light exercise on an ergometer. During the ensuing recovery phase, the ejection fraction then rose, overshooting the resting value. This was probably the result of sympathetic stimulation caused by the exercise test, which carried over into the ensuing recovery phase. Here, prior administration of gallopamil did not modify the response in the various situations. We may therefore conclude that, because of the severe ventricular damage, there was no scope for an increase in the ejection fraction under volume load or during an exercise test at work loads of up to 50 watts. However, there was no evidence from this parameter or from the stroke volume of any adverse effect on left ventricular function. Since, in view of the severe ventricular damage, in many patients there was no further scope for any increase of contractility, we have to consider a change in the properties of the ventricle and a reduction of oxygen demand or of the oxygen supply as possible causes. The results show that 100 mg gallopamil reduced heart rate and systolic and diastolic blood pressure both at rest and during exercise, with the result of a significant reduction of

Table 4. Rapid filling time as a percentage of the period of diastole: changes in the values under volume loading and during the exercise tests. Comparison of the values obtained before and under treatment with 100 mg gallopamil orally

	At rest	under volume load.	1st–2nd min 25 watts	3rd–4th min 50 watts*	5 min	10 min after exercise	15 min
Before gallopamil							
x̄	58	64	72	74	62	63	65
s	13	13	10	10	14	14	16
After gallopamil (100 mg orally)							
x̄	53	58	63	60	57	56	55
s	13	13	10	13	12	10	12
Comparison of the values (Wilcoxon's test)							
p =	ns	0.07	0.02	0.01	0.05	ns	0.04

n = 15, except for * n = 8

the double product during exercise. Oxygen demand was therefore reduced and this indicated that the heart worked more economically.

Pump function of the left ventricle is affected by the factors mentioned above and by the change in the compliance of the left ventricle during systole and diastole, resulting in a change of systolic emptying and diastolic filling (3, 5). Under gallopamil there was no change of systolic ventricular motion, and as far as this parameter indicates, no change of systolic contraction. On the other hand, during diastole, the values for rapid filling time as a percentage of the period of diastole and for the percentage filling during the first half of diastole indicated faster ventricular filling. Both these parameters indicated an improvement of left ventricular compliance during diastole (3, 5, 9, 10).

We know from the literature that calcium antagonists can produce very disparate clinical results, particularly in patients with compromised left ventricular function. There has been some debate as to whether calcium antagonists which exhibit an intrinsic reflex sympathomimetic effect might offer advantages in this situation. However, from the results reported here, under the stated conditions gallopamil did not impair cardiac function. In fact, as has been reported in the literature, we found that any reduction of contractility was offset by a reduction of afterload, of the double product and hence of oxygen demand. Moreover, ventricular compliance improved, particularly during diastole, and this improvement of the compliance of the left ventricle benefited coronary perfusion. Published reports (7, 8, 12) also indicate that in patients with severe coronary heart disease gallopamil reduces myocardial oxygen demand and has a beneficial effect on the stenosed coronary vessels. Thus, altogether, the haemodynamic changes we found indicate that even in patients with severe coronary heart disease, the calcium antagonist gallopamil does not reduce left ventricular pump function, and that it improves myocardial oxygen balance and left ventricular compliance.

References

1. Brugger P (1985) Zur Bestimmung des Herzminutenvolumens mit einem neuen nichtinvasiven nuklearmedizinischen Verfahren. Herz/Kreislauf 4:192–196
2. Brugger P (1985) Zur nichtinvasiven nuklearmedizinischen Beurteilung der linksventrikulären Funktion bei Patienten mit koronarer Herzkrankheit. Wien Med Wochenschr 135:407–413
3. Burgger P Th (1986) Left ventricular diastolic function in patients with coronary artery disease. Nuc Compact 17:191–198
4. Brüggemann Th, Schwietzer U, von Leitner ER, Kruck L, Krupenhagen K, Reuter E, Biamino G (1983) Nichtinvasive Bestimmung der linksventrikulären Ejektionsfraktion mit einer mobilen EKG-getriggerten Szintillationsmeßsonde. Korrelation zu Cineventriculographie, Echokardiographie und Radionuklidventrikulographie. Z Kardiol 72:1–6
5. Brutsaert DL, Rademakers FE, Sys SU, Gillebert TC, Housmans PR (1985) Analysis of relaxation in the evaluation of ventricular function of the heart. Progr Cardiovasc Dis 23:143–163
6. Eichstädt H (1985) Calciumantagonisten, In: Handbuch der Inneren Medizin Volume IX/3. Springer, Berlin Heidelberg New York, pp. 1069–1113
7. Eichstädt H, Gutmann M, Schmutzler H, Felix R (1983) Nachweis verbesserter Mikroperfusion unter intravenöser und oraler Gabe des Calciumantagonisten Gallopamil. Z Kardiol 72:24–30
8. Fleckenstein A, Fleckenstein B, Späh F, Byon YK (1983) Gallopamil (D 600) – ein Calciumantagonist von hoher Wirkungsstärke und Spezifität. Effekt auf Myokard und Schrittmacher. In: Kaltenbach M, Hopf R (eds) Gallopamil: Pharmakologisches und klinisches Wirkungsprofil eines Calciumantagonisten. Springer, Heidelberg New York Tokio, pp. 1–35
9. Maini CL, Antonelli Incalzi R, Bonetti MG, Valle G, Montenero AS (1985) Left ventricular diastolic performance at rest in patients with angina and normal systolic function – assessment by equilibrium radionuclide angiography. Nuklearmedizin 24:159–163

10. Mauser M, Karsch KR, Wagner S, Seipel L (1985) Änderung der diastolischen Ventrikeleigenschaften durch intravenöse Nifedipininfusion bei Patienten mit instabiler Angina pectoris. Z Kardiol 74: 590–597
11. Raschack M, Gries J, Bühler V, Maurer R (1983) Untersuchungen zur kardialen und vasalen Wirksamkeit von Gallopamil. In: Kaltenbach M, Hopf R (eds) Gallopamil: Pharmakologisches und klinisches Wirkungsprofil eines Calciumantagonisten. Springer, Berlin Heidelberg New York Tokyo, pp. 75–83
12. Sesto M, Ivancic R, Custovic F (1983) Die Wirkung von Gallopamil auf die Hämodynamik bei Patienten mit KHK. In: Kaltenbach M, Hopf R (eds) Gallopamil: Pharmakologisches und klinisches Wirkungsprofil eines Calciumantagonisten. Springer, Berlin Heidelberg New York Tokyo, pp. 97–101.

Author's address:

Prof. Dr. med. B. Brisse
Med. Univ.-Klinik
Abt. Innere Medizin C
Albert-Schweitzer-Straße 33
D–4400 Münster
West Germany

Discussion

N. N.

Can you extend your results to long-term treatment?

BRISSE

Of course, several other effects have to be taken into account concerning long-term treatment. If we assume that the drug concentration is comparatively high at the 2-hour measurement and hence that the response is very pronounced, then we might conclude that neither the desired nor the undesired changes will exceed beyond this during long-term medication. Naturally there are variations during the interval between doses, but systematic measurement is needed here and we would like to do this. However, there are technical problems because patients with such severe coronary heart disease rarely remain on single-drug therapy for long, so other medications are added, and this makes it difficult to measure the effect of a single drug.

FLEISCHMANN

You gave 100 mg gallopamil. It is always said that gallopamil is 2.5 times more potent than verapamil; 50 mg gallopamil is equivalent to about 120 mg isoptin. This means that you would have given more than 300 mg verapamil equivalent, and that to a patient with that degree of impairment of ventricular function. I would not dare to do that.

BRISSE

It is not intended to give this medication three times a day. Short-term medication is of course given to investigate the mechanism of action and to see what has to be expected during continuous treatment; the level of the response will depend on the dose selected.

BENDER

Range-finding studies to ascertain the dose for the various grades of coronary heart disease have yet to
be completed.

STAUCH

There was a fairly marked fall of EF during the predrug investigation. Did the patients show clear-cut
signs of ischaemia? There are not usually any major changes when the EF is at this level; the patients
have a large infarction, but no signs of ischaemia. If they did show signs of ischaemia, one would
anticipate a marked improvement, and maybe after giving an anti-ischaemia drug as well.

BRISSE

We did not go into these interrelationships in more detail here because they have been dealt with by
other speakers. The patients showed typical ischaemic changes of the ST-segment and there were
improvements under the medication.

STAUCH

Is it not possible to attribute at least some of these changes in the parameters, particularly during
diastole, to the reduction of heart rate in relation to the period of diastole?

BRISSE

This is why we also calculated the rapid filling time as a percentage of the period of diastole. This
changes the absolute value into a relative one and then, in relation to this cardiac phase, rapid filling is
shorter. On this basis, we concluded that compliance improved.

STAUCH

Was that only during exercise, or at rest too?

BRISSE

Both.

BALA SUBRAMANIAN

With regard to the ejection fraction and these studies, we must be very sure about the technique.
Radionuclide ventriculography does not give a very accurate value for stroke volume or ejection
fraction and the reproducibility in various studies is very poor. I believe that the low ejection fraction
which we observed during exercise was not due to an actual reduction of ejection fraction, but probably
to the use of the nuclear probe.

BRISSE

As I am sure you are aware, this instrument was developed at the John Hopkins Institute by Dr.
Wagner, who is well versed in nuclear cardiology. Once the method had been developed, he and his
colleagues compared the results with those obtained by other techniques and they found a correlation of
0.9 between the values obtained by cardiac catheterization and by radionuclide ventriculography. So, I
believe that this is a very good technique and gives good reproducibility. We have made some
comparisons and on this basis we cannot accept your objections.

BALA SUBRAMANIAN

During my last visit to the John Hopkins, The National Institute of Health, I found that the radionuclide
ventriculograph was not being used since, after various experiments, the results initially published by
Dr. Wagner have not been confirmed by other authors. We ourselves have abandoned radionuclide

140

ventriculography as a way of determining the ejection fraction. It is very useful for determining systolic filling time, diastolic filling time and other variables, but for measuring the ejection fraction it was found that the reproducibility achieved with this instrument is very poor because the beam is set over a very small area.

BRISSE

There are a whole range of measuring instruments in the John Hopkins Institute and they compare the results obtained with every instrument. I believe that the feature of this method is that it enables volumes to be compared at very short time intervals; these measurements can only be done by radionuclide *stethoscopy,* and not by means of a camera. So, I believe that the various instruments are suitable for different measurements. Even if a team which has developed a technique is not using it at a particular moment, that does not mean that the technique or the instrument is regarded as unsuitable. Whether or not it is in use depends on what they happen to be researching at the time.

STAUCH

We too have stopped taking measurements by radionuclide *stethoscopy,* although Dr. Wagner visited us and was very enthusiastic about this instrument and put his at our disposal. However, we were not able to use it because the results were not reproducible. We would like to use it, because it is so simple to operate and very portable, so that measurements can be taken under different conditions. However, our Nuclear Medicine Department stopped us using the instrument because the technical staff and doctors say that it is not suitable for us to use. However, it may be quite a different matter if you are using the instrument for specific purposes and operate it yourself the whole time.

BENDER

Mr. Stauch, what do you think of the possibility to observe the within-patient changes over a short period rather than the absolute values. Are these data comparable? Do you think it is feasible to compare measurements taken within a few minutes of each other from the same patient?

STAUCH

I cannot remember a situation of this sort. It is so long now since we carried out these investigations. Perhaps you have more experience. I cannot really answer this question.

BRISSE

I would like to add something here. The ejection fraction cannot be measured by radionuclide ventriculography in a patient with a cardiomegaly. This is well known. However, if these patients are excluded, the determinations are easy to carry out and they are reproducible.

EICHSTÄDT

Dr. Bender, if I understand your question correctly, you want to know whether the results obtained within a few minutes by the same investigator are reproducible. They certainly are. However, we must distinguish between investigations carried out like this and those carried out at an interval of weeks. We carried out investigations by radionuclide ventriculography between 1981 and 1983. All the other advantages of radionuclide ventriculography have already been mentioned. I certainly believe, Dr. Stauch, that the results obtained within minutes are reproducible. I have very often found this myself.

BRISSE

The investigations were carried out at many different locations before this instrument was used at all for any investigations in hospitals. The most important results came not only from the Americans, but also from studies carried out by members of Brunner's team, at the Cardiac Centre in Munich and in Berlin. They all found a correlation of 0.9 between the different methods and I know of no publication which refutes this result.

ZEHENDER

A question about the double product. You found that the double product rises less under gallopamil than under placebo. Comparing the 25-watt work load with the 50-watt work load, the rise under gallopamil from 4000 to 8000 was smaller than the rise under placebo from 6000 to 9000. Do you have any experience regarding the change in these values at higher levels of loading? Does the difference between placebo and gallopamil become even smaller? A second question about the ejection fraction: on an average in all the patients this was slightly lower under gallopamil, although the difference was not significant. The same applies to the ejection volume in the first half of systole. Was this value very low in a few patients, or were the values for the patients fairly similar?

BRISSE

To answer your second question first, the values for the patients were fairly similar. As regards to your first question, with the heart failure which developed during the exercise tests as a result of the coronary heart disease, concerning the overall clinical picture we were only able to stress a few patients at work loads above 50 watts. This is why we only carried out a statistical analysis on the data obtained up to the 50-watt stage.

Effects of intravenous and oral treatment with calcium antagonists on myocardial microperfusion

H. Eichstädt, O. Danne, H. P. Koch, M. Langer, M. Cordes, C. Schubert, R. Felix, H. Schmutzler

Departments of Cardiology and Radiology, University Hospital Rudolf Virchow, Free University of Berlin

Introduction

The introduction of computerized methods for data quantification (1, 2, 3) and tomographic techniques to improve spatial resolution has made computerized emission tomography of the myocardium an available tool for the control of therapy (7, 8). We demonstrated the value of this methods for therapy control in patients with coronary artery disease in earlier publications (4, 5). This paper gives a summary of our investigations on calcium antagonists over the last five years.

Patients and methods

Various calcium antagonists were investigated in a multicrossover-study design with a study population of 56 patients. 21 (20 women and 1 man, with an average age of 53 years) of the original 56 patients completed the trial, and were treated successfully with the calcium antagonists gallopamil, verapamil, diltiazem, nifedipine, bepridil, prenylamine and fendiline. Separate studies were also carried out with other substances and single parameters were also tested for nisoldipine and nitrendipine. The study population comprised patients with angiographically proven coronary artery disease and hemodynamically relevant stenoses. Coronary angiography was carried out twice, with an interval of at least two years between examinations, to confirm that no changes in the hemodynamically relevant coronary artery stenosis occurred. Most of the patients had multi-vessel-disease (13 patients had three-vessel-disease and 2 patients had two-vessel-disease); only 6 patients had single-vessel-disease. The maximum exercise tolerance in the run-in placebo phases was limited to 75 watts.

The following parameters were registered for every patient and each calcium antagonist at the end of the therapy phases in a multicrossover-study design: Frequency of anginal attacks, nitroglycerine consumption, ST-segment deviation and exercise tolerance, blood pressure, heart rate, quantification of systolic and diastolic functional parameters by radio-nuclid-ventriculography and measurement of microperfusion by computerized emission tomography of the myocardium with high resolution multiplanar imaging. The majority of investigations were carried out with an Elscint large field camera and an Apex 415 computer. For some studies we used an Ohio sigma 410 large field camera with a seven-pinhole collimator. Acquisition time was 2×550 sec and aperture was 5.5 mm with an overall storage of at least $2 \times 375\,000$ counts. The myocardium of the left ventricle was reconstructed into 12 slices at maximum with the seven pinhole collimator and into 64 slices at maximum with the rotating gamma camera by means of a negative reciprocal arithmetic computer algorithm. The impulses were registered as counts per matrixpoint on the 64×64 computer matrix. The interpolated subtracted background of the lungs and the ventricular cavity constitute the reference points for measurement of count density (6).

Thallium-201 was used as the radiopharmaceutical. The quantitative distribution of Thallium-201 in the myocardium is directly proportional and linear related to blood flow, so analysis of count density provides a suitable parameter for measurement of regional myocardial microperfusion. Other factors determining Thallium uptake, such as myocardial mass and membrane activity were regarded as constant. The study protocol for each calcium antagonist consisted of a treatment-free run-in placebo phase of 1 week, followed by baseline examination. During this run-in period patients were only permitted to take fast acting nitrates. A scintiscan of the myocardium was performed at the end of this wash-out phase. An average of 110 MBq Thallium-chloride was injected intravenously about 1 minute before the anticipated end of the exercise test. Computerized emission tomography was immediately started after exercise. A scintiscan at rest was performed 3 hours after termination of exercise to obtain information about the redistribution. The effect of each calcium antagonist was studied after four weeks of oral treatment. Some calcium antagonists were also investigated after intravenous injection (Table 1).

Table 1. Dosages of the calcium antagonists tested

	Injection	Oral medication
Gallopamil	2 × 2 mg i. v.	50 mg t. i. d.
Verapamil	2 × 5 mg i. v.	80 mg t. i. d.
Diltiazem		2 × 90 mg t. i. d.
Nifedipine	2 × 5 mg/50 ml	20 mg t. i. d.
Bepridil		100 mg t. i. d. – q. i. d.
Prenylamine		60 mg t. i. d.
Fendiline		100 mg t. i. d.

Results

During the run-in placebo phases there were 4 anginal attacks per day on average. The frequency of anginal attacks decreased to 1–3 attacks per day after 4 weeks of oral treatment. There was a significant reduction to about 1 attack per day under gallopamil, verapamil, diltiazem and bepridil, whereas reduction under nifedipine, prenylamine and fendiline was less obvious. The consumption of fast acting nitrates was reduced in parallel to the frequency of anginal attacks (Fig. 1). At the end of the run-in placebo phases, maximum exercise capacity ranged from 50 to 65 watts. Maximum exercise tolerance increased to 75–100 watts after therapy. A mean maximum exercise tolerance of 100 watts was achieved only under gallopamil and bepridil (Fig. 2). ST-segment depression was 0.25 mV during the run-in placebo phases which preceded medication with each of the calcium antagonists. Treatment with gallopamil, bepridil, diltiazem and verapamil reduced ST-segment depression to 0.1 mV or less. Under treatment with nifedipine and prenylamine the mean ST-segment depression was still 0.13 mV and 0.17 mV respectively (see Fig. 2).

Under long-term treatment with each of the calcium antagonists heart rate was about 80 beats per minute and systolic blood pressure was about 120 mm Hg at rest. After termination

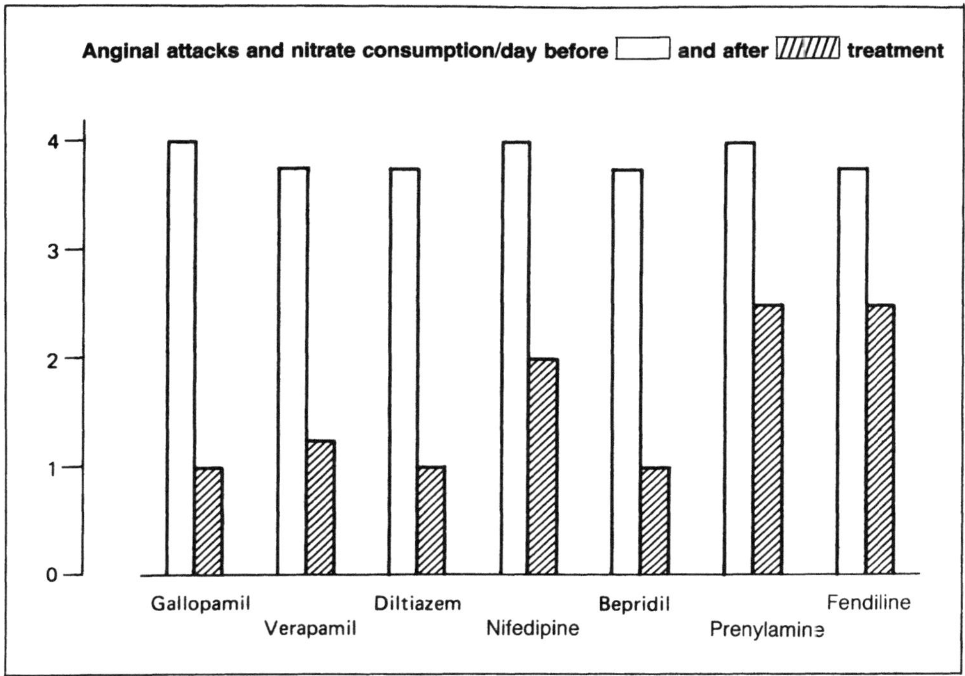

Figure 1

of exercise heart-rate reached the highest level under nifedipine with 170 beats per minute and lowest under gallopamil, verapamil and prenylamine with 130 to 140 beats per minute (Fig. 3). Systolic blood pressure increased to about 158 mm Hg under nifedipine and 175 to 180 mm Hg under gallopamil, bepridil, diltiazem and verapamil (see Fig. 3). All the stated differences were statistically significant ($p < 0.001$).

The count rates obtained by computerized emission tomography of the myocardium were evaluated separately for the anterolateral, septal, inferior, and posterolateral segments of the myocardium and also for the whole ventricular circumference. Gallopamil was one of the three drugs which were also investigated after intravenous application. Two injections of 2 mg gallopamil were given i. v. over a period of 10 min before exercise. Figure 4 shows the count density distribution over 4 segments in 10 patients with septal defects.

In the septal segment which demonstrated low perfusion the absolute count rate increased from 225 counts per matrixpoint to 384 counts per matrixpoint after the intravenous injection. At the end of the 4 weeks oral treatment, further improvement to 474 counts per matrixpoint was observed in these patients.

In order to obtain an overall picture of all the calcium antagonists tested, the count rates were expressed as percentages and absolute values over the whole ventricular circumference; these data are shown in Fig. 5. Some of the values for individual segments differed significantly from the value for the whole circumference. The histogram shows the results obtained after four weeks of oral treatment with each calcium antagonist. Gallopamil increased the count rate by 33%. Verapamil, diltiazem and nifedipine also increased the count rates, which varied at about 30% or more around the whole circumference. Increases

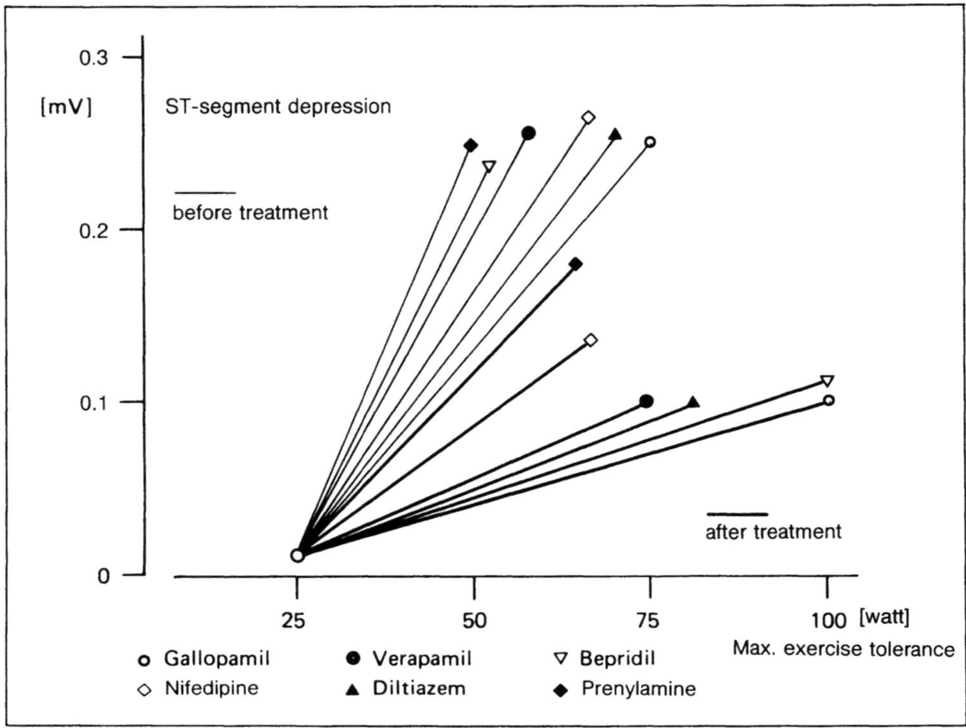

Figure 2

in count density were much smaller with the other drugs, bepridil, prenylamine and fendiline. With bepridil there was a discrepancy in that it exhibited a marked antianginal effect but the increase in count density was not as clearly demonstrable as with the first group of drugs.

The improvements in perfusion are illustrated even more clearly by the unquantified imaging results than by the above analysis of absolute count rates. Figure 6 shows the improvement of microperfusion in a patient with severe 3-vessel-disease. Alongside the predrug image there are images of the same slice of the myocardium after oral treatment with each of the calcium antagonists at a work load of 75 watts. Drugs may be devided into two groups based on the improvement in microperfusion. Gallopamil, nifedipine, verapamil and diltiazem produced significant improvement whereas under bepridil, prenylamine, and fendiline the improvement was not so pronounced.

The regional and global function of the left ventricle under these calcium antagonists was measured by radionuclide ventriculography. Calcium antagonists with the most powerful vasodilator effects (lowering of the total peripheral resistance) reduced the ejection time in comparison to normal values obtained from healthy volunteers. This response was observed under gallopamil and nifedipine (Fig. 7). The other drugs used in this multicrossover trial increased the ejection time. However, this did not diminish global ejection fraction.

146

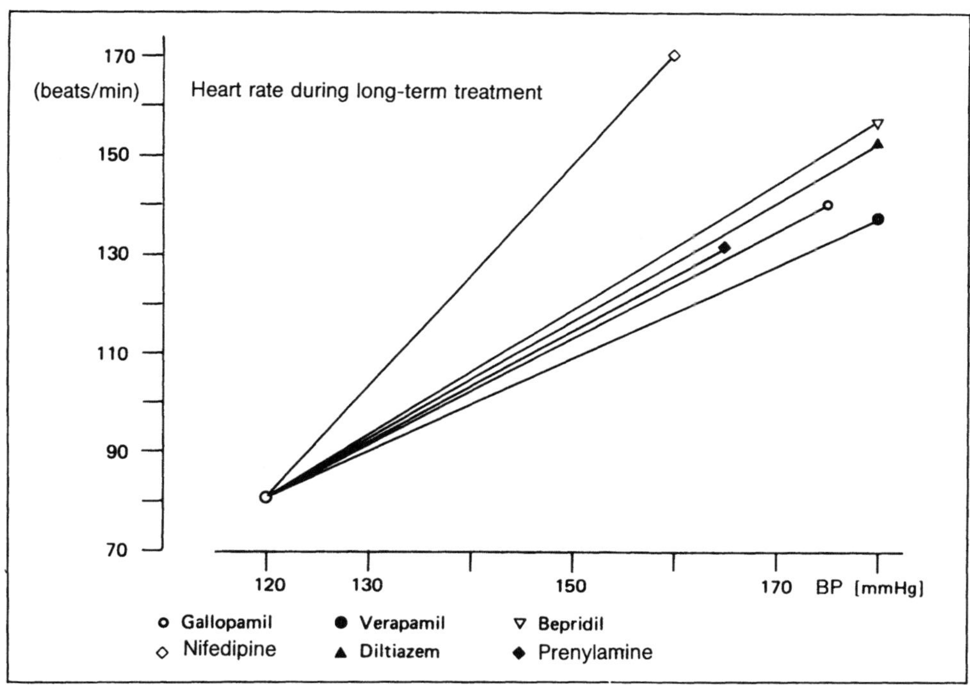

Figure 3

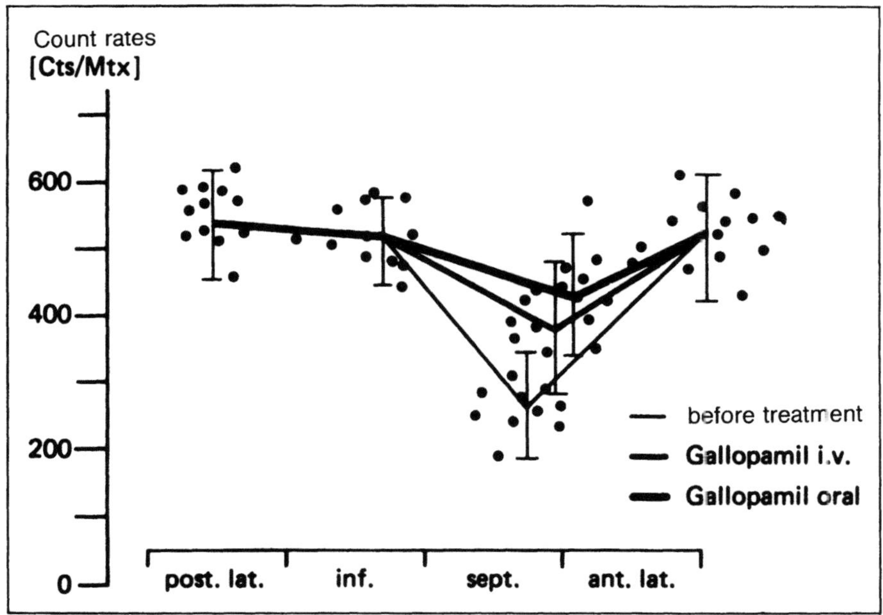

Figure 4

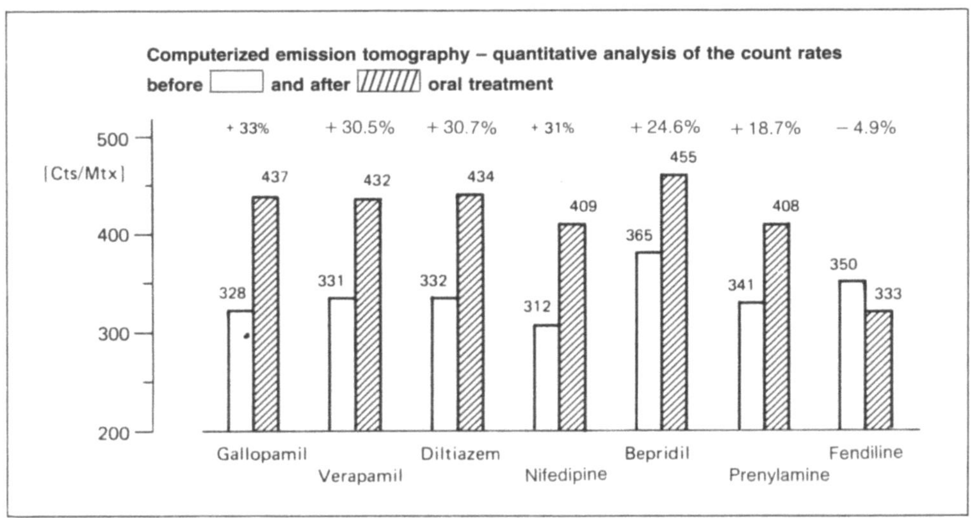

Figure 5

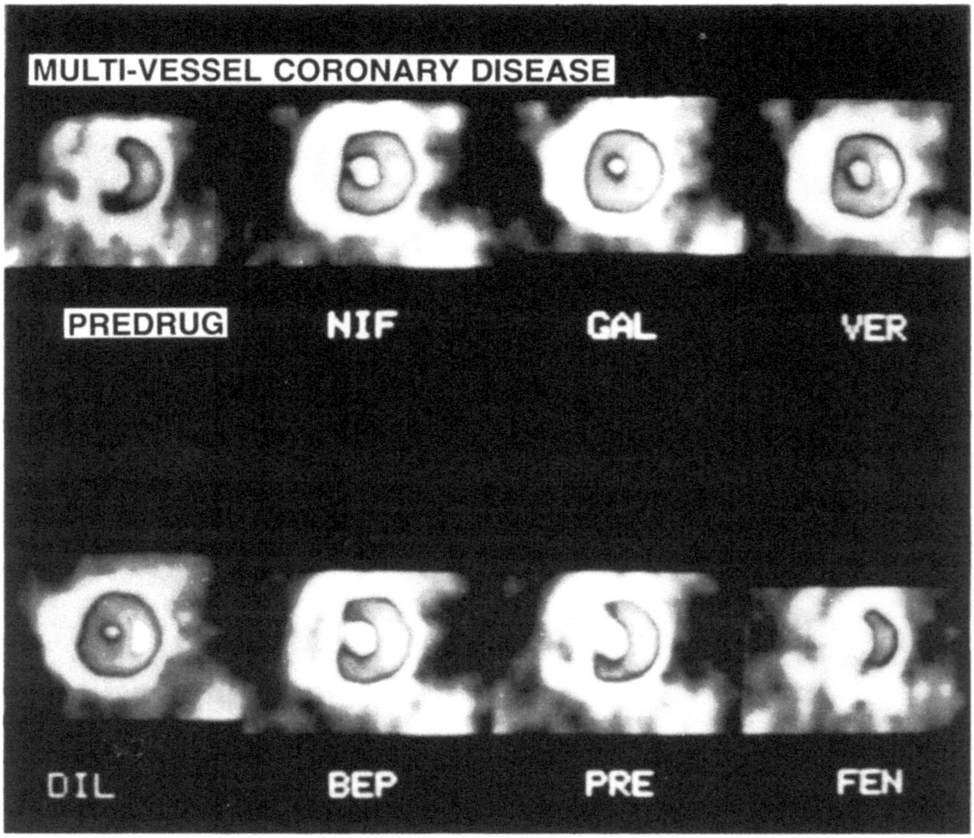

Figure 6

148

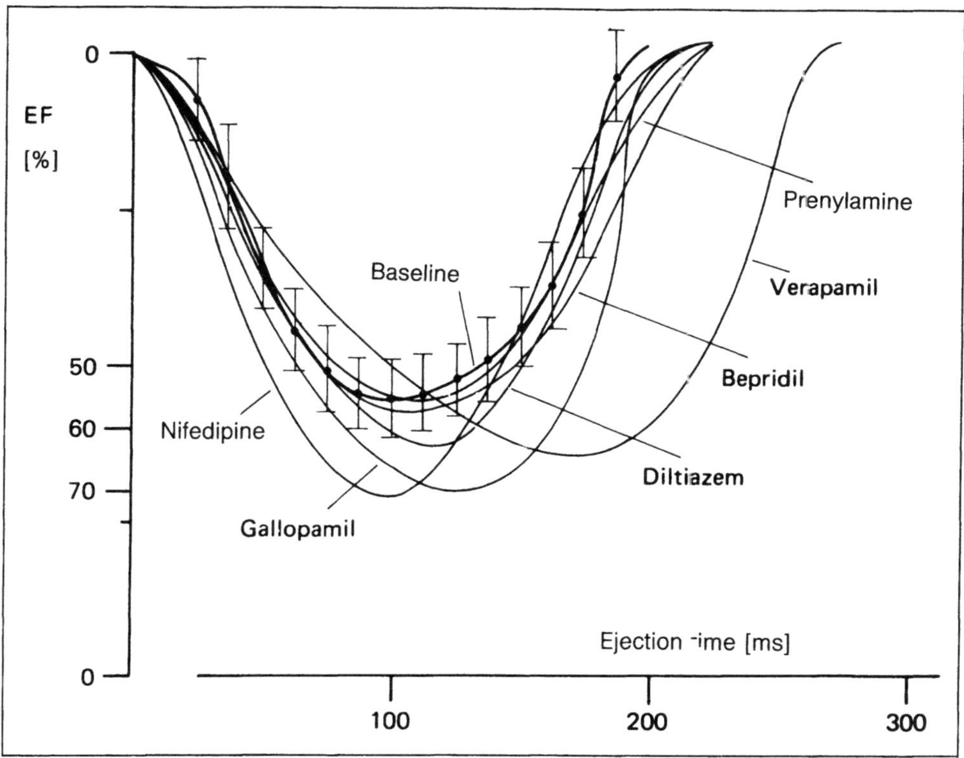

Figure 7

Discussion

Exercise tolerance, heart rate, blood pressure and especially the patients reports on anginal attacks are comparatively unreliable parameters, whereas reduction of ST-segment depression is a parameter with acceptable reproducibility. Computerized emission tomography, as the method we used, allows non-invasive imaging of myocardial perfusion with good correlation to the areas of coronary artery supply. Therefore the method provides additional information as to the quantification of improvement in myocardial microperfusion under calcium antagonists. Both after intravenous administration and after long term oral treatment practically all drugs tested produced a significant increase in count density. According to all measurements, gallopamil was the top at the list in this respect. At the other end of the scale prenylamine still exhibited an antianginal effect, whereas there was no improvement in the count rates under fendiline.

Our studies could be relative to some extent, in that we did not carry out dose titration with each calcium antagonist in each patient. However, we based dosage on the records of anginal attacks of the patients. If the patient reported the same reduction in angina pectoris at the doses we used, we felt justified in assuming that these doses were clinically equivalent.

149

Summary

In a multicrossover-study design 56 patients were treated with various calcium antagonists from 1983 to 1986. At the end of the study there was a complete set of data for the calcium antagonists gallopamil, verapamil, diltiazem, nifedipine, bepridil, prenylamine, and fendiline for 21 of these patients. Each of the 21 patients was examined by coronary angiography twice with an interval of at least two years between examinations to confirm that there have been no changes in the hemodynamically relevant coronary stenoses. In this multicrossover-study design the following parameters were registered during the treatment with each calcium antagonist: Frequency of anginal attacks, nitroglycerine consumption, ST-segment depression, exercise tolerance, blood pressure, heart rate, quantitative determination of filling and ejection parameters and microperfusion. Notably gallopamil, but also diltiazem and nifedipine, increased the count rate in previously ischemic areas of the left ventricle by more than 30%. Verapamil and bepridil improved the count rate by 20–25%. Prenylamine and fendiline increased the count rate by less than 20%. Measurements of healthy areas showed that there were apparently no relevant steal effects with any of the calcium antagonists.

References

1. Büll U, Strauer BE, Hast B, Niendorf HP (1976) Die 201-Thallium-Szintimetrie des Herzens als neues Verfahren zur funktionellen Differenzierung der koronaren Herzkrankheit. Fortschr Röntgenstr 124:434
2. Eichstädt H, Schumacher M, Feine U, Kochsiek K (1978) Computergesteuerte Auswertung der 201-Tl-Myokardszintigraphie bei koronarer Herzerkrankung. In: Schaper W (ed) Proceedings of the Deutsche Gesellschaft für Herz- und Kreislaufforschung 44, Steinkopff Darmstadt
3. Eichstädt H, Maisch B, Feine U, Kochsiek K, Felix R, Schmutzler H (1980) Verbesserung quantitativer Aussagemöglichkeiten bei der Thallium-Myokardszintigraphie durch den Einsatz von Auswertungsrechnern. Verh Dtsch Ges Inn Med 86:573
4. Eichstädt H, Krämer R, Gutmann M, Felix R, Schmutzler H (1983) Schichtszintigraphische Darstellung der Hypertrophieregression bei Hypertonikern unter chronischer Betarezeptorenblokkade. Therapiewoche 33:5964
5. Eichstädt H, Gutmann M, Schmutzler H, Felix R (1983) Nachweis verbesserter Mikroperfusion unter intravenöser und oraler Gabe des Calciumantagonisten Gallopamil. Z Kardiol 72(Suppl 2):24
6. Eichstädt H (1984) Quantitative Myokardszintigraphie bei Koronaroperationen. Springer-Verlag Berlin–Heidelberg–New York–Tokyo
7. Parker JA, Uren RF, Jones AF, Maddox DF, Zimmermann RE, Holeman BL (1977) Radionuclide left ventriculography with the Slant Hole Collimator. J Nucl Med 8:250
8. Zaret BL, Strauss HW, Martin ND (1973) Non-invasive regional myocardial perfusion with radioactive potassium: study of patients at rest, exercise and during angina pectoris. N Engl J Med 288:809

Author's address:

Prof. Dr. H. Eichstädt
Universitätsklinikum Charlottenburg
Spandauer Damm 130
1000 Berlin 19

Incidence and importance of silent myocardial ischaemia – treatment with gallopamil

M. Zehender, T. Meinertz, A. Geibel, S. Hohnloser, C. Weiss, H. Just

Medical Department III, Freiburg University Hospital

Introduction

In view of the prevalence of coronary heart disease, diagnosing and treating myocardial ischaemia is a major challenge. It has been demonstrated in recent years that some patients with proven coronary heart disease may be partially or completely free from the cardinal symptom, angina pectoris. Routine ECGs revealed previous myocardial infarction as an incidental finding in 708 of the 5127 volunteers who took part in the Framingham study (1). When their history was taken, 15% of these volunteers reported that they had never experienced any cardiac symptoms. Recently, many other studies have confirmed that silent myocardial ischaemia is much more frequent than was once thought (2–6). This is all the more important in the light of recent evidence that the effect of brief episodes of ischaemia in the development of larger areas of myocardial necrosis (7) and bioelectrical instability is cumulative (8). In this paper we shall consider the qualitative and quantitative aspects of silent myocardial ischaemia in comparison with symptomatic episodes. We shall also touch on the problems posed by the techniques and methods used and report the first results of treating patients who have silent myocardial ischaemia.

Detection of symptomatic and silent myocardial ischaemia

The most reliable method for detecting reduced myocardial perfusion is to measure myocardial blood flow. In 30 patients with proven coronary heart disease Deanfield et al. demonstrated silent myocardial ischaemia by intravenous administration of rubidium-82 (9). As during episodes of symptomatic ischaemia, during silent myocardial ischaemia there are disorders of regional wall motion which can be demonstrated by ventriculography (10) and this dysfunction may cause an intermittent rise of end diastolic pressure (11). Non-invasive techniques such as echocardiography and radionuclide angiography reveal similar findings (12). The exercise ECG, which gives very reliable results in symptomatic patients, is a much more widely used technique for diagnosing reduced myocardial perfusion (13, 14). On the other hand, if the ST segment during exercise is pathological but there are no analogous anginal symptoms, there is inevitably the quandary as to whether this is a "false positive" finding or silent myocardial ischaemia. Coronary angiography reveals significant coronary stenosis in 22%–72% of these patients (15, 16). Exercise scintiscanning appears to show higher specificity (17). To summarize the published results, silent myocardial ischaemia was confirmed by ventriculography in 29%–75% of patients with coronary heart disease, by the exercise ECG in 17%–47% and by perfusion scintiscanning in 29%–75%. However, this must be qualified by adding that some of these studies did not include the use of invasive procedures to confirm the diagnosis of the underlying cardiac disease (13, review in 18). Long-term electrocardiographic monitoring is being used increasingly for diagnosing silent myocardial ischaemia. This technique enables the patient's ST segment to be analysed continuously during daily life. Although in terms of the method used this technique still poses a number of problems, which will be discussed below, the first published results are very encouraging; altogether 197 patients with coronary heart disease were examined and the frequency of silent ST-segment changes was reported to be 20%–60% (19–21).

Comparison of asymptomatic and symptomatic myocardial ischaemia

It was assumed early on that the underlying pathophysiological processes in symptomatic and asymptomatic myocardial ischaemia are comparable, namely "stable" coronary stenosis, with inadequate myocardial blood flow during exercise, and "dynamic" coronary stenosis, in which the coronary lumen is narrowed as a result of an increase in vessel tone (22, 23). In view of the high incidence of silent myocardial infarction in diabetics (17), it was thought that the lack of symptoms in silent myocardial ischaemia may be because the warning system has failed or is defective (24). However, it was also shown that the majority of patients with coronary heart disease have episodes of symptomatic and of asymptomatic myocardial ischaemia (2, 3, 6, 21). Surprisingly episodes of silent myocardial ischaemia appear to be more prevalent than symptomatic episodes. They occur mainly during the day (25), do not last so long and are of less haemodynamic relevance than symptomatic episodes (2). Nevertheless, we should not underestimate the importance of silent myocardial ischaemia since, among other effects, it has ben observed to raise the left ventricular end diastolic pressure to more than 30 mm Hg. So, there is also the prognostic importance of the two types of compromised myocardial perfusion to consider.

According to published data, annually 7%–65% of patients with coronary artery disease and silent myocardial ischaemia are potential candidates for treatment (12, 18, 20). Systematic studies verify a one-year mortality rate of 0% amongst patients with silent myocardial ischaemia in whom cardiac catheterization was not considered to be indicated (20). On the other hand, the mortality rate was 2.7% amongst patients with angiographically confirmed coronary heart disease and 5% amongst patients with proven three-vessel disease (12, 26). In order to improve the appraisal of the risks and the treatment, Cohn (26) therefore suggested dividing the patients into three groups according to whether or not the silent myocardial ischaemia was associated with simultaneous episodes of symptomatic ischaemia and to whether the patient had had a myocardial infarction.

In the MRFIT study, which included altogether 12 866 patients, the 6-year mortality rate for the 165 patients who only had silent myocardial ischaemia was less than 1%/year (27). However, 3.5% of asymptomatic patients showed angiographic evidence of main-stem stenosis and amongst these patients the one-year mortality rate (10%) was virtually the same as that in a comparison symptomatic group (28).

There are no comparable data for groups of patients with both symptomatic and asymptomatic myocardial ischaemia. The latter type of myocardial ischaemia was not apparent until the introduction of modern long-term electrocardiographic monitoring indicated that 60%–90% of all episodes of myocardial ischaemia appear to be silent (11, 19–21). It is also difficult in prognostic analyses to consider the very different quantitative effect of the symptomatic episodes seperately. However, initial results obtained from this group of patients indicate the appreciable prognostic importance of silent myocardial ischaemia, particularly amongst patients who had also experienced a myocardial infarction.

For example, according to Theroux et al. the one-year mortality rate may be up to 27% in a group of patients of this sort (29).

Techniques and methods for detecting asymptomatic and symptomatic myocardial ischaemia by long-term electrocardiographic monitoring

Thus, clearly it is not adequate for the majority of patients with coronary heart disease to consider completely asymptomatic, coronary patients with silent ischaemia on their own. On the other hand, it is appropriate to detect both forms of ischaemia during daily life and this can be done by means of long-term electrocardiographic monitoring. As was mentioned above, problem-oriented ST-segment analysis had to wait for technical improvements in the recording and analysis equipment. There is no doubt that the long-term ECG systems developed for detecting arrhythmias are only of limited use for analysing ST segments (6, 20, 29, 30). Problems in recording and analysing the ST segment arise firstly because signal transmission in the low-frequency range, which covers most of the ST segment, is often inadequate, and secondly because there is a filter-induced phase shift in the frequencies and there are technical problems in limiting artefacts in the ST-segment analysis. Here, we shall not discuss which has been done to try to optimize the position and stability of the electrodes. With respect to the above problems associated with recording the ST segment on magnetic tape, from the technical point of view, frequency-modulated systems are preferable to amplitude-modulated systems (31). However, since these systems have distinct disadvantages for detecting arrhythmias, amplitude-modulated systems with improved ST-analysis units have also been on trial recently (32–35). These improved amplitude-modulated systems also detect arrhythmias reliably.

Currently we use the amplitude-modulated MK 4 system from Cardiodata. The features of this system which improve ST-segment analysis are a specific ST-segment algorithm, modified "all-pass" frequency filtering and the inclusion of "logical" criteria in the evaluation (32–35). The frequency response of the recording and analysis unit covers ranges from 0.05 to 60 Hertz, and studies by Andresen et al. indicate that the linearity is comparatively high, particularly in the low-frequency range (0.06–20 Hertz, ±3 dB); this complies with the 1985 requirements of the American Heart Association and in some respects it is even superior to frequency-modulated systems (32).

For ST-segment analysis, the investigator fixes two points corresponding to the iso-electric line and the position immediately after the J point. To determine the time course of the ST segment a third measuring point is fixed 60 ms after the second measuring point. Only "dominant" QRS complexes (±10% deviation from the shape of the QRS complex classed as normal) are detected for the analysis (33). A wandering window, containing in each case four QRS-ST complexes, eliminates beat-to-beat ST deviations larger than 0.2 mV and sums up the course of the ST segment over one minute, as long as at least 16 QRS complexes recognized as "dominant" are included. This analysis can be monitored continuously by the investigator or can be done entirely automatically and the results are printed out. Figure 2 shows the trend towards a change in the ST segment detected by this method, with and without the clinical symptoms. Currently, we rate changes in the ST segment of at least 3 minutes duration and a deviation from the iso-electric line of at least 0.15 mV as pathological. The reliability of these criteria has been checked in the exercise ECG and in patients before, during and after PTCA (36).

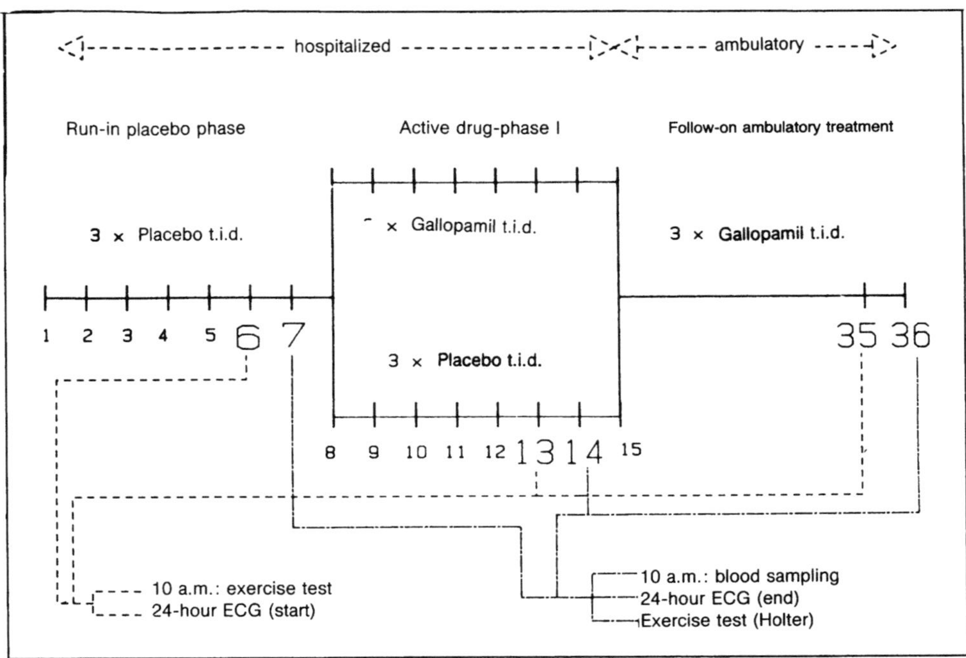

Fig. 1. Trial protocol

Drug treatment of silent and symptomatic myocardial ischaemia

There are only a few published studies on the treatment of silent myocardial ischaemia. Initial results obtained with beta-blockers (review in 26) and nitrates (6) show a clear-cut reduction in the incidence of asymptomatic episodes of ischaemia. The calcium antagonists are amongst the most promising of drugs in this respect and there are reports that patients with asymptomatic myocardial ischaemia respond well to nifedipine (37, 38) and verapamil (38, 39), and to the combination with nitrates (40).

In our study, altogether 21 patients with symptomatic and asymptomatic episodes of ischaemia in the long-term ECG and in the exercise ECG should be treated in a randomized, double-blind placebo vs. gallopamil comparison. All the patients had coronary heart disease confirmed by angiography. Concomitant medication was maintained during the study, but long-acting nitrates and digitalis preparations were not permitted. All the patients received placebo for 7 days, then half of the patients were treated for 7 days with gallopamil 50 mg t.i.d. and the other half of the patients with placebo (Fig. 1). In a third treatment phase, all the patients received gallopamil 50 mg t.i.d. At the end of each of the three treatment phases a 24-hour ECG was recorded and all the patients underwent a standardized exercise test with ECG monitoring. The plasma concentration of gallopamil was also determined at this time.

The trial is still in progress and, up to now, 9 patients have taken part. Compared with placebo, they have shown a clear-cut increase in exercise tolerance under gallopamil. The 24-hour ECG showed a clear-cut reduction of about 40% in the incidence of both symptomatic and asymptomatic myocardial ischaemia (Fig. 3) and the duration of the episodes was reduced.

154

These parameters showed a better response in respect to silent myocardial ischaemia than in symptomatic myocardial ischaemia. Since the trial as a whole has not yet been evaluated, we shall describe the results from one of our patients as an example.

This 59-year-old patient with two-vessel coronary disease (90% stenosis of the interventricular branch of the left coronary artery and 70% stenosis of the circumflex branch) confirmed

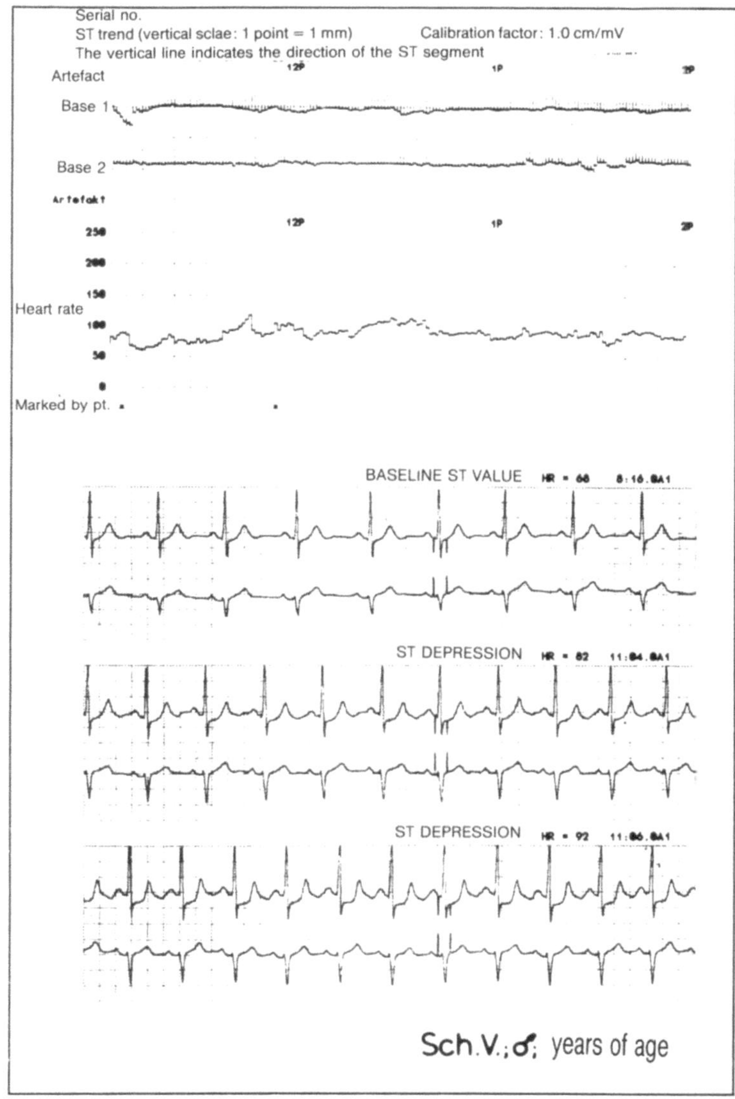

Fig. 2. ST trend in two ECG channels in comparison with the heart rate (top half of Figure). The recording covers a period from 11.00 a.m. to 2.00 p.m. Symptomatic episodes of ischaemia have been marked by the patient below the heart rate. In the plot of the ST trend a downward deviation of 1 cm corresponds to an ST-segment depression of 1 mV. The change in the ST segment is marked by a vertical line. The bottom half of the Figure shows the ECG during exercise, at heart rates of 68, 82 and 92 beats/min. The measurement markers are shown in position.

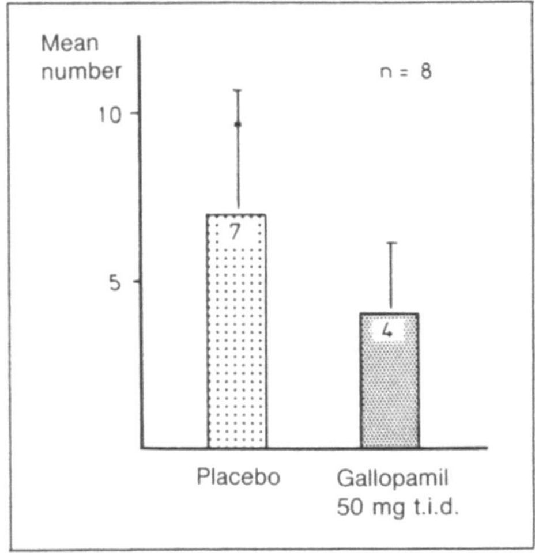

Figure 3. Mean number of episodes with an ST depression of > 0.1 mV and lasting more than 3 minutes in the long-term ECG under placebo and under 50 mg gallopamil t.i.d.

by angiography reported definite anginal symptoms at a low work load. In the exercise ECG there was a pathological ST-segment depression of maximum 0.25 mV while he was exercising at a work load of 100 watts for 2 minutes. The patient did not report any symptoms. The long-term ECG showed altogether 16 episodes in 24 hours with an ST-segment depression of more than 0.15 mV, and each episode lasted for at least 3 min. Nine of these episodes were asymptomatic and the patient marked 7 of the episodes as symptomatic. The mean heart rate during the episodes of silent myocardial ischaemia, 92.5 beats/min, was on average 9.8 beats/min lower than during the symptomatic episodes, when it was 102 beats/min. Overall, the heart rates were distinctly higher than in the phases without myocardial ischaemia, when it was 76 beats/min. Fifteen of the 16 ischaemic episodes occurred during the day.

Under 50 mg gallopamil t.i.d. the patient's exercise tolerance increased from 100 watts for 2 min to 125 watts for 1.5 min, while the maximum heart rate increased from 112 to 120 beats/min. The medication abolished the exercise-related depression of the ST segment (Fig. 4).

Summary

With the improvements in the techniques for ST-segment analysis, long-term electrocardiography is now an important and very promising alternative for detecting silent and symptomatic myocardial ischaemia during daily life. In view of the high incidence of silent myocardial ischaemia in patients with coronary heart disease, this technique will also be used in future for assessing the response to treatment. This application was demonstrated in this study, in which gallopamil was used as the medication.

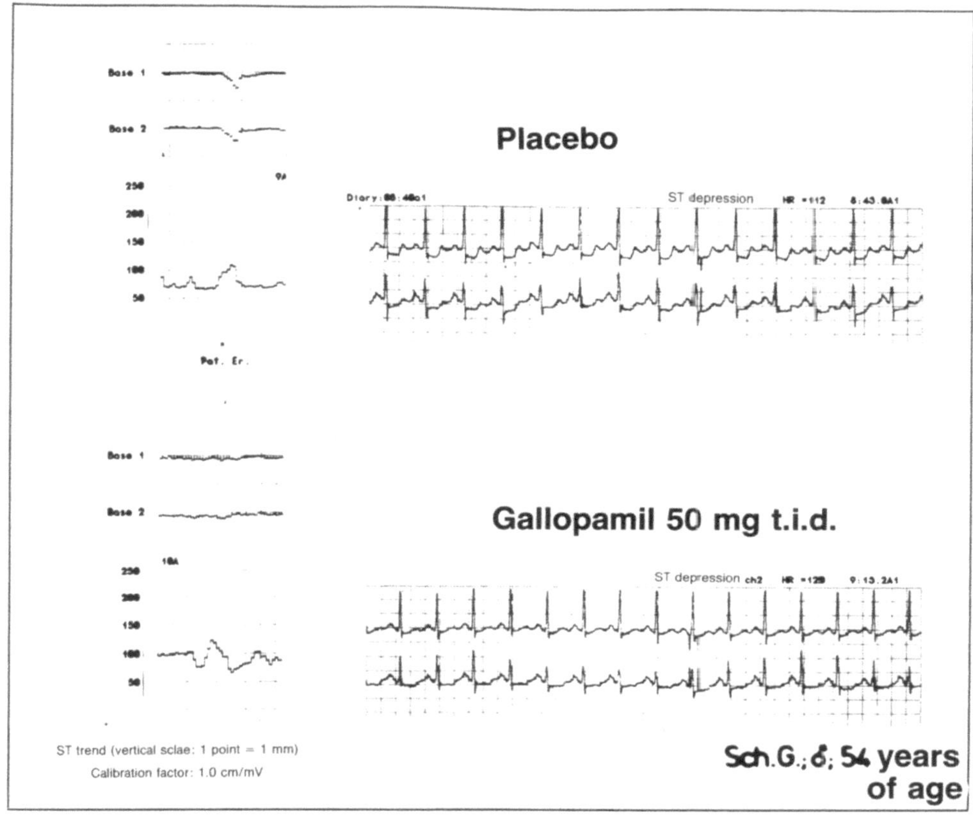

Figure 4. Comparison of the ST trend plot and the heart rate (on the left) and the ST changes during exercise (on the right) under placebo and under gallopamil (50 mg t.i.d.). The work load was 100 watts for 2 minutes (placebo) and 125 watts for 1.5 minutes (gallopamil). In each case the ECG changes were asymptomatic.

References

1. Kannell WB, Abott RD (1984) Incidence and prognosis of unrecognized myocardial infarction: An update on the Framingham study. N Engl J Med 311:1144–1147
2. Cecchi AC, Dovellinie EV, Marchi F, Pucci P, Santoro GM, Fazzini PF (1983) Silent ischemia during ambulatory electrocardiographic monitoring in patients with effort angina. J Am Coll Cardiol 1:934–939
3. Cocco G, Braun S, Strozzi C, Leishman B, Chu D, Rochat N (1982) Asymptomatic myocardial ischaemia in patients with stable and typical angina pectoris. Clin Cardiol 5:403–408
4. Cohn PF (1980) Silent myocardial ischemia in patients with a defective anginal warning system. Am J Cardiol 45:697–702
5. Resnelov I (1985) Silent myocardial ischemia: Therapeutic implications. Am J Med 79:3A.30–34
6. Schang SJ, Pepine CJ (1977) Transient asymptomatic ST-segment depression during daily activity. Am J Cardiol 39:396–402
7. Geft H, Fishbein MC, Ninomiyal K, Hashida J, Chaux E, Yano J, Y-Rit J, Shell W, Ganz W (1982) Intermittent brief periods of ischemia have a cumulative effect and may cause myocardial necrosis. Circulation 66:1150–1153

8. Opie LH (1985) Products of myocardial ischemia and electrical instability of the heart. JACC 5:162B–165B

9. Deanfield JE, Shea M, Ribeiro P, Landsheere CM de, Wilson RA, Horlock P, Selwyn AP (1984) Transient ST-segment depression as a marker of myocardial ischemia during daily life. Am J Cardiol 54:1195–1200

10. Hirzel HO, Leutwyler R, Krayenbuehl HP (1985) Silent myocardial ischemia: Hemodynamic changes during dynamic exercise in patients with proven coronary artery disease despite absence of angina pectoris. J Am Coll Cardiol 6:275–284

11. Grossmann W (1985) Why is left ventricular diastolic pressure increased during angina pectoris? JACC 5:607–608

12. Cohn PF, Harris P, Barry WH, Rosati RA, Rosenbaum P, Waternaux C (1981) Prognostic importance of anginal symptoms in angiographically defined coronary artery disease. Am J Cardiol 47:227–237

13. Bermann JL, Wynne J, Cohn PF (1978) A multivariate approach for interpreting treadmill exercise tests in coronary artery disease. Circulation 52:619–626

14. Lindsey HE, Cohn PF (1978) Silent myocardial ischemia during and after exercise testing in patients with coronary artery disease. Am Heart J 95:441–447

15. Froehlicher VF, Thompson AJ, Longo MR jr., Triebwasser JH, Lancaster MC (1976) Value of exercise testing for screening asymptomatic men for latent coronary artery disease. Prog Cardiovasc Dis 18:265–267

16. Erikssen J, Enge J, Forfang K, Storstein O (1976) False positive diagnostic tests and coronary angiographic findings in 105 presumably healthy males. Circulation 54:371–376

17. Caralis DG, Baley I, Kennedy HL, Pitt B (1979) Thallium-201 myocardial imaging in evaluation of asymptomatic individuals with ischemic ST-segment depression on exercise electrocardiogram. Br Heart J 42:562–567

18. Silber S, Vogler A (1986) Die stumme Myokardischämie: Dimensionierung eines Problems, Intensivmed 23, 2:52–63

19. Ciariello M, Indolfi C, Cotecchia MR, Sifola C, Romano M, Condorelli M (1985) Asymptomatic transient ST changes during ambulatory ECG monitoring in diabetic patients. Am Heart J 110:529–534

20. Stern S, Tzivoni D (1974) Early detection of silent ischemic heart disease by 24-hour electrocardiographic monitoring of active subjects. Br Heart J 36:481–486

21. Wolf E, Tzivoni D, Stern S (1974) Comparison of exercise tests and 24-hour ambulatory electrocardiographic monitoring in detection of ST-T-changes. Br Heart J 36:90–95

22. Freeman IJ, Nixon PGF (1985) Dynamic causes of angina pectoris. Am Heart J 110:1087–1092

23. Maseri A, Chierchia S, Davies G, Glazier J (1985) Mechanism of ischemic cardiac pain and silent myocardial ischemia. Am J Med 79 (Suppl. 3A):7–11

24. Cohn PF (1980) Silent myocardial ischemia in patients with a defective anginal warning system. Am J Cardiol 45:697–702

25. Ouyyumi AA, Mockus L, Wright C, Fox K (1985) Morphology of ambulatory ST-segment changes in patients with varying severity of coronary artery disease. Investigation of the frequency of nocturnal ischemia and coronary spasm. Brit Heart J 53:186–193

26. Cohn PF (1985) Silent myocardial ischemia: Classification, prevalence and prognosis. Am J Med 79 (Suppl 3A):2–6

27. Giagnoni E, Secchi MB, Wu SC, Morabito A, Oltrona I, Mancarella S, Volpin N, Fossa I, Bettazi L, Arangio G, Sachero A, Folli G (1983) Prognostic value of exercise ECG testing in asymptomatic normotensive subjects: A prospective matched study. N Engl J Med 309:1085–1089

28. Deumite NJ, Chaitman BR, Davis KB, Killip T, Frommer PL, Rogers WJ (1985) Asymptomatic left main coronary artery disease (CASS). J Am Coll Cardiol 5:518

29. Bragg-Remschel DA, Anderson CM, Winkle RA (1982) Frequency response characteristics of ambulatory ECG monitoring systems and their implications for ST-segment analysis. Am Heart J 103:20–31

30. Bethge KP, Gonska BD (1985) ST-Segment-Analyse im Langzeit-Elektrokardiogramm: Ist die Methode ausgereift? Dtsch med Wochenschr 26:1023–1024

31. Armin TH (1985) ST-Segment-Analyse im Langzeit-EKG. Dtsch Med Wochenschr 110:1047–1051

32. Brueggemann T, Andresen D, Erbherr G, Schroeder R (1987) Frequenzantwort verschiedener Langzeit-EKG-Systeme im Vergleich zum Standard-EKG. In the press

33. Hubelbank M, Feldman CL, Glasser SP, Clarp PI, Polan BA. ST-Analysis of Holter tapes (1984) IEEE Computers in Cardiology, 269–272

34. Shook TL, Balke W, Kotilainen PW, Selwyn AP, Stone PH (1986) Accuracy of detection of myocardial ischemia by amplitude-modulated and frequency-modulated Holter techniques. JACC 7,2:104A

35. Hubelbank M, Feldman CL, Kotilainen P (1985) The use of computer aided Holter monitoring for detection of ST-changes. IEEE Computers in Cardiology, 515–517

36. Zehender M, Bonzel T, Geibel A, Weiss C, Hohnloser S, Kasper W, Meinertz T, Just H (1986) ST-Strecken und Arrhythmiemonitoring vor, während und nach PTCA. Z Kardiol (Abstract). In the press

37. Cocco G, Strozzi C, Chu D, Amrein R, Castagnoli E (1979) Therapeutic effects of pindolol and nifedipine in patients with stable angina pectoris and asymptomatic resting ischemia. Eur J Cardiol 10:59–69

38. Johnson SM, Mauritson DR, Corbett JR, Woodward W, Wilerson JT, Hillis LD (1981) Doubleblind, randomized, placebo-controlled comparison of propranolol and verapamil in the treatment of variant angina pectoris: Preliminary observations in 10 patients. Am J Cardiol 47:1295–1258

39. Parodi O, Simonetti I, Labbate A, Maseri A (1982) Verapamil versus propranolol for angina at rest. Am J Cardiol 50:923–928

40. Winniford MD, Gabliani G, Johnson SM, Mauritson DR, Fulton KL, Hillis LD (1985) Calcium antagonists for acute ischemic heart disease. Am J Cardiol 55: 116E–124B.

Author's address:

Dr. med. M. Zehender
Innere Medizin III
Hugstetter Str. 55
7800 Freiburg
West Germany

Discussion

BRISSE

If you use these stringent criteria, what percentage of patients with severe or proven coronary heart disease are suitable for this investigation?

MEINERTZ

Not very many. Firstly, not all patients are candidates for angiography and, secondly, even fewer have a normal ECG. We would not use this technique as a method of screening for coronary heart disease. We are of course still at the stage of having to validate the technique and we are using this therapeutic approach, as it were, as a validation method. To answer your question in one sentence, no more than 20% of all our coronary patients are suitable candidates for the examination in this form. No patient with bundle-branch block, with major ECG abnormalities or with absolute arrhythmia associated with atrial fibrillation can be considered, because the problem of eliminating artefacts from the traces of these patients is disproportionately large. Of course, ST-segments analysis is also a problem in patients with frequent, severe arrhythmias.

BENDER

To be quite clear, Dr. Meinertz, please confirm that you analyse the data manually and you only use the long-term ECG to locate points at which the ST is altered?

MEINERTZ

That is what we do at the moment. We can use automatic analysis and we can determine the areas under the ST segment automatically, but to play safe and to check out the system, up to now we have been analysing these data manually. We have measured the times and the amount of change in the ST segment; the computer system can also do this, but in my view it needs checking out beat by beat.

BENDER

Can you say roughly how often you get a false positive from your equipment or from the Oxford system which you usually advocate?

MEINERTZ

I cannot say anything about the Oxford system. The FM system is certainly very good, and published reports corroborate this. This frequency-modulated system has other problems. Quite frankly, to me an amplitude-modulated system is too much like a black box. Admittedly it produces the histograms of the ST segments, but with this system we are neither able to intervene in the automatic analysis, nor can we reproduce all the data rapidly and reliably from the original ECG. We have come across false positive results in a few patients. With the computer, the software is so flexible that we can instruct it to show simply ST-segment changes which persist for 30 seconds, one minute or 3 minutes. This is a very good way of eliminating some of the beat-to-beat artefacts associated with ST-segment changes. We have not observed any false positive results using the 3-minute criteria, although there have been some questionable positive findings. However, this also depends on the programming of the system, on which ST-segment criteria are used; that too is flexible with this system. The analysis points can also be modified. For example, the measurements can be taken at 80 milliseconds after the J point or 60 milliseconds.

FLEISCHMANN

But as a general principle would you not be able to do that with any long-term ECG system? And I am sure you had to have a particular way of positioning the electrodes, didn't you? If they are in the optimum positions, it is possible to use other long-term ECG systems.

MEINERTZ

You have brought up the two most important, critical points, the technical and the physiological. In reply to your second question, certainly the electrodes have to be in the optimum positions. For example, the electrode positions for monitoring ischaemia in the diaphragm region differ from the positions for ischaemia in the anteriolateral region and the shape of the patient's chest also has to be considered. We locate the optimum electrode positions by means of the exercise ECG, and so we have also selected these patients. We know what their ischaemia looks like and we assume, as a hypothesis, that silent ischaemia appears in the ECG exactly as exercise-induced, symptomatic ischaemia. If it is quite different in other ECG leads, then we do not detect it. We have to be quite clear about this; we only detect the ischaemia which resembles exercise-induced ischaemia, but is asymptomatic. There are other problems associated with positioning the electrodes which I do not want to go into now. As regards your first point, about the technique, not all systems give really good reproduction of the ST segment, because with some systems there may be a frequency drop, or at 1 Hz transfer is not linear in terms of the input-output ratio and there may be enormous distortion of the ST segments if there is an overshoot at 40 Hz. You may not determine the J point correctly and if the frequencies above 30 Hz are cut off the amplitude of the QRS complex is reduced. In my opinion, most amplitude-modulated systems are unusable. Certainly they show striking phenomena, enormous rises and falls of the ST segment, but far more often one is hoodwinked by artefacts.

160

Anti-anginal effect of gallopamil versus nifedipine

G. Rettig, S. Sen

Medical Department III, University Hospital and Outpatient Department,
Homburg/Saar
(Director: Prof. Dr. med. L. Bette)

Introduction

Gallopamil is a methoxy derivative of verapamil. It is only in recent years that the anti-anginal properties of verapamil have been systematically researched (4, 5, 7, 9, 10). In previous studies conducted by our group (10) under controlled conditions gallopamil exhibited a dose-dependent anti-ischaemic effect; at a dosage of 50 mg t.i.d. it was both effective and well tolerated. For the trial reported here we therefore used the same dosage schedule to compare the antianginal effect of gallopamil with that of nifedipine, another calcium antagonist used for treating angina.

Patients and method

The study was carried out as a random, double-blind, cross-over trial with altogether 30 patients with stable angina pectoris. It was originally planned to compare 50 mg gallopamil t.i.d. with 20 mg nifedipine t.i.d. However, when 9 patients had participated, the trial had to be stopped because of adverse events in the nifedipine phase (see below). Subsequently, the trial was restarted with a lower dose of nifedipine (10 mg t.i.d.). Twenty-one patients took part in this restarted trial. All the details on method and evaluation of the trial reported below relate to this second trial.

These 21 patients, 20 men and one woman, who were from 42 to 73 years old, average age 56 ± 8, all had angina of effort which had been stable for at least 6 months, with a reproducible horizontal or descending ST-segment depression of at least 0.1 mV in the exercise ECG. Two patients had had an infarction and one patient had had a bypass operation. Coronary heart disease was confirmed by angiography in 16 of the 21 patients. The criteria for exclusion were unstable ischaemic syndromes, such as unstable angina pectoris and/or an infarction within the last 6 months, overt heart failure, bradycardic arrhythmias, sick sinus syndrome and AV blocks, valvular and hypertensive heart disease, disorders of renal function and hepatic function, ECG abnormalities (left ventricular hypertrophy, left bundle-branch block, Wolff-Parkinson-White syndrome) and medications such as digitalis glycosides, beta-blockers, long-acting nitrates, other calcium antagonists and anti-arrhythmic agents which might have resulted in a false positive or false negative interpretation of the ischaemic response in the exercise ECG. The patients were permitted to take nitroglycerin capsules p.r.n. to relieve attacks.

The trial lasted 11 weeks, with 3 one-week single-blind placebo phases separated by the two 4-week active-drug phases. In the active-drug phases the patients received 50 mg gallopamil t.i.d. or 10 mg nifedipine t.i.d. orally in random sequence and then, after the cross-over, the alternative medication. The double-dummy technique was used for administering the

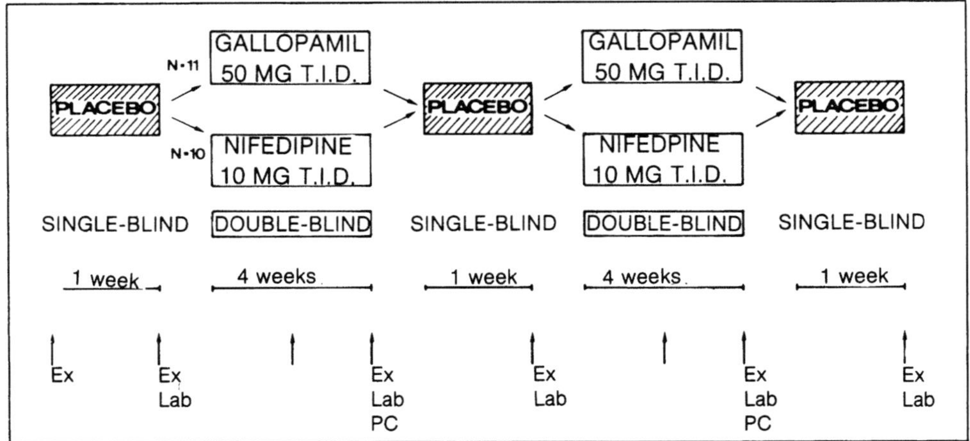

Figure 1. Design of the trial. Ex = exercise, Lab = laboratory tests, PC = plasma concentrations of gallopamil or nifedipine. Arrows = check-up times

medications. There were regular check-ups at the times indicated by the arrows in Figure 1. Exercise tests and the most important laboratory tests were performed at the end of each trial phase. The patients kept a record of when they took their medication, of anginal attacks and of other events, particularly those which may have been adverse reactions to the medication.

The exercise tests, which were symptom-limited, were carried out with the patients seated on a bicycle ergometer. They were performed in the morning, 1–2 h after the last dose of the medication, starting at a work load of 50 W and increasing in 25 W increments every 2 minutes. The ST-segment depression was determined in chest leads V4–V6 0.08 s after the J point, from 5 successive cycles with a stable iso-electric line. The sum of the ST-segment depressions in these leads was used for assessing the data.

The Kruskal-Wallis non-parametric rank test was used to compare the two test drugs. They were considered to be significantly different if the null hypothesis, i.e. the hypothesis that the treatments had the same effect, was rejected with a probability of error of $p < 0.05$.

Results

At the dosage of 20 mg nifedipine t.i.d. selected initially, there was appreciable worsening of the angina in three of the patients and one of them died. Apparently, this patient died suddenly on his way to see his general practitioner because of increasing anginal symptoms. Opening the emergency envelopes containing the randomization codes showed that all 3 patients had experienced these adverse events under nifedipine. The trial, for which 9 patients had already been recruited, was then stopped and a new trial was started with the lower nifedipine dosage of 10 mg t.i.d.

Two of the 21 patients recruited for this trial dropped out because of unstable angina pectoris, one during the initial placebo phase and the other during the nifedipine phase. The results reported here are therefore for the 19 patients who completed the second trial.

162

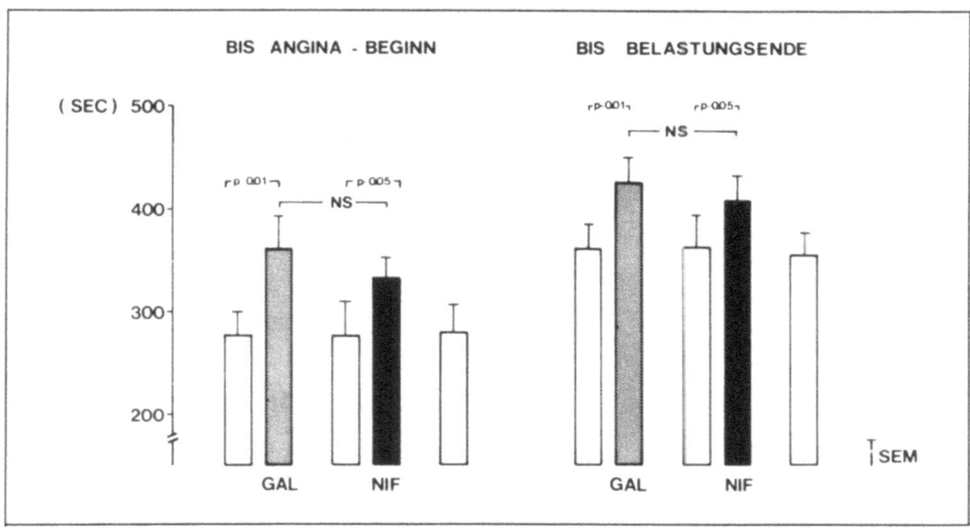

Figure 2. Period of exercising up to the onset of angina and up to the end of the exercise test. The unshaded columns represent the three placebo phases. GAL = gallopamil, NIF = nifedipine, NS = not significant

In the placebo phases the end point of the exercise tests for all 19 patients was angina pectoris. Under gallopamil 4 patients and under nifedipine one patient did not experience angina during exercise and so the test was stopped when the patient was exhausted and/or short of breath.

In terms of the preceding placebo phase, gallopamil increased the period of exercising up to the onset of angina by 30% and up to the discontinuation of the test by 18%; the corresponding figures for nifedipine were 20% and 13% respectively. There was no significant difference between the two medications (Figure 2). As the exercise test protocol was identical in each case, the period of exercising is also representative of the work done. An ischaemic ST-segment depression appeared later under the anti-anginal medication than under placebo and it was less marked, particularly at higher levels of loading (Figure 3). Here again, the trend was for the anti-ischaemic effect of gallopamil to be rather more marked than that of nifedipine.

Comparison of the ST-segment depression at the highest comparable work load, that is to say at the highest level of loading achieved in all phases, revealed a significant, 75% reduction of the ischaemic response under gallopamil and a 51% reduction under nifedipine (Figure 4). By disregarding the placebo phase we can make a direct comparison of the two trial drugs at a higher maximum comparable level of loading. Figure 4 shows that the anti-ischaemic effect of gallopamil was more marked than that of nifedipine, and the difference almost reached the 5% level of statistical significance.

The number of anginal attacks and nitroglycerin consumption were reduced by both medications. However, because these data showed a large variation, neither the comparisons with placebo nor the comparison of the two medications with each other revealed any statistically significant differences.

The blood pressure readings at rest and during exercise were virtually identical in all phases of the trial, whereas the heart rate was somewhat lower under gallopamil than in any other

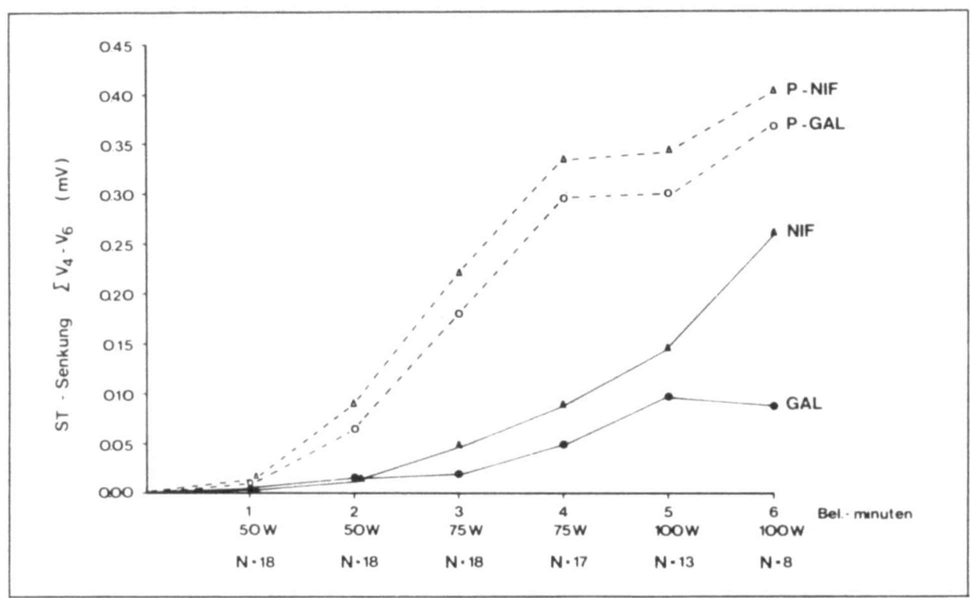

Figure 3. Mean ST-segment depression during the exercise tests. P-NIF and P-GAL = placebo before nifedipine and gallopamil respectively

phase of the trial. Consequently, direct comparison of the trial drugs at the highest comparable work load revealed that the heart rate and the rate-pressure product were significantly lower under gallopamil than the mean values under nifedipine (Figure 5). Altogether, there were fewer reports of adverse reactions (Table 1) under gallopamil (3 specific reports by 3 patients) than under nifedipine (6 patients/13 reports) and under

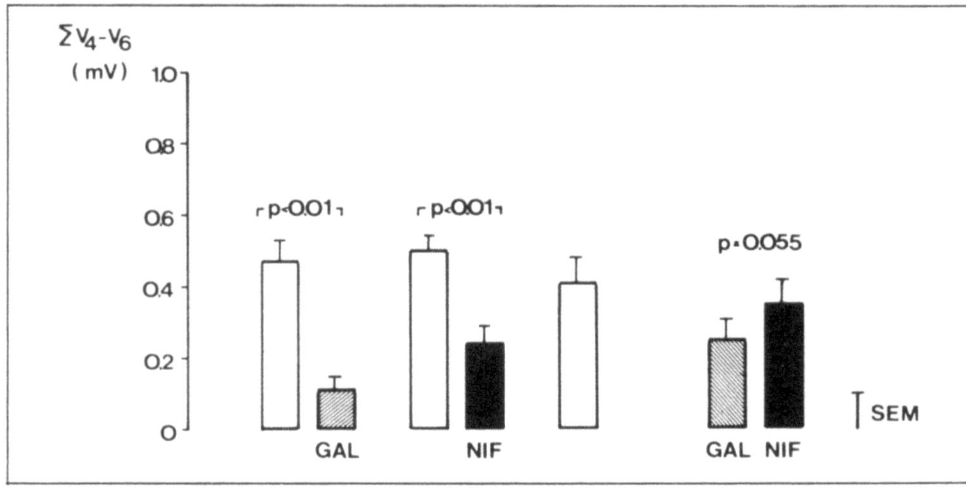

Figure 4. ST-segment depression at the highest comparable work load. On the left including the placebo (unshaded columns), and on the right a direct comparison of gallopamil (GAL) with nifedipine (NIF)

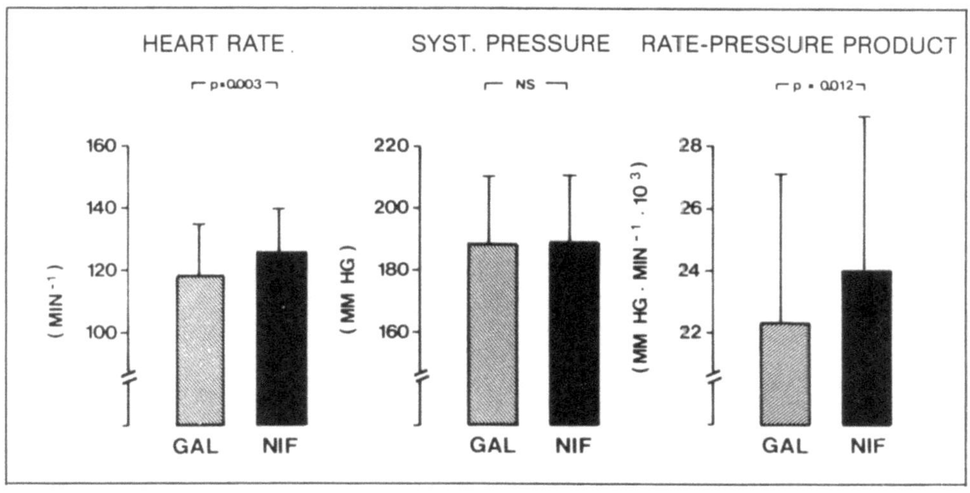

Figure 5. Heart rate, systolic pressure and rate-pressure product at the highest comparable work load under gallopamil (GAL) and nifedipine (NIF). NS = not significant

placebo (10 reports by 6 patients in 3 weeks). If we rule out, as unrelated to the medication, all adverse reactions in the active-drug phases which were also reported by the same patient under placebo the only remaining adverse reaction reported under gallopamil was constipation; the remaining adverse reactions under nifedipine (10 mg t.i.d.) were those known to be associated with peripheral vasodilation, namely leg oedema, headache, restlessness, dizziness, tachycardia and, as mentioned above, exacerbation of the angina. None of the laboratory values were pathological.

Discussion

The results of this study verify the anti-anginal and anti-ischaemic effect of gallopamil, although the trial was not designed to demonstrate the efficacy of gallopamil versus placebo, which has been reported elsewhere (10). The relative merits of gallopamil for treating stable angina pectoris were to be verified by comparing it with an established calcium antagonist. The study showed that gallopamil had a rather more marked effect on the angina and ST-segment depression than nifedipine, the difference between the two medications being on the borderline of statistical significance, and it caused far fewer adverse reactions, so that, overall, gallopamil exhibited an appreciably larger therapeutic index.

Dosage is an important consideration when comparing two anti-anginal drugs, particularly if fixed dosage schedules are used, as was the case in this study. While a single dose of 50 mg gallopamil has been shown to be both effective and well-tolerated (4, 5, 7, 9, 10), there are problems in finding the optimum dose for nifedipine. For example, Bala Subramanian et al. (1, 2) reported that the anti-anginal effect of 10 mg nifedipine t.i.d. was not significant versus placebo, but at the more effective dosage of 20 mg t.i.d, 22% of the patients had to drop out of the study prematurely because of adverse reactions, one notable one being

Table 1. Adverse reactions

	Nifedipine	Gallopamil	Placebo A	C	E	Total, placebo
Pat./adverse reaction	6/13	3/3	3/4	3/5	2/3	6/10
Weakness	1					
Blushing	1					
Headache	1					
Restlessness	1			1		
Dizziness	1					
Sensation of heat	1		1			
Racing heart	1				1	
Leg oedema	1					
Angina pectoris	1		1			
Nervousness	2	1		1		
Sleep disorders				1		
Tiredness		1		1	1	
Constipation		1				
Irregular stool	1					
Stomach pain	1					
Impotence			1			
Neck pain			1		1	
Stress syndrome				1		

exacerbation of the angina. Similar observations have been reported by other groups (3, 6, 8, 12); in addition to the familiar reflex tachycardia, redistribution involving the withdrawal of blood from the region supplied by blocked coronaries bypassed by collaterals has been postulated as a possible explanation for this paradoxical effect of nifedipine (11). We too have observed alarming aggravation of the anginal symptoms under nifedipine and this may actually have been responsible for the death of one of our patients. Although the patient who died had not undergone coronary angiography, blocked vessels bypassed by collaterals were present in all the other patients and, according to Schulz et al. (11), it is this pathological change which increases the risk of paradoxical responses to nifedipine. Also, all the patients showed sometimes pronounced sinus tachycardia at rest and during the exercise tests. Although in itself desirable, for practical reasons we did not carry out dose titration. However, the fact that even the lower dosage of 10 mg nifedipine t.i.d. aggravated the angina of one patient shows that even dose titration would not absolutely guarantee that there would be no adverse reactions of this type.

In contrast, all the patients tolerated gallopamil without any problems. In agreement with the results of Hopf et al. (5), the smaller increase in the rate-pressure product during exercise under gallopamil relative to that under nifedipine suggests that the trend towards a more marked anti-anginal effect under gallopamil may be because, relative to nifedipine, gallopamil reduces myocardial oxygen uptake.

Conclusions

1. The anti-ischaemic effect of gallopamil in patients with stable angina pectoris is at least on a par with that of nifedipine.

2. There is a high incidence of adverse reactions under nifedipine, some of which are serious; consequently, nifedipine has a distinctly smaller therapeutic index.
3. It is therefore rational to combine nifedipine with a beta-blocker, whereas gallopamil may be prescribed as single-drug treatment.

References

1. Bala Subramanian V, Bowles MJ, Khurmi NS, Davis AB, Raftery EB (1982) Rationale for the choice of calcium antagonists in chronic stable angina. An objective double-blind placebocontrolled comparison of nifedipine and verapamil. Am J Cardiol 50:1173–1179
2. Bala Subramanian V, Bowles MJ, Khurmi NS, Davies AB, Raftery EB (1982) Randomized double-blind comparison of verapamil and nifedipine in chronic stable angina. Am J Cardiol 50:696–703
3. Dawson JR, Whitaker NHG, Sutton GC (1981) Calcium antagonist drugs in chronic stable angina. Comparison of verapamil and nifedipine. Br Heart J 46:508–512
4. Hopf R, Becker HJ, Kober G, Dowinsky S, Kaltenbach M (1982) Therapie der Angina pectoris mit Calcium-Antagonisten. Herz/Kreisl 4:221–234
5. Hopf R, Drews H, Kaltenbach M (1983) Die antianginöse Wirkung von Gallopamil im Vergleich zu Nifedipin. In: Kaltenbach M, Hopf R (eds) Gallopamil. Springer Berlin Heidelberg New York Tokyo, pp. 126–135
6. Jariwalla AG, Anderson EG (1978) Production of ischemic pain by nifedipine. Br Med J 1:1181–1182
7. Khurmi NS, O'Hara MJ, Bowles MJ, Bala Subramanian V, Raftery EB (1984) Randomized double-blind comparison of gallopamil and propranolol in stable angina pectoris. Am J Cardiol 53:684–688
8. Müller HS, Chahine RA (1981) Interim report of multicenter double-blind placebo-controlled studies of nifedipine in chronic stable angina pectoris. Am J Med 71:645–657
9. Niemelä L, Mitrovic V, Neuss H, Schlepper M (1982) Zur antianginösen Wirkung des Calcium-Antagonisten Gallopamil. Herz/Kreisl 14:611–616
10. Rettig G, Sen S (1983) Akut- und Langwirkungen von Gallopamil (D 600) bei stabiler Angina pectoris – eine randomisierte Doppelblindstudie. Z Kardiol 72:746–754
11. Schulz W, Jost S, Kober G, Kaltenbach M (1985) Relation of antianginal efficacy of nifedipine to degree of coronary arterial narrowing and to presence of coronary collateral vessels. Am J Cardiol 55:26–32
12. Uusitalo A, Arstila M, Bac EA, Härkönen R, Keyriläinen O, Rytkönen U, Schjeldrup-Mathiecsen PM, Wendelin H (1986) Metoprolol, nifedipine and the combination in stable effort angina pectoris. Am J Cardiol 57:733–737

Author's address:

Prof. Dr. med. G. Rettig
Medizinische Universitäts- und Poliklinik
Lehrstuhl Innere Medizin III
Landeskrankenhaus
D–6650 Homburg/Saar
West Germany

Discussion

FLEISCHMANN

How long after administration was the exercise ECG recorded?

RETTIG

Two to 3 hours after the morning dose of the medication.

FLEISCHMANN

Adverse reactions are invariably our problem, too. Each patient has to be seen individually and it is sometimes dangerous to allocate a patient like this to a nifedipine group by slavishly following the schedule. You have to pick out the suitable patients.
There are always patients with a comparatively high heart rate and if they are given nifedipine there is the risk of provoking angina.

RETTIG

That is the disadvantage of trials with a rigid schedule. Of course, you can also do it the other way round, starting with 10 mg t.i.d., like Bala Subramanian find nothing and then go on to 20 mg t.i.d. We chose the reverse approach. These adverse reactions can occur even with 10 mg t.i.d. But you are quite right, a patient should not be prescribed single-drug treatment with nifedipine without due consideration and care. Of course, there is the possibility of combined treatment.

BENDER

The problem you have discussed besets many double-blind trials.

HEUSCH

In my talk yesterday I pointed out that there are two key mechanisms, particularly in exercise-induced angina pectoris. These are tachycardia and putative alpha-adrenoceptor-mediated coronary constriction of the ischaemic vessels. The tachycardia redistributes the flow of blood from the ischaemic vessels to the non-ischaemic vascular bed. There is no withdrawal of blood as you put it; the blood flow is redistributed. If we base our arguments on these two mechanisms, gallopamil and nifedipine have a completely different mechanism of action and it is quite by chance that they both have an anti-anginal effect. In fact we must assume that the underlying effect of nifedipine is that it prevents coronary constriction. If tachycardia is the predominant mechanism it is likely that there will be deleterious effects of this sort. Conversely, with gallopamil, I would assume, without having done any studies of my own, that the negative chronotropic effects predominate. So, looked at in pathophysiological terms, I do not believe that a comparative study of this sort is very felicitous. Either the drugs must be compared at the same heart rate or they must be used in different patients with a different indication. Comparing them at the same levels of loading does not solve the problem.

RETTIG

Based on our results, I agree entirely with your conclusions. In fact, it will not be possible just to prescribe the two drugs for treating angina pectoris; distinctions will have to be made. I believe that the value of a study of this sort is that it shows that you can not make an all-embracing comparison of different calcium antagonists; you have to be much more discriminating.

BENDER

Dr. Heusch, do you think this also applies at a lower heart rate, in other words in circumstances in which nifedipine will probably increase the heart rate more than gallopamil? Or ought one always to set a mean heart rate? Is an absolutely identical heart rate the correct basis on which to make a comparison?

HEUSCH

I am no clinician. I would assume that under clinical conditions the decision whether to prescribe nifedipine or gallopamil must be based on the patient's needs, in other words, whether the primary objective is to bring down the heart rate or whether the underlying pathology is not considered to be related to the heart rate, in which case nifedipine is prescribed. When comparing the two drugs we must consider whether the comparison is being made at the same work load or at the same heart rate. Gallopamil will come out better at the same work load, because it reduces the heart rate. At the same heart rate nifedipine will probably come out better, because it has anti-ischaemic effects which do not rely on reducing the heart rate. So, it depends on what you are actually comparing and, in the final analysis, it is so difficult to draw any conclusions that in my opinion it is impossible to see in them any therapeutic implications apart from the fact that the drugs can not be regarded as interchangeable when you are prescribing for a specific patient.

BENDER

Another question for Dr. Heusch. Is it always correct to assume that when there is an increase in heart rate there is also an increase in alpha-adrenoceptor-mediated coronary tone? In other words, is the heart rate such a reliable guide?

HEUSCH

The heart rate is not a reliable guide. But the heart rate is easy to measure and, generally speaking, is a prominent feature, that is to say if the patient presents with pronounced tachycardia associated with exercise-induced ischaemia it is rational to start by doing something to control the tachycardia. However, if there is no response there is a definite alpha-adrenergic component. In my paper there is a Figure which shows that, at an identical heart rate, phentolamine reduced the ischaemic ST-segment depression in a patient.

KLEIN

Could you have anticipated which patients would deteriorate under nifedipine, from an excessively low blood pressure or from their heart rate, or was this actually a complete surprise? Secondly, did the patients in whom there was an increase in the incidence of angina show a better response to other calcium antagonists of the verapamil type?

RETTIG

It would not have been possible to identify these patients, even in retrospect. One does not just have patients with very slow or fast heart rates. These patients complain of angina at a heart rate of 115 and 130/min and so are in the grey area which we so often come across. We did not treat these patients with other calcium antagonists; we followed on with beta-blockers.

BALA SUBRAMANIAN

I do not believe that the gulf between the theoretical and practical is so large as regards nifedipine. I would like to add some data to the facts discussed by Dr. Heusch. We have clearly identified three mechanisms as possible causes of the increased incidence of angina under nifedipine. One of them is tachycardia, the second is marked hypotension and the third is inadequate perfusion in narrowed coronary vessels owing to coronary steal. In my talk I will also quote typical examples. However, it is not possible to predict how the patient will respond, on the basis of the heart rate. The simplest way is to give a low dose such as 10 mg nifedipine and observe whether the incidence of angina reported by the patient increases in the ensuing 6 hours. The cause is hastened absorption from the intestine; this produces extremely high serum levels of nifedipine in these patients. Secondly, in a verapamil-versus-nifedipine study, we took a very detailed look at the ST-segment responses in relation to heart rate. One point which we looked at more closely was the beat-to-beat increase in the heart rate during exercise. We calculated the overall ST-segment changes per increase in each beat. In this analysis, drugs such as verapamil and diltiazem came out much better than nifedipine and nicardipine. The conclusion to be drawn, as has been quite rightly stated already, is that the calcium antagonists act by more than one or two mechanisms and that the mechanism of action of drugs like diltiazem and verapamil is probably multimodal, which explains their superior effect on parameters of both silent and exercise-induced ischaemia.

Clinical and electrocardiographic effects of gallopamil and nifedipine in patients with coronary heart disease receiving basic treatment with ISDN

G. Bachour

Outpatient Department (Internal Medicine and Cardiology), Ahlen

Introduction

Unfortunately, an anti-anginal medicine often fails to satisfy the clinical and pharmacological needs, namely oral administration and patient-specific dosage, a long-lasting and reproducible effect with no untoward effects on regulator systems and, if at all possible, no adverse effects on the patient's general well-being. The increase in the effectiveness of a drug, or the "response curve", becomes increasingly flat at higher doses. However, raising the dosage markedly increases the incidence of adverse reactions.

Nitrates, calcium antagonists and beta-adrenoceptor blockers are the main groups of drugs used to treat coronary heart disease. It is often necessary to combine two or all three of these types of drugs to achieve a satisfactory therapeutic response. One advantage of combined therapy is that it may make it possible to increase efficacy by exploiting the synergistic effects of different drugs. Avoiding the need to use very high dosages of single drugs may also substantially reduce the incidence of substance-specific complications.

We therefore set out to investigate the efficacy of calcium antagonists in patients who did not show a satisfactory response to single-drug treatment with nitrates.

Patients and method

Twenty patients with coronary heart disease (CHD), confirmed by clinical examination and electrocardiography, took part in the trial. The treatment was stopped prematurely in two patients because of adverse reactions. Thus, the data from 18 patients were evaluated. Six of these patients were women and 12 were men. They were from 40 to 64 years of age, between 165 and 183 cm tall and weighed between 67 and 96 kg (Table 1).

Nine patients had had a myocardial infarction, but not in the 6 months before the start of the study. Another patient had an aortocoronary bypass operation. Six patients had arterial hypertension, which was well controlled by diuretics. Three patients had had NYHA class II myocardial failure. Many of the patients were known to have metabolic disorders: 9 had hyperlipidaemia, 4 had diabetes mellitus and one had hyperuricaemia. Two patients had moderately severe bronchopulmonary diseases and 2 had a strumectomy or radio-iodine

Table 1. Information about the patients (n = 18; 6 f, 12 m)

	Mean	Min.	Max.
Age [years]	56	40	64
Height [cm]	173	165	183
Weight [kg]	79	67	96

therapy for hyperthyroidism. One patient had a rheumatoid condition and one had nephrolithiasis.

Accordingly, the patients were receiving very different concurrent medications. However, patients taking drugs with electrocardiographic effects, particularly digitalis glycosides or beta-adrenoceptor blockers, were excluded from the trial, as were patients with an ionic imbalance between intracellular and extracellular fluid, severe kidney or liver disease or class III or IV myocardial failure.

All the patients were receiving 20 mg slow-release isosorbide dinitrate t.i.d., but nevertheless still experienced exercise-induced angina pectoris. In an exercise test they showed a pathological horizontal to descending ST-segment depression of more than 0.1 mV. The exercise tolerance of the patients in the study was always limited by angina pectoris. The frequency of anginal attacks and nitroglycerin consumption were determined over a period of one week and the baseline data were then measured. In a within-patient, double-blind, randomized, cross-over study the data were obtained under the same standardized conditions with the patients in the recumbent position on the same ergometer, after 4 weeks' add-on treatment with 50 mg gallopamil t.i.d. or 10 mg nifedipine t.i.d. (Table 2).

Table 2. Trial design

ISDN retard	20 mg t.i.d.
Gallopamil	50 mg t.i.d.
Nifedipine	10 mg t.i.d.
Run-in phase:	2 weeks on ISDN retard
Trial phase A:	4 weeks add-on gallopamil or nifedipine
Cross-over trial	
phase B:	4 weeks add-on gallopamil or nifedipine
Check-ups at the end of the	run-in phase:
	Trial phase A
	Trial phase B

Results

In the week prior to the baseline exercise test the patients had on average 6.6 *anginal attacks* and took on average 8.3 *buccal doses* of 0.8 mg *nitroglycerin.* Under the add-on treatment with the calcium antagonists gallopamil or nifedipine, in the 4th week there was, on average, a highly significant reduction of more than 60% in the two parameters, to 2.6 anginal attacks and to 2.9 or 3.2 doses of nitroglycerin (Table 3).

The *average ST-segment depression* in the 3 chest leads V3, V4 and V5 was used as a measure of the ischaemic response in the exercise test. The means and standard deviations calculated from these data for each group were analysed statistically. At a comparable work load, that is to say for the same level and duration of exercise, at all check-ups the mean ST-segment was reduced to on average 0.16 ± 0.05 mV under the treatment with ISDN retard alone. At the maximum work load, that is to say at the end of the exercise test, which was always defined by the occurrence of angina pectoris, the ST-segment depression was on average 0.20 ± 0.05 mV under single-drug treatment with ISDN retard. Immediately after the exercise test there was on average no change in the ischaemia. In the second minute of recovery the ischaemia showed a clear-cut tendency to reverse (Fig. 1).

172

Table 3. Frequency of anginal attacks and nitroglycerin consumption reduced by combining ISDN retard with gallopamil or nifedipine

	Angina pectoris [attacks/week]	Nitrate consumption [doses/week]
ISDN retard 20 mg t.i.d.	6.6	8.3
Gallopamil 50 mg t.i.d. + ISDN retard 20 mg t.i.d.	2.6	2.9
Nifedipine 10 mg t.i.d. + ISDN retard 20 mg t.i.d.	2.6	3.2

After add-on treatment with gallopamil or nifedipine for 4 weeks there was on average a significant reduction in the mean ST-segment depression of about 37% at a comparable work load ($\bar{x} \pm s = 0.10 \pm 0.05$ mV) and of about 30% at the maximum work load ($\bar{x} \pm s = 0.14 \pm 0.06$ mV). There was no difference in the effect of the two calcium antagonists.

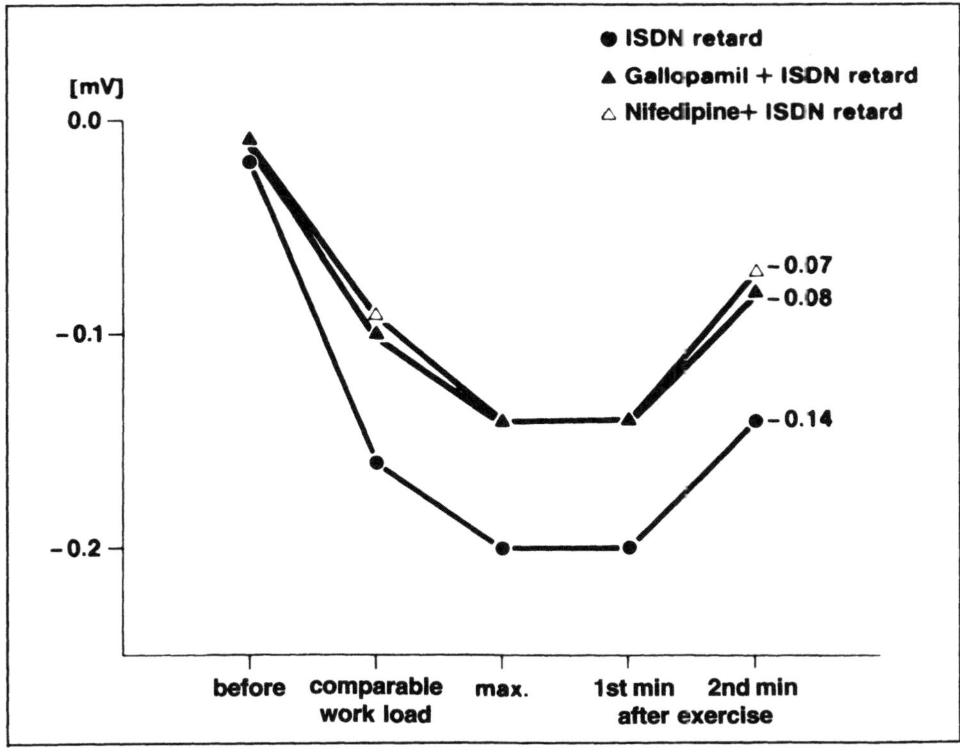

Figure 1. ST-segment depression during exercise tests reduced by combining ISDN retard with gallopamil or nifedipine

The severity of the coronary heart disease in our group of patients is more obvious if we consider the maximum ST-segment depressions in one of the chest leads. Under treatment with ISDN retard alone, at the end of the exercise test the depressions were 0.16–0.42 mV ($\bar{x} \pm s = 0.25 \pm 0.06$ mV). Under the add-on treatment with gallopamil or nifedipine, the beneficial effect on the ST-segment response during exercise was in the same ratio as the average ST-segment changes.

The *heart rate,* at rest or during the exercise tests, was the same under the single-drug treatment with ISDN retard and under the combined treatments with gallopamil or nifedipine (Fig. 2).

Under ISDN retard, the *systolic pressure* was normal at rest and during the exercise tests. After add-on treatment with gallopamil or nifedipine, there was a slight reduction in systolic pressure; there was no appreciable difference in the effect of the two calcium antagonists (Fig. 3)

Indirect measurements of the exertional *diastolic pressure* taken with the aid of a cuff and the Korotkoff sounds are liable to large errors. Consequently, the reliability of this parameter is a very vexed question, particularly if drugs which modify vascular tone have been administered. We shall not, therefore, discuss this parameter here.

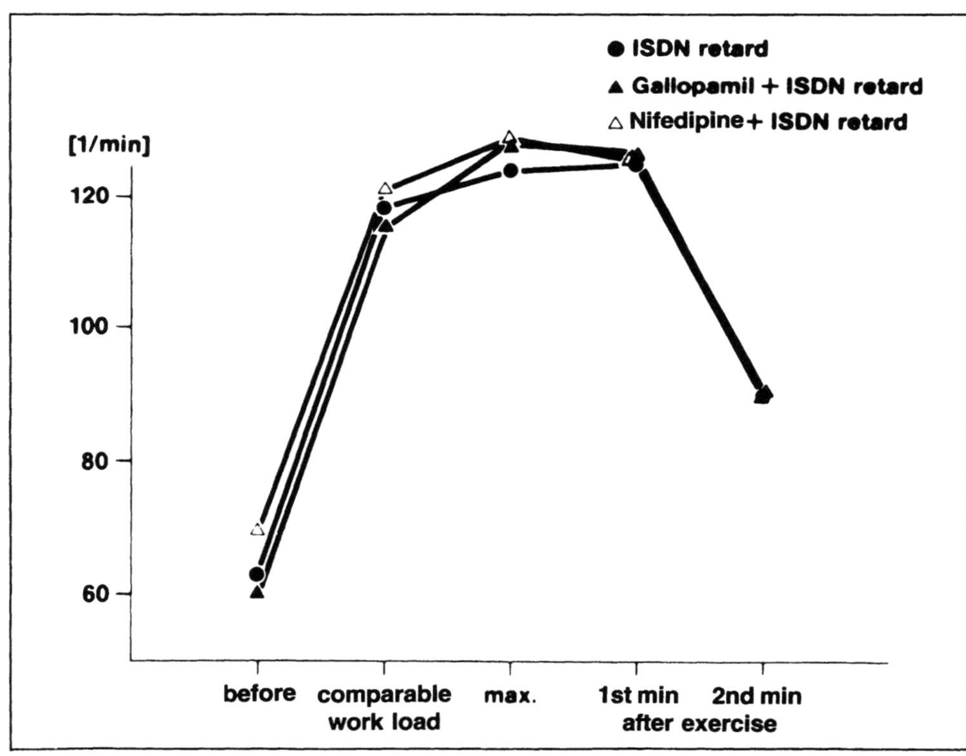

Figure 2. Heart rate at rest and during exercise on an ergometer under single-drug treatment with ISDN retard and under ISDN retard combined with gallopamil or nifedipine

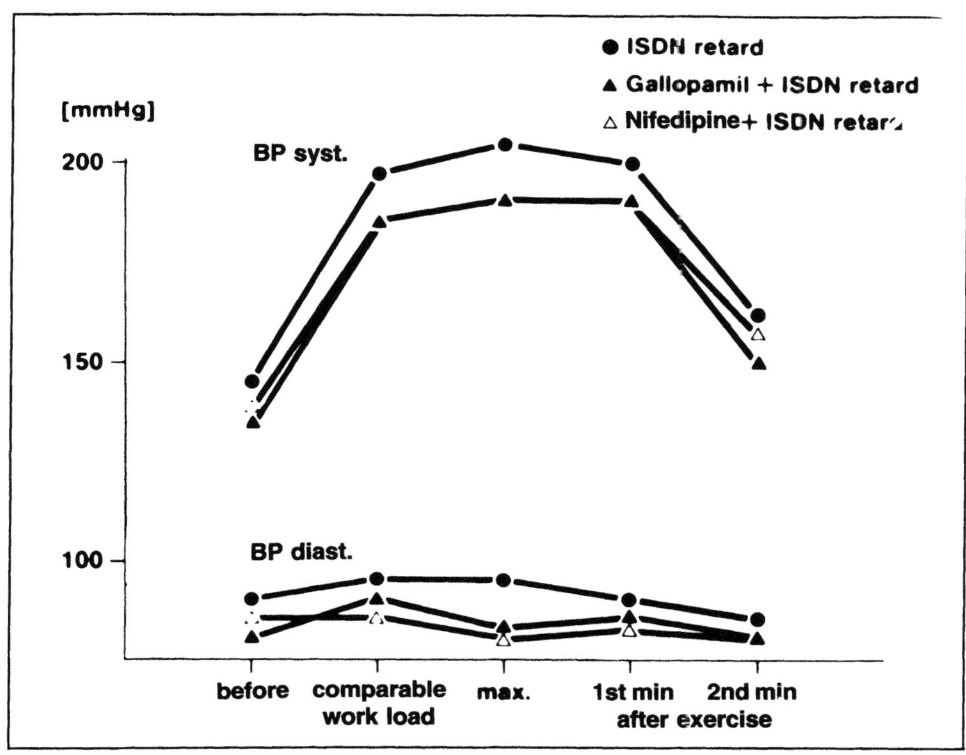

Figure 3. Systolic pressure at rest and during exercise on an ergometer moderately reduced by combining ISDN retard with gallopamil or nifedipine

The supplementary use of gallopamil or nifedipine only caused a minimal, non-significant reduction of about 5%–11% in the *rate-pressure product* as compared with the data obtained under the single-drug treatment with ISDN retard. Here too, there was no evidence of any difference in the effectiveness of the two calcium antagonists. From a mean baseline of 486 ± 177 watts/min, there was a clear-cut, 13% increase in the *work done* under add-on treatment with gallopamil and an increase of 21% under nifedipine (Fig. 4).

In two patients, during the first week of treatment there were *adverse reactions* which necessitated stopping the trial prematurely. About 1–2 hours after taking gallopamil, one 64 year-old patient reported inner unrest, more frequent exertional dyspnoea and that he tired rapidly, although he did not experience his familiar anginal attacks. He stopped the medication on the 4th day, whereupon these symptoms disappeared. Another male patient, who was 66 years old, experienced headaches, a sensation of heat, palpitations, unrest and smarting of the skin on his arms and legs about 30 minutes to one hour after taking 10 mg nifedipine. When the single dose was reduced to 5 mg he experienced no adverse reactions and they did not recur when the dose was increased two weeks later to 10 mg t.i.d. Both patients were excluded from the study. No other significant or persistent adverse reactions were observed.

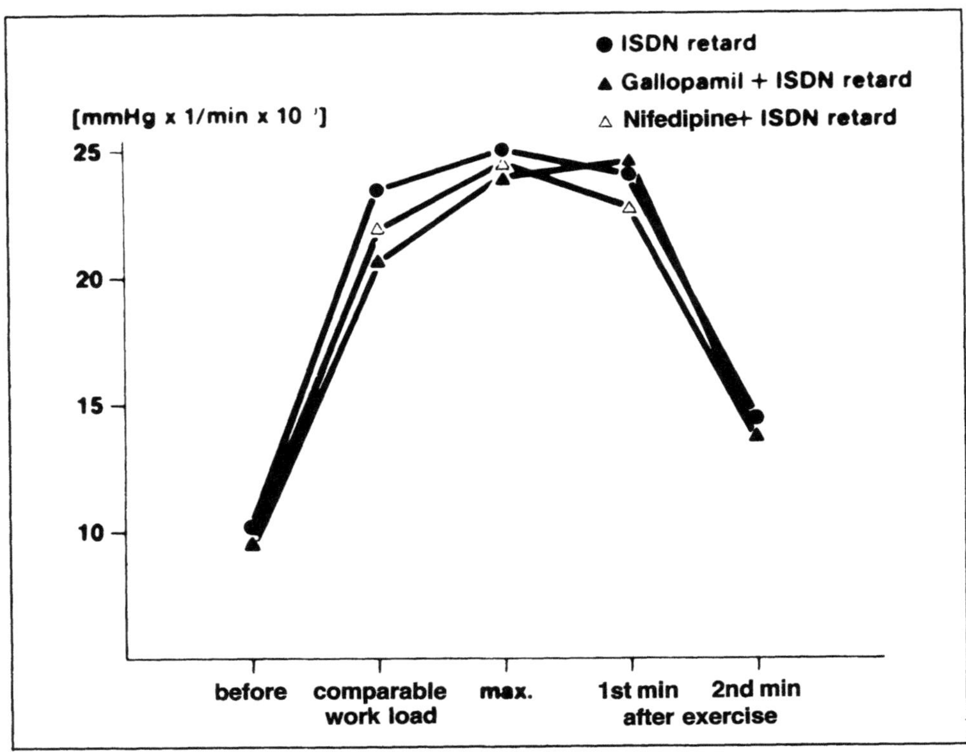

Figure 4. Rate-pressure product at rest and during exercise on an ergometer under single-drug treatment with ISDN retard and under ISDN retard combined with gallopamil or nifedipine

Discussion

In a within-patient, double-blind, randomized, cross-over trial the anti-anginal efficacy of 4 weeks' add-on treatment with the calcium antagonists gallopamil (50 mg t.i.d.) or nifedipine (10 mg t.i.d.) was investigated in 18 patients with coronary heart disease confirmed by clinical examination and electrocardiography. All the patients were receiving basic medication with a slow-release isosorbide dinitrate preparation (20 mg t.i.d.), but they still experienced frequent, exercise-induced angina pectoris and showed reproducible ischaemia responses in exercise tests.

The add-on treatment with a calcium antagonist resulted in a highly significant reduction of more than 60% in the weekly incidence of anginal attacks and in the weekly nitroglycerin consumption. This is consistent with the results of trials to investigate the efficacy of gallopamil or nifedipine used on their own for the treatment of coronary heart disease; as a rule, single-drug treatment was investigated in these trials (1, 2, 3, 5).

The add-on treatment with the calcium antagonists gallopamil or nifedipine resulted in a highly significant reduction in the ST-segment depression which still occurred under the single-drug treatment with ISDN retard during the exercise tests. At a comparable work load, that is to say at the same level and duration of exercising, both drugs reduced the ST-segment depression by about 37%. At the maximum work load, which was always defined

176

by the occurrence of angina pectoris, the add-on treatment with the calcium antagonists resulted in a reduction in the ST-segment depression of about 30%. Bearing in mind all the differences in method, this is consistent with the results obtained by Kaltenbach's team, who found no significant difference between gallopamil and nifedipine in terms of their effect on the ST-segment depression (1). Add-on treatment with gallopamil increased the work done by 13% and add-on nifedipine treatment increased it by 21%. Treatment with the calcium antagonists gallopamil or nifedipine resulted in a minimal reduction of the systolic pressure at rest and during exercise on the ergometer. The heart rate and the rate-pressure product were in the main unchanged; this is consistent with the results of Rettig et al. (4).

For patients with coronary disease, in terms of anti-anginal efficacy the combined use of a nitrate and calcium antagonist was preferable to single-drug treatment with a nitrate. There was no difference in the efficacy of the two trial combinations, namely gallopamil plus ISDN retard and nifedipine plus ISDN retard.

References

1. Hopf R, Drews H, Kaltenbach M (1983) Die antianginöse Wirkung von Gallopamil im Vergleich zu Nifedipin. In: Kaltenbach M, Hopf R (eds) Gallopamil. Springer, Berlin Heidelberg New York Tokyo, p. 127
2. Jansen W, Osterspey A, Schell U, Hombach V, Fuchs M, Tanchert M, Hilger HH (1983) Hämodynamik und Belastbarkeit von Koronarpatienten unter akuter und chronischer Behandlung mit Nifedipin. Herz/Kreislauf 15:159
3. Niemelä L, Mitrovic V, Neuss H, Schlepper M (1982) Zur antianginösen Wirkung des Kalziumantagonisten Gallopamil. Herz/Kreislauf 14:611
4. Rettig G, Sen S, Schieffer H, Bette L (1983) Akut- und Langzeitwirkungen von Gallopamil (D 600) bei stabiler Angina pectoris – Eine randomisierte Doppelblindstudie. Z. Kardiol 72:746
5. Bala Subramanian V (1985) Vergleichende Untersuchung von Gallopamil und 6 weiteren Ca^{++} Antagonisten mit Placebo und Propranolol bei Patienten mit chronisch stabiler Angina pectoris. Z Kardiol u Angiol 17:20

Author's address:

Prof. Dr. med. George Bachour
Internistisch-kardiologische Ambulanz
Karlstr. 4
D–4730 Ahlen
West Germany

Discussion

BENDER

Dr. Bachour, with combined treatments you always have to bear in mind the question of dosage. You used 10 mg nifedipine three times a day. Had you previously tried a higher dosage of nifedipine for these patients?

BACHOUR

We know, and it was clear just now from the discussion about the talk given by Dr. Rettig, that adverse reactions are more frequent with a higher dosage of nifedipine. The dose is normally 10 mg. Some of the patients had already had calcium antagonists, but not in the last two weeks.

Assessment of gallopamil (D 600) in patients with chronic stable angina pectoris
Results of a placebo-controlled single-blind study

G. Specchia, F. Cobelli*, L. Tavazzi**, S. De Servi, M. Ferrario, S. Ghio, C. Opasich*, G. Riccardi*

Divisione di Cardiologia Policlinico S. Matteo (IRCCS) Pavia
* Fondazione Clinica Lavoro di Pavia (IRCCS): Centro Medico di Montescano (PV)
** Fondazione Clinica Lavoro di Pavia (IRCCS): Centro Medico di Veruno (NO)

The anti-anginal effects of calcium antagonists are due to a reduction of myocardial oxygen uptake and/or an improvement of oxygen supply to the myocardium, depending on the affinity of the drug to specific sites of action and differences in the pathogenesis of the myocardial ischaemia.

D 600 is a new calcium antagonist which differs from verapamil only by the addition of a methoxyl group. As a result of this modification of the molecule, D 600 is five to six times more potent than verapamil (1, 2).

D 600 has been shown to increase the exercise tolerance of patients with stable, exercise-induced angina (3, 4, 5, 6, 7). The anti-anginal effect of D 600 appears to be related to an improvement in the myocardial oxygen balance. However, the mechanisms responsible for the anti-ischaemic effect, and the tolerance in D 600 in patients who had suffered an acute myocardial infarction (AMI) still required investigation.

A multicentre study on exercise-induced angina pectoris was carried out on collaboration with the Cardiology Department of the Policlinico S. Matteo, Pavia (IRCCS) and the Cardiology Departments of the Medical Rehabilitation Centres in Montescano and Veruno (Fondazione Clinica Lavoro di Pavia IRCCS).

Twenty-nine patients, 28 men and one woman, who had had an acute moyocardial infarction were recruited for the study. They were between 41 and 65 years of age (on average 54 ± 5.3).

Thirty days after the acute myocardial infarction, the patients underwent an initial symptom-limited exercise test in the sitting position on a bicycle ergometer. The initial work load was 25 watts and this was increased in 25-watt increments every 3 minutes. Part of the study was a wash-out phase for which beta-blockers and verapamil were withdrawn 7 days, and nifedipine and nitrates 24 hours before the first exercise test.

During the exercise tests, all the patients showed an ST-segment depression of at least 1 millimetre. This was associated with pain in 12 patients and was asymptomatic in 17.

A second exercise test was carried out within 2 days, in order to verify the stability of the ischaemia threshold, which was expressed as a variability of not more than maximal ± 20% of the double product at 1-mm ST-segment depression from two exercise tests.

In the cross-over single-blind trial all the patients were to undergo two treatment phases, either with the trial medication (50 mg t.i.d.) or with placebo. Further exercise tests were carried out on the 7th day and 14th day after the administration of D 600 or placebo (Figure 1).

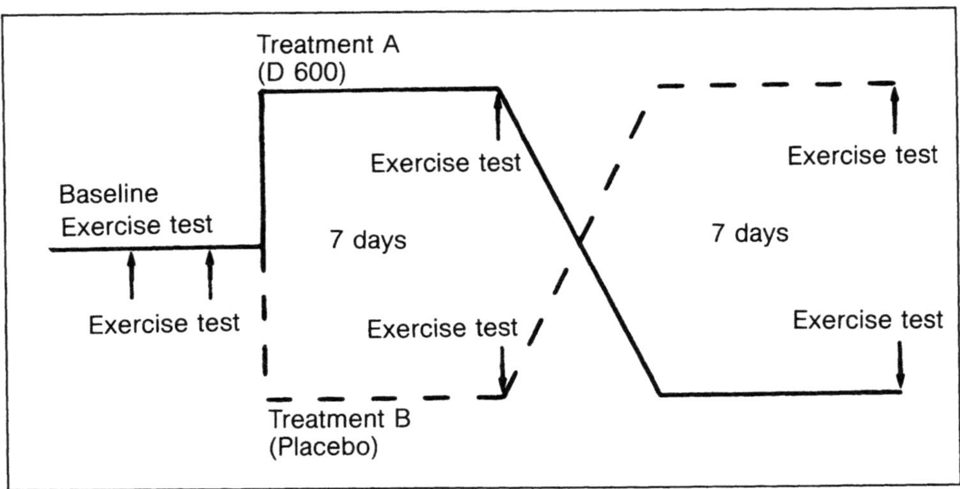

Figure 1. Protocol for single-blind study

Altogether 4 patients dropped out of the study, 2 because of a skin rash, one because of anginal pain under placebo and the fourth because of 1st degree AV block after gallopamil. During the run-in phase none of the 25 patients who completed the study showed significant changes of heart rate, blood pressure or in the double product, either at rest or during exercise. Nor were there any significant changes in the exercise time, the mean ST-segment depression at the maximum work load or in the double-product ischaemia threshold. Thus, the response to D 600 could be assessed by comparison with the mean values for the parameters measured in the two exercise tests in the run-in phase (Table 1).

In comparison with placebo, treatment with D 600 did not alter the resting heart rate, systolic blood pressure or double product.

However, D 600 significantly increased the exercise time (12.6 ± 0.5 vs 10.9 ± 0.7; $p < 0.01$) and the elapsed time before the ischaemia threshold was reached (ST depression $= 1$ mm), (9.4 ± 1.1 vs 7 ± 1; $p < 0.01$). At the maximum work load, D 600 reduced the maximum ST depression (1.2 ± 0.2 vs 1.7 ± 0.1) without significantly altering the double-product ischaemia threshold (249 ± 20 vs 213 ± 14; ns).

A provisional conclusion from analysing these data is that D 600 increased the exercise tolerance of patients with chronic stable angina pectoris following acute myocardial infarction, probably by reducing myocardial oxygen uptake.

This conclusion appears to be confirmed by the results of another study on the effect of D 600 on blood flow in the coronary sinus during myocardial ischaemia induced by atrial pacing (8).

Ten patients with chronic stable angina pectoris and angiographically proven coronary heart disease (stenosis $\geq 75\%$), in all cases involving the proximal portion of the interventricular branch of the left coronary artery, took part in the study.

Blood flow in the coronary sinus was measured by the thermodilution technique using a triple thermistor catheter which was advanced into the sinus from a peripheral vein.

Arterial blood pressure was recorded continuously via a Teflon cannula inserted in a brachial artery.

180

Table 1. Parameters at rest and during exercise (mean ± SE) before and after administration of D 600 or placebo

	At rest			At maximum work load (MWL)			$\downarrow$ ST	Exercise time (ET)	ET at	$DP \times 10^2$
	HR	sBP	$DP \times 10^2$	HR	sBP	$DP \times 10^2$	at MWL		$\downarrow$ ST = 1 mm	$\downarrow$ ST = 1 mm
P-t	79 ± 2	144 ± 3	115 ± 5	135 ± 3	199 ± 5	270 ± 10	1.9 ± 0.1	10.2 ± 0.6	6.9 ± 0.7	229 ± 12
P	74 ± 3	140 ± 4	104 ± 6	133 ± 3	191 ± 6	250 ± 12	1.7 ± 0.1	10.9 ± 0.7	7 ± 1	213 ± 14
D	75 ± 2	135 ± 4	102 ± 5	136 ± 3	199 ± 6	212 ± 12	1.2 ± 0.2	12.6 ± 0.5	9.4 ± 1.1	249 ± 20

P-t = before treatment   P = Placebo   D = D 600
HR = heart rate   sBP = systolic blood pressure   DP = double product
* = $p < 0.05$; ** = $p < 0.01$.

Measurement of the baseline values was followed by control pacing during which the rate was increased in 10-beat increments every 2 minutes. The end-points selected were chest pain or an ST-segment depression of ≥ 2 mm or a maximum paced heart rate of 170/min. All the measurements were repeated at maximum pacing.

After a recovery phase of 40 minutes, D 600 was administered as a bolus (0.03 mg/kg) followed by an infusion of 0.0005 mg/kg/minute.

Ten minutes later all baseline values were obtained and a second phase of atrial pacing was started.

After D 600, a higher heart rate (158 ± 5.4 vs 142 ± 4.7; $p < 0.001$) and a longer pacing time (14.8 vs 11 minutes) were observed in all the patients. In contrast, there was a reduction of the mean blood pressure from 133 ± 5.4 mm Hg to 116 ± 5.3 mm Hg ($p < 0.005$) and a modest, although not significant, change in the double product. There were no changes in blood flow in the coronary sinus (134 ± 18 vs 113 ± 12; ns) or in resistance in the coronary vessels (1.15 ± 0.16 vs 1.18 ± 0.17; ns) in comparison with pacing in the pharmacological wash-out phase. These results confirm that D 600 mainly improves exercise tolerance by reducing myocardial oxygen uptake.

It is known that calcium antagonists can reduce oxygen uptake by reducing myocardial contractility and this can, theoretically, have adverse effects by impairing myocardial performance (9, 10).

The second part of our study was to discover whether the anti-ischaemic effect of D 600 is associated with relevant negative inotropic effects and whether it is safe to administer this drug to patients who have had an acute myocardial infarction but who had no clinical symptoms of left ventricular failure.

We started by investigating the effects of an intravenous bolus of D 600 on the systolic and diastolic left ventricular function of 10 male patients who had had an acute myocardial infarction in NYHA classes I and II (11).

Left ventriculography was performed, with simultaneous high-fidelity measurement of pressure in the left ventricle using a microtip catheter transducer, before and after administration of D 600 as a bolus of 0.03 mg/kg followed by infusion of 0.0005 mg/kg/minute.

D 600 caused a slight, but significant, reduction in the contractility index DP/Dt/P (25.8 ± 1.8 vs 28 ± 2; $p < 0.01$) and a slight increase in end diastolic ventricular volume (129 ± 8.2 vs 125 ± 9.2; $p < 0.01$) without any change in the ejection fraction (0.54 ± 0.02 vs 0.55 ± 0.02; ns) or left ventricular end diastolic pressure (18.7 ± 1.8 vs 18.8 ± 1.7; ns). The haemodynamic effects of an intravenous bolus of D 600 were also assessed at rest and during exercise.

Ten male patients, on average 42.7 ± 7 years of age, who had had an acute myocardial infarction (posterior-wall infarction in 7 patients and anterior-wall infarction in 3) in NYHA classes I and II in whom exercise tests did not confirm exercise-induced ischaemia, underwent right-heart catheterization 30 to 40 days after the infarction. Using Seldinger's percutaneous approach with fluoroscopic monitoring, a Swan-Ganz thermodilution catheter (Charrière size 7) was advanced through the basilic or femoral vein via the right ventricle into a branch of the pulmonary artery.

After catheterization, the baseline haemodynamic data were obtained at rest with the patient supine and on the bicycle ergometer with legs raised to the pedals. The pulmonary capillary pressure in this position had to be less than 20 mm Hg.

There was then a 6-minute warming-up phase at a work load of 20 watts. After 25 minutes' rest the patients underwent their first exercise test under the same clinical conditions, with the work load being increased in 75-watt increments every 3 minutes (Figure 2).

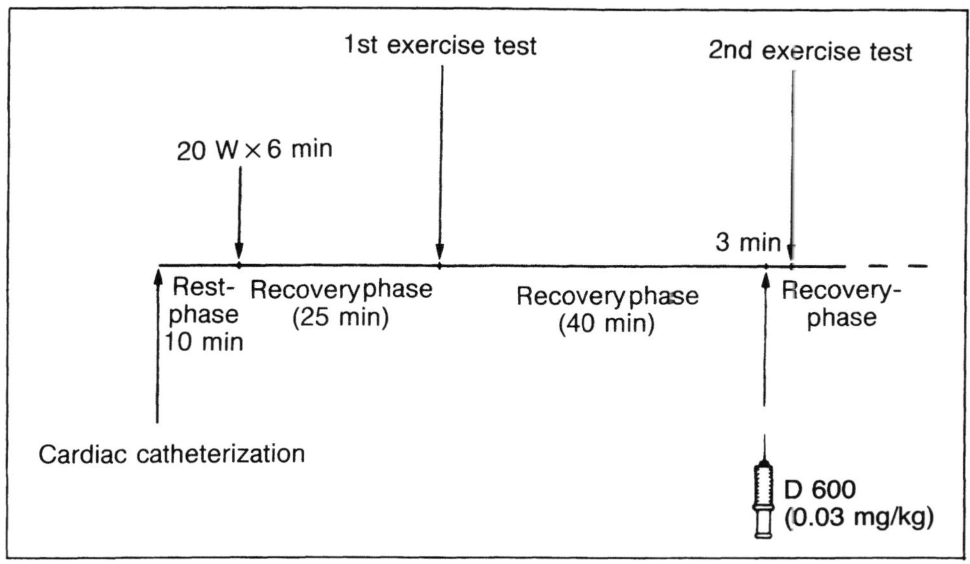

Figure 2. Protocol for haemodynamic study

The following haemodynamic parameters were monitored continuously at rest and during exercise with an HP 38805 A preamplifier: mean atrial pressure, pulmonary artery pressure (PAP), pulmonary capillary wedge pressure (PWP) and arterial blood pressure (measured by percutaneous catheterization of the brachial or radial artery). Cardiac output (CO) was determined by the thermodilution technique with the aid of an Edwards 9520A Cardiac Output Computer. A 12-lead electrocardiogram was recorded, and the heart rate was calculated, with the aid of a MAC 1 Marquette Recorder.

Forty minutes after the first exercise test, 0.03 mg/kg D 600 was injected in one minute, and after 3 minutes the haemodynamic parameters were again determined at rest with the patient's legs raised to the pedals of the ergometer, and during exercise (see Figure 2).

At rest, D 600 caused a significant reduction in systolic blood pressure (SBP) (from 153 ± 6 to 141 ± 5; $p < 0.05$), it increased pulmonary artery pressure (from 15.8 ± 0.8 to 18.2 ± 1; $p < 0.05$) and increased pulmonary capillary wedge pressure (from 8.9 ± 0.8 to 11.2 ± 1.2; $p < 0.01$), while cardiac output was unchanged (Table 2). At the same work load (25 watts $\times$ 3 minutes), D 600 caused a significant reduction in systolic blood pressure (from 199 ± 10 to 184 ± 9; $p < 0.05$), in pulmonary artery pressure (from 26.4 ± 2.1 to 24.8 ± 2; $p < 0.05$) and in pulmonary capillary wedge pressure (from 15.6 ± 2.6 to 13.2 ± 2; $p < 0.05$), while cardiac output and the heart rate were virtually unchanged (see Table 2).

These data are evidence that the trial medication had a weak negative inotropic effect without it reducing left ventricular function during exercise in patients who had had an acute myocardial infarction but who had no clinical signs or symptoms of heart failure.

To sum up, in patients with stable, exercise-induced angina pectoris D 600 exhibited a good anti-ischaemic effect, mainly as a result of a reduction of myocardial oxygen uptake.

Table 2. Parameters at rest and during exercise (75 watts $\times$ 3 min), (mean $\pm$ SE) before and after administration of D 600

		HR	sBP	PAP	PWP	CO	TPR	SVR
at rest	W.O.	80 ± 3	153 ± 6	15.8 ± 0.8	8.9 ± 0.8	7.3 ± 0.4	172 ± 14	1170 ± 72
	D 600	85 ± 3	141 ± 5	18.2 ± 1	11.2 ± 1.2	7.6 ± 0.5	193 ± 15	1076 ± 73
		ns	p<0.05	p<0.05	p<0.01	ns	ns	p<0.05
75 watts × 3 min	W.O.	124 ± 6	199 ± 10	26.4 ± 2.1	15.6 ± 2.6	12.9 ± 0.4	168 ± 17	786 ± 30
	D 600	126 ± 5	184 ± 9	24.8 ± 2	13.2 ± 2	12.9 ± 0.6	158 ± 15	728 ± 37
		ns	p<0.05	p<0.05	p<0.05	ns	ns	ns

W.O. = pharmacological wash-out phase; HR = heart rate; sBP = systolic blood pressure; PAP = pulmonary artery pressure; PWP = pulmonary capillary wedge pressure; CO = cardiac output; TPR = pulmonary vascular resistance; SVR = systemic vascular resistance

D 600 increased exercise tolerance without significantly impairing left ventricular function. Therefore, this drug can safely be given to patients who have had an acute myocardial infarction and who do not have severe left ventricular dysfunction, without jeopardizing cardiac function.

References

1. Fleckenstein A, Tritthart HA, Fleckenstein B, Herbst A, Grün G (1969) Eine neue Gruppe kompetitiver Ca-Antagonisten (Iproveratril, D 600, Prenylamin) mit starken Hemmeffekten auf die elektromechanische Koppelung im Warmblütermyokard. Pflügers Arch Physiol 307:R25
2. Fleckenstein A, Fleckenstein B, Sparth F, Byon YK (1983) Gallopamil (D 600) ein Calcium-Antagonist von hoher Wirkungsstärke und spezifischem Effekt auf Myocard und Schrittmacher. In: Kaltenbach M, Hopf R (eds.): Gallopamil, pharmacologisches und klinisches Wirkungsprofil eines Kalziumantagonisten, Springer, Berlin Heidelberg New York
3. Hopf R, Drews H, Kaltenbach M (1983) Die antianginöse Wirkung von Gallopamil – Vergleich zu Nifedipin. In: Kaltenbach M, Hopf R (eds.) Gallopamil, pharmakologisches und klinisches Wirkungs-Profil eines Kalziumantagonisten. Springer, Berlin Heidelberg New York Tokio
4. Mitrovich K, Nimela L, Neuss N, Shepher M (1984) Zur antianginösen Wirkung des Kalzium-antagonisten Gallopamil. In: Kaltenbach M, Hopf R (eds.) Gallopamil, pharmakologisches und klinisches Wirkungsprofil eines Kalziumantagonisten. Springer, Berlin Heidelberg New York Tokio
5. Rettig G, Sen S (1984): Akut- und Langzeiteffekte von Gallopamil mit stabiler Angina pectoris. In: Kaltenbach M, Hopf R (eds.) Gallopamil, pharmakologisches und klinisches Wirkungsprofil eines Kalziumantagonisten. Springer, Berlin Heidelberg New York Tokio, p. 136.
6. Sučić MJ, Schiemann J (1984) Ergebnisse einer offenen multicentrischen Studie bei 455 Patienten mit KHK, die über ein Jahr mit Gallopamil behandelt wurden. In: Kaltenbach M, Hopf R (eds.) Gallopamil, pharmakologisches und klinisches Wirkungsprofil eines Kalziumantagonisten. Springer, Berlin Heidelberg New York Tokio, p. 132
7. Khurmi NS, O'Hara MJ, Bowles MJ, Bala Subramanian V, Raftery EB (1984) Randomized double-blind comparison of gallopamil and propranolol in stable angina pectoris. Am J Cardiol 53:684
8. De Servi S, Ferrario M, Angoli L, Ghio S, Bramucci E, Mussini A, Specchia G (1987) Effects of Gallopamil on regional coronary hemodynamics during an atrial pacing in patients with stable exertional angina. Br Heart J, in press
9. Mitchell LB, Schroeder JS, Mason JW (1982) Comparative clinical electrophysiologic effects of diltiazem, verapamil and nifedipine: a review. Am J Cardiol 49:629
10. Nayler WG, Horowitz JD (1983) Calcium antagonists: a new class of drugs. Pharmac Ther 20:203
11. Ghio S, Poma E, Ferrario M, De Servi S, Bramucci E, Angoli L, Mussini A, Montemartini C, Specchia G (1986) Effetti del Gallopamil sulla funzione ventricolare sinistra in pazienti con infarto miocardico pregresso. G Ital Cardiol 16 (Suppl 1): 110

Author's address:

Prof. Guiseppe Speccia
Divisione di Cardiologica
Policlinico S. Matteo
27100 Pavia
Italy

Discussion

FLEISCHMANN

How does intravenous injection of gallopamil correlate with an oral dosage? Is it possible to estimate the oral dosage for these patients like this?

SPECCHIA

By giving the drug intravenously we were studying the short-term effects, so it is very difficult to relate this intravenous dosage to long-term, therapeutic use of the drug and to oral doses. We based our use of the drug on determinations of gallopamil in plasma, and we decided to use this as the criterion for monitoring. The plasma level was 50 to 60 ng/ml.

Gallopamil and six other calcium antagonists in stable angina pectoris and a within-patient comparison of gallopamil with diltiazem

V. Bala Subramanian

Brunel Institute for Bioengineering, Uxbridge, Middx., UK

Introduction

Ca^{2+} antagonists are well-proven and valuable drugs for the treatment of unstable and stable angina pectoris (1, 3, 5, 6, 9, 13). Nifedipine, verapamil and diltiazem are used medicinally the world over. At present gallopamil is available in the Federal Republic of Germany.
Ca^{2+} antagonists are now amongst the drugs of first choice for the treatment of angina pectoris (10, 14). The second generation and third generation Ca^{2+} antagonists are at present undergoing clinical trials (2, 7, 12).
There is a distinction between cardiovascular and vascular Ca^{2+} antagonists. Cardiovascular Ca^{2+} antagonists such as verapamil, diltiazem and gallopamil act on the vascular system and on the heart and its nodal structures. Vascular Ca^{2+} antagonists, of which nifedipine is the prototype, exert their effect solely by causing vascular dilation.
The purpose of the trial was to investigate the anti-anginal efficacy of seven Ca^{2+} antagonists, irrespective of type.

Patients and methods

All the patients were between 30 and 70 years of age and complied with the following criteria for inclusion:
1. A history (at least 3 months) of stable exercise-induced angina;
2. Pain alleviated by stopping exercise and/or sublingual nitroglycerin;
3. Taking nitroglycerin at least four times a week;
4. Classic anginal pain induced by exercising on a treadmill;
5. Exercise-induced descending ST-segment depression of at least 1 mm in two bipolar ECG leads;
6. CHD confirmed by thallium scintiscan, coronary angiography or evidence of recent myocardial infarction.

There was a two-week, single-blind phase with placebo before each test phase. The patient was then treated using a randomized, double-blind, cross-over procedure. Each treatment phase lasted for 2 or 4 weeks.
Maximal exercise tests on a treadmill conducted before recruitment for the trial and at 2-week intervals after treatment were used to assess the efficacy of treatment with placebo or active drug. The exercise tests were carried out with the aid of a microcomputer system linked to a Quinton treadmill. The tests were timed with a built-in digital clock with a maximum variation of 6s. The exercise tests were symptom-limited. Two bipolar ECG derivations were recorded continuously at rest and during the exercise tests for calculating the ST-segment depression. The ST-segment depression and heart rate were printed out

automatically for both leads at the end of each minute. At the end of the tests, the computer printed out the period of exercising, work load, heart rate and ST-segment depression.

Results

Exercise time

Table 1 shows the symptom-limited increase in exercise tolerance under treatment with seven different Ca^{2+} antagonists at different dosages, in comparison with placebo and propranolol. With an increase in exercise tolerance of 4.7 min versus placebo, gallopamil proved to be the most effective drug.

Table 1. Maximal exercise time on a treadmill ergometer under treatment with propranolol and seven Ca^{2+} antagonists, versus placebo

Drug	Dose (mg)	Number of patients	Exercise time (min) Placebo	Active drug	p	Increase in exercise tolerance (min)
Propranolol	80, 3×1 t.i.d.	22	5.5	7.8	<0.001	2.3
	80, 3×1 t.i.d.	15	5.8	9.6	<0.001	3.8
	80, 3×1 t.i.d.	15	5.4	8.2	<0.001	2.8
	80, 3×1 t.i.d.	18	5.4	9.4	<0.001	4.0
Diltiazem	60, 3×1 t.i.d.	10	5.5	7.9	<0.001	2.4
	60, 3×1 t.i.d.	15	5.8	9.0	<0.001	3.2
	90, 3×1 t.i.d.	20	5.5	8.0	<0.001	2.5
	120, 3×1 t.i.d.	20	5.5	9.5	<0.001	4.0
	120, 3×1 t.i.d.	15	5.4	8.3	<0.001	2.9
Gallopamil	50, 3×1 t.i.d.	18	5.4	10.1	<0.001	4.7
KB 944	100, 1×1 o.d.	16	6.5	9.4	<0.001	2.9
	200, 1×1 o.d.	16	6.5	10.0	<0.001	3.5
Nicardipine	10, 3×1 t.i.d.	20	6.4	7.4	<0.001	1.0
	20, 3×1 t.i.d.	20	6.4	7.8	<0.001	1.4
	30, 3×1 t.i.d.	17	7.3	8.9	<0.001	1.6
	40, 3×1 t.i.d.	17	7.3	9.4	<0.001	2.1
Nifedipine	10, 3×1 t.i.d.	20	6.8	6.9	ns	0.1
	20, 3×1 t.i.d.	28	5.7	7.9	<0.001	2.2
PY 108	25, 3×1 t.i.d.	18	6.1	9.3	<0.001	3.2
	50, 3×1 t.i.d.	18	6.1	9.2	<0.001	3.1
Verapamil	120, 3×1 t.i.d.	28	6.6	11.2	<0.001	4.6
	120, 3×1 t.i.d.	22	5.5	9.1	<0.001	3.6
	120, 3×1 t.i.d.	28	5.7	10.0	<0.001	4.3

Changes in the ST segment

An objective parameter of the anti-anginal efficacy of a drug is the exercise time required to produce a specific ST-segment depression. In Table 2, the parameter used is the time required to produce a ST-segment depression of 1 mm in two bipolar leads, during treatment with seven different Ca^{2+} antagonists and propranolol.

188

Table 2. 1-mm time in lead CM_5 under propranolol and seven Ca^{2+} antagonists versus placebo, in minutes after starting to exercise

Drug	Dose (mg)	Number of patients	1-mm time under Placebo	Active drug	p	Difference
Propranolol	80, 3×1 t.i.d.	22	3.3	5.7	<0.001	2.4
	80, 3×1 t.i.d.	15	3.3	5.3	<0.001	2.0
	80, 3×1 t.i.d.	15	3.6	5.8	<0.001	2.2
	80, 3×1 t.i.d.	18	3.7	7.2	<0.001	3.5
Diltiazem	60, 3×1 t.i.d.	20	3.4	4.8	<0.001	1.4
	60, 3×1 t.i.d.	15	3.3	5.3	<0.001	2.0
	90, 3×1 t.i.d.	20	3.4	5.0	<0.001	1.6
	120, 3×1 t.i.d.	20	3.4	5.5	<0.001	2.1
	120, 3×1 t.i.d.	15	3.6	4.8	<0.001	1.2
Gallopamil	50, 3×1 t.i.d.	18	3.7	6.4	<0.001	2.7
KB 944	100, 1×1 o.d.	16	4.3	6.2	<0.001	1.9
	200, 1×1 o.d.	16	4.3	6.6	<0.001	2.3
Nicardipine	10, 3×1 t.i.d.	20	4.8	5.4	ns	0.6
	20, 3×1 t.i.d.	20	4.8	5.6	ns	0.8
	30, 3×1 t.i.d.	17	4.9	6.6	<0.001	1.7
	40, 3×1 t.i.d.	17	4.9	7.0	<0.001	2.1
Nifedipine	10, 3×1 t.i.d.	20	4.8	4.6	ns	− 0.2
	20, 3×1 t.i.d.	28	3.9	5.8	<0.001	1.9
PY 108	25, 3×1 t.i.d.	18	4.4	5.7	<0.05	1.3
	50, 3×1 t.i.d.	18	4.4	5.9	ns	1.5
Verapamil	120, 3×1 t.i.d.	28	4.4	7.2	<0.001	2.8
	120, 3×1 t.i.d.	22	3.3	5.5	<0.001	2.2
	120, 3×1 t.i.d.	28	3.9	7.1	<0.001	3.2

Heart rate

Table 3 shows that propranolol caused a clear-cut reduction of the resting heart rate. The Ca^{2+} antagonists had different effects on the heart rate. The resting heart rate was reduced by the cardiovascular Ca^{2+} antagonists verapamil, diltiazem and gallopamil, whereas it rose under the vascular Ca^{2+} antagonists of the nifedipine type.

Adverse reactions and tolerance

All the Ca^{2+} antagonists were well tolerated, with slight differences between the classes of compounds. Flush, headache, oedema of the feet, palpitations and, occasionally, paradoxical angina pectoris were observed during treatment with the vascular Ca^{2+} antagonists. As regards the cardiovascular Ca^{2+} antagonists, constipation was frequently reported under verapamil; constipation was not reported by any of the patients under gallopamil. Left ventricular failure did not occur in any of the patients under treatment with Ca^{2+} antagonists, whereas under propranolol two patients developed signs of left ventricular dysfunction which made it necessary to stop the treatment prematurely.

Table 3. Resting heart rate under propranolol and seven Ca^{2+} antagonists, versus placebo

Drug	Dose (mg)	Number of patients	Resting heart rate (beats/min) Placebo	Active drug	p	Decrease or increase
Propranolol	80, 3×1 t.i.d.	22	76	56	<0.001	−20
	80, 3×1 t.i.d.	15	78	57	<0.001	−21
	80, 3×1 t.i.d.	15	80	56	<0.001	−24
	80, 3×1 t.i.d.	18	81	57	<0.001	−24
Diltiazem	60, 3×1 t.i.d.	20	75	65	<0.01	−10
	60, 3×1 t.i.d.	15	78	78	ns	> 0
	90, 3×1 t.i.d.	20	75	65	<0.01	−10
	120, 3×1 t.i.d.	20	75	64	<0.01	−11
	120, 3×1 t.i.d.	15	80	73	<0.01	− 7
Gallopamil	50, 3×1 t.i.d.	18	81	74	<0.01	− 7
KB 944	100, 1×1 o.d.	16	68	63	<0.05	− 5
	200, 1×1 o.d.	16	68	66	ns	− 2
Nicardipine	10, 3×1 t.i.d.	20	71	75	ns	+ 4
	20, 3×1 t.i.d.	20	71	79	<0.01	+ 8
	30, 3×1 t.i.d.	17	69	73	ns	+ 4
	40, 3×1 t.i.d.	17	69	76	<0.001	+ 7
Nifedipine	10, 3×1 t.i.d.	20	74	76	ns	+ 2
	20, 3×1 t.i.d.	28	74	77	ns	+ 3
PY 108	25, 3×1 t.i.d.	18	82	86	ns	+ 4
	50, 3×1 t.i.d.	18	82	85	ns	+ 3
Verapamil	120, 3×1 t.i.d.	28	74	65	<0.01	− 9
	120, 3×1 t.i.d.	22	76	71	<0.01	− 5
	120, 3×1 t.i.d.	28	74	68	<0.01	− 6

Within-patient comparison of gallopamil with diltiazem

In the previous studies, seven Ca^{2+} antagonists, a beta-blocker and placebo were tested by between-patient comparisons. Within-patient comparisons are necessary to confirm trends indicated by these between-patient comparisons. The anti-anginal efficacy of gallopamil, 50 mg t.i.d., was therefore compared on a within-patient basis with that of diltiazem, 60 mg t.i.d., in 20 patients with stable angina pectoris, by means of standardized exercise tests on a treadmill and a 24-h ECG. Table 4 shows the results of this study.

Discussion – therapeutic conclusions

It seemed appropriate to compare the efficacy of the familiar Ca^{2+} antagonists with that of a beta-blocker (propranolol) and placebo in the treatment of coronary heart disease. The beta-blockers were, after all, the drugs of choice in the 1970s. In the meantime, however, direct blockade of the Ca^{2+} channels by Ca^{2+} antagonists has become an increasingly accepted method of treatment.

The results show that, if we spotlight their efficacy in coronary heart disease and disregard co-existing diseases, cardiovascular Ca^{2+} antagonists are superior both to the beta-blockers and to the vascular Ca^{2+} antagonists (15). This naturally raises the question as to the

Table 4.

	Placebo	Diltiazem	Gallopamil
Average exercise time before occurrence of angina	8.5 min	10.8 min	11.9 min
1-mm time	5.3 min	8.1 min	8.7 min
Number of anginal attacks/week	6.9	4.7	3.2
Nitroglycerin tablets/week	4.3	3.2	2.1
Number of symptomatic and silent episodes of ischaemia in the long-term ECG with ST-segment depression more than 1 mm and lasting longer than 1 min	5.5	3.0	2.0

difference between the cardiovascular Ca^{2+} antagonists as regards therapeutic efficacy. The investigations, including the within-patient comparison of gallopamil with diltiazem, show that gallopamil is the most effective drug for increasing exercise tolerance. A dosage of 50 mg gallopamil t.i.d. produces a distinctly more marked increase in the exercise tolerance of patients with coronary heart disease than clinically acceptable, high doses of diltiazem (60 mg t.i.d.) or verapamil (120 mg t.i.d.); (4, 8, 11, 16, 17). The dose-limiting factor with diltiazem here is its depressant effect on the sino-atrial node and the associated risk of clinically significant bradycardia. The dose-limiting factor with verapamil is the increase in the incidence of constipation, which is proportional to dose.

Thus, in the between-patient study the trend was for gallopamil to show the best benefit-to-risk ratio. In the within-patient study, gallopamil was more effective than diltiazem in the clinically acceptable dose range. It would be desirable to carry out more within-patient studies to compare the various Ca^{2+} antagonists and other coronary drugs and to investigate the benefit-to-risk profile.

Summary

The anti-anginal effect of seven Ca^{2+} antagonists was investigated in patients with stable exercise-induced angina, with the aid of quantitative exercise tests on a treadmill ergometer and identical protocols. The trial parameter was the increase in the duration of exercising in symptom-limited exercise tests on the treadmill. The ECG was recorded on an online digital computer which enabled ST-segment depressions and changes in heart rate during the treatment to be calculated. The trial drugs were gallopamil, diltiazem, KB 944, nicardipine, nifedipine, PY 108 and verapamil. The efficacy and profile of action of all the drugs were compared with those of placebo and propranolol. Subjective differences and observer bias were eliminated by using identical criteria for inclusion and exclusion and computer analysis of the data.

In this trial, gallopamil proved to be the most effective drug for increasing exercise tolerance: under gallopamil, at a dosage of 50 mg t.i.d., the period of exercising was 4.7 minutes longer than under placebo. In the within-patient study, in a clinically acceptable dose range gallopamil was more effective than diltiazem. In general terms cardiovascular calcium antagonists, which are capable of lowering the resting heart rate, are more potent anti-anginal drugs than calcium antagonists which only exhibit vascular effects.

References

1. Bala Subramanian V, Bowles MJ, Khurmi NS, Davis AB, Raftery EB (1982) A randomized double-blind comparison of verapamil and nifedipine in chronic stable angina. Am J Cardiol 50: 696
2. Bala Subramanian V, Bowles MJ, Khurmi NS, Raftery EB (1982) Comparative evaluation of four slow channel blockers with propranolol in stable angina pectoris. Circulation 66:72 (Abstr)
3. Bala Subramanian V, Bowles MJ, Lahiri A, Davis AB, Raftery EB (1981) Long-Term antianginal action of verapamil assessed with quantitated serial treadmill stress testing. Am J Cardiol 48:529
4. Bala Subramanian V, Khanna PK, Narayanan GR, Hoon RS (1976) Verapamil in ischaemic heart disease – quantitative assessment by serial multistage treadmill exercise. Postgrad Med J 43
5. Bala Subramanian V, Khurmi NS, Bowles MJ, O'Hara M, Raftery EB (1983) Objective evaluation of three dose levels of diltiazem in patient with chronic stable angina. J Am Coll Cardiol 1:1144
6. Bala Subramanian V, Pramasivan R, Lahiri A, Raftery EB (1980) Verapamil in chronic stable angina: a controlled study with computerized treadmill exercise. Lancet I, 841
7. Bowles MJ, Bala Subramanian V, Khurmi NS, Davies AB, Raftery EB (1982) Efficacy of a new calcium blocking agent nicardipine in chronic stable angina. Br J Clin Pharmacol 13:590 (Abstr)
8. Burkart F, Nager F (1984) Stable angina pectoris and calcium antagonists in International Symposium on calcium-antagonism. In: Althaus U, Burckhardt D, Vogt E (eds), Frankfurt, p. 62
9. Corbalan R, Gonzales R, Chamono G, Munoz M, Rodriquez JA, Casanegra P (1981) Effects of a calcium inhibitor, nifedipine, on exercise tolerance in patients with angina pectoris. Chest 79:302
10. Frishman W, Klein NA, Strom JA et al. (1981) Superiority of verapamil to propranolol in stable angina pectoris: a double blind randomized cross-over trial. Circulation 65 (Suppl 1):1
11. Go, M jr., Hollenberg M (1984) Improved efficacy of high-dose versus medium and low-dose diltiazem therapy for chronic stable angina pectoris. Am J Cardiol 53:669
12. O'Hara MJ, Bala Subramanian V, Khurmi NS, Bowles MJ, Raftery EB (1983) Diltiazem compared with propranolol for the treatment of stable angina pectoris using serial quantitated treadmill tests (abst). J Am Coll Cardiol 1:680
13. Krikler DM, Rowland E (1983) Clinical value of calcium antagonists in treatment of cardiovascular disorders. J Am Coll Cardiol 1:355
14. Leon MG, Rosing DR, Bonow RO et al (1981) Clinical efficacy of verapamil alone and combined with propranolol in treating patients with chronic stable angina. J Am Cardiol 48:131
15. Mueller HS, Chahine RA (1981) Interim report of multicenter double-blind, placebo controlled studies in chronic stable angina. Am J Med 71:645
16. Petru MA, Crawford MH, Sorensen SG, Chaudhuri TK, Levine S, O'Rourke RA (1983) Short- and long-term efficacy of high-dose oral diltiazem for angina due to coronary artery disease: a placebo-controlled, randomized double-blind cross-over study. Circulation 68:139
17. Pine MB, Citron PD, Baily DJ, Butman S, Plascencia GO, Landa DW, Wong RK (1982) Verapamil versus placebo in relieving stable angina pectoris. Circulation 65:17

Author's address:

Dr. V. Bala Subramanian
52, Harley Street
London
United Kingdom

Discussion

SPECCHIA

As regards the anti-anginal effect of nifedipine, Maseri's group showed that it is practically impossible to induce an occlusion experimentally in a very severely stenosed vessel by reducing the prestenotic pressure. On the other hand, nifedipine very rarely triggers an attack of angina, while a very large number of patients with severe stenosis are treated with nifedipine. Don't you think that the drug may elicit a violent spasm in some patients and may induce non-spastic occlusion where there is a reduction of the dynamic stenosis due to a reduction of prestenotic pressure?

BALA SUBRAMANIAN

We considered this possibility when we observed these patients in our group and heard of three other patients reported by a German group and one patient from an American group. However, whatever clinical investigations were carried out, and whenever nifedipine was instilled experimentally on the stenotic side, all the investigations showed that there was no individual fall of blood pressure and that this spasm was only provoked in one patient. Since, as a rule, the patients were angiographed, I think that these interrelationships ought to be investigated. Whenever this occurs, I would ask the physician preparing the angiograph to administer a small dose of nifedipine at the site of the obstruction so that we may learn more about this very interesting problem.

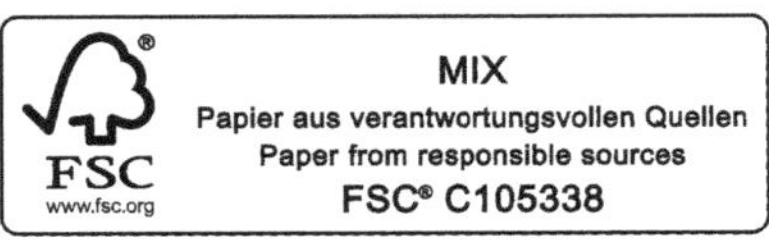

If you have any concerns about our products,
you can contact us on
ProductSafety@springernature.com

In case Publisher is established outside the EU,
the EU authorized representative is:
Springer Nature Customer Service Center GmbH
Europaplatz 3, 69115 Heidelberg, Germany

Printed by Libri Plureos GmbH
in Hamburg, Germany